BECOMING OBJECT

BECOMING OBJECT

The Sociopolitics of the Samuel George Morton Cranial Collection

Pamela L. Geller

UNIVERSITY OF FLORIDA PRESS

Gainesville

Cover: Letter, Richard Harlan to Samuel George Morton, 9 December 1831. Mss.B.B843. Samuel George Morton Papers. American Philosophical Library.

Copyright 2024 by Pamela L. Geller
All rights reserved
Published in the United States of America

29 28 27 26 25 24   6 5 4 3 2 1

ISBN 978-1-68340-459-0 (hardback)
ISBN 978-1-68340-472-9 (pbk.)

A record of cataloging-in-publication data is available from the Library of Congress.

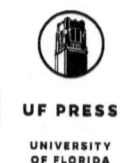

University of Florida Press
2046 NE Waldo Road
Suite 2100
Gainesville, FL 32609
http://upress.ufl.edu

Barbara and Sidney . . . thanks for humoring me

Nothing is more misleading than the illusion created by hindsight in which all the traces of a life, such as the works of an artist or the events at a biography, appear as the realization of an essence that seems to preexist them.
　　　　　—Pierre Bourdieu, *The Logic of Practice* (1990, 55)

No, no, we can surely do better, we can surely stop the downward slide and retrace our steps, retaining both the history of humans' involvement in the making of scientific facts and the sciences' involvement in the making of human history.
　　　　　—Bruno Latour, *Pandora's Hope* (1999, 10)

Yet how does one recuperate lives entangled with and impossible to differentiate from the terrible utterances that condemned them to death, the account books that identified them as units of value, the invoices that claimed them as property, and the banal chronicles that stripped them of human features?
　　　　　—Saidiya Hartman, "Venus in Two Acts" (2008, 3)

CONTENTS

List of Figures xi

List of Tables xiii

Preface xv

Acknowledgments xxiii

List of Abbreviations xxviii

Introduction 1

1. The Friend 27
2. "Licence to Kill and Cure" 53
3. "Your Obedient Servant" 79
4. Border Making, Border Crossing 111
5. The Beloved Woman 141
6. Legacy 171

Notes 209

References 229

Index 271

FIGURES

I.1. Illustrated portrait of Samuel George Morton   2

1.1. *Friends' boarding school, West-town, PA*, by John Taylor French   33

1.2. Portrait of John Jay Smith, ca. 1880   37

1.3. Oil painting of Thomas Hodgkin   47

3.1. *Euchee*, a lithograph, 1839   85

3.2. "Tanner's Florida, 1823"   93

3.3. *Foke-Luste-Hajo a Seminole*, 1842   99

3.4. *General View of Laurel Hill Cemetery*, 1847   110

4.1. Service record for Dr. Edward S. Aldrich   116

4.2. Portrait of Colonel John James Abert, 1886   118

4.3. "Map of the seat of war in Florida," 1838   120

4.4. Page from the 1850 Census about Samuel Morton's household   130

4.5. *Massacre of the Whites by the Indians and Blacks in Florida*, 1836   136

5.1. Portrait of Rebecca Pearsall Morton, or Mrs. Samuel George Morton   142

5.2. Portrait of Rachel Pearsall Smith   144

5.3. The sisters Charlotte and Susan Cushman as Romeo and Juliet   158

5.4. Lithograph of *Dacota, N.W. Territory*, plate 39   162

5.5. *A Seminole Woman*, 1838, by George Catlin   166

5.6. Tombstone for James St. Claire Morton   169

5.7. Grave markers of Rebecca P. Morton and Samuel G. Morton   170

6.1. Stone monument with panels engraved in Samuel's memory   173

6.2. Naturalization papers of Abraham Geller   191

6.3. World War II dog tags for Jerome Sirkin   192

TABLES

3.1. Creek Skulls with Information   87

3.2. Cherokee Skulls with Information   89

3.3. Seminole Skulls with Information   96

PREFACE

Samuel G. Morton and the skulls he collected have long been on my mind. In the early 1990s, I was an undergraduate anthropology major at the University of Pennsylvania. Some thirty years prior, in 1966, the Academy of Natural Sciences (then of Philadelphia, now of Drexel University, and shortened here as ANS) had loaned the Samuel George Morton Cranial Collection to the University of Pennsylvania Museum of Archaeology and Anthropology (more recently rebranded as Penn Museum). Many of the skulls were placed in storage. But a number of "specimens" had found their way into the glass cabinets running the perimeter of my classroom walls. (The Department of Anthropology's classrooms are located in a building that is attached to the museum.) During lectures, my gaze wandered from projected slides and handwritten notes to empty eye-socketed skulls. Occasionally, my professors pulled the latter from their resting places. Curios transformed briefly into objects with educational value. Despite passage of the Native American Graves Protection and Repatriation Act (NAGPRA) in 1990, I presumed that the collection was no longer controversial. Stephen Jay Gould (1978, 1981) had laid bare Samuel's scientific racism more than a decade earlier. (Shortly, I explain my intentional usage of his first name in lieu of his surname.) Rather than serving as morphological evidence of racial differences, the skulls now functioned pedagogically as historic artifacts.

But, in the years that followed, my academic interest became tempered by anxiety and ambivalence. After returning to Penn for doctoral studies, I was hired as a NAGPRA project assistant at the museum. As one of my tasks, I inventoried "Samuel's" skulls—a possessive descriptor that I now use with irony. A year prior, in 1997, the ANS had transferred formal ownership to Penn, and the institution was now required to comply with NAGPRA. During the inventory process, I discovered that ownership obfuscates the past and is ever conditional. The dynamism of this legacy collection became readily apparent. Skulls had moved—between individuals, across landscapes, from institution to institution—effacing information about decedents' proveniences and biographies. Many separate archives housed pertinent materials, which had also traveled over time.

Cultural affiliation was then established based on a preponderance of evidence. Next, notifications were dutifully sent to federally recognized tribes. Thereafter, the repatriation process became idiosyncratic, informed by the complex inner workings of major institutions like Penn and the unique histories and present-day politics of each tribe. In some cases, tribes came to reclaim their ancestors' remains; repatriation then involved reburial. Other tribes did not pursue repatriation, for varied reasons; beliefs about the dead deterred responses or ongoing crises forestalled them, the latter being a legacy of settler colonialism, forced relocation, and inherited trauma. And so, Penn Museum continued to care for these decedents. This process impressed on me the culturally and politically sensitive nature of human remains, as well as the need to conduct research in a respectful manner. I took these lessons in hand as I completed doctoral work on pre-columbian Maya burials.

Years after my initial repatriation work, in 2011, I returned to the Morton Collection, having secured permission from Penn Museum. I intended to confirm the anecdotal. Previously, I had heard that Black Indians and warrior women were among the collection's decedents (later in this book, I discuss both in greater detail). Their biohistorical study, I thought, could counter narrow, categorical framings of racialized and gender identities. Exactly *who* composed the Morton Collection, I initially wondered. Next, as my research proceeded, *how* began to puzzle me. Little by little, I realized that Samuel's sizeable collection of skulls was made possible by an extensive network of men. When *why* came to nag, I turned my attention to context—those economic, political, social, religious, and ideological conditions in which Samuel lived and the individuals making up his collection died.

What I have since come to understand is that during the nineteenth century the scientific study of bodies and their biopolitical regulation by physicians and ethnologists—and Samuel was an exemplar—cannot be disentangled from US nation-building. Living bodies were racialized or gendered and then associated with disease; incarcerated in the almshouse, restricted to the plantation, or forcibly relocated to the reservation; slain on battlefields; fragmented and included in natural historical or anatomical collections; and morphed into pedagogical specimens. As national and scientific agendas changed, these bodies became forgotten relics that gathered dust in storage cabinets. With a postcolonial turn, controversy ensued. For anthropology, Samuel's and colleagues' complicity was undeniable. Atonement for the past sins of intellectual ancestors was imperative. Hence, legislation like NAGPRA. And now, historically fraught legacy collections are publicized as a flashpoint in twenty-first-century debates about decoloniality and decolonization, two related concepts that I distinguish between in chapter 6. *Becoming Object* attempts to track this "history of the present" (a phrase articulated by Michel Foucault [1977]).

While I do not see a direct equivalency between yesterday and today, I do acknowledge a relationality. Like Samuel, my formative years and formal schooling took place in Philadelphia and its surrounding suburbs. To situate archival descriptions of his nineteenth-century world, which was defined by increasing urbanization and a shifting physical and human landscape, I drew from my mental map of the city. As a graduate student at Penn, I lived within city blocks of the various houses and institutions associated with the people who populate this book. Yet, apart from basic cartography, my personal experiences have imparted an unexpected sensory window into the past. Take, for instance, the passage authored by John Jay Smith (b. 1798, d. 1881), Samuel's brother-in-law, in his memoir *Recollections:*

> [My uncle's neighbor,] Joseph Parker Norris, and his large family, occupied a fine old house opposite, where now stands the customhouse. It was surrounded by a large garden extending to Fifth Street and to the Philadelphia Library. Hide and seek, in this garden and in the streets, the latter almost deserted in the evenings, were among my amusements. (Smith 1892, 83)

Having walked this same street at dusk, I am well acquainted with its smells in the green-deep of summer. I am familiar with the sound leaves make when they rust orange and descend to city sidewalks in the autumn's cooling. I know how the grayness dims out the sun too early on February afternoons. Or how the light diffuses gold as the days start to extend in early spring. Places I encountered from an early age onward have developed a more layered history and physicality. Street names, public parks, buildings erected and demolished all acquired nuances. My research has had the feel of homecoming with the familiar's evocation of comfort and frustration.

But I now live in Miami, and tracking skulls as they moved from south to north has revealed the Morton Collection's darker and far more tragic dimensions. For this reason, inclusion of personal reflections is only part indulgent nostalgia. While my family has an immigrant tale that includes decisions constrained by circumstance and antisemitism, it does not involve colonial usurpation of ancestral land or enslavement.

Homecoming is still very much a part of the Florida story, however. Repatriation has allowed others' narratives about retribution, compassion, and reunion to surface. Such outcomes were reiterated by the Seminole Tribe of Florida's chief justice of Tribal Court, Willie Johns. On 12 October 2015, the tribe repatriated the remains of ancestors that had been included in the Morton Collection. Within days, they buried them at Okeechobee Battlefield. "Welcome home, welcome home," Johns eulogized at the funeral ceremony. "And, oh, by the way, did you hear? We won! Your people are still here in Florida. And they are doing well" (Gallagher 2015). As his words testify, there is a connection between historic human remains and living descendant communities.

Given the relationality between the past and present, researchers' due diligence must extend beyond legal requirements to deliberate about ethical issues. As I have come to learn (and am still learning), in addition to asking for institutional permissions, engaging with living descendants of the ancestors composing legacy collections may also be necessary. I collected the osteological data discussed in this book—skulls in the Morton Collection from the southeastern US are its focus—more than a decade ago. Then bioarchaeologists were not expected to collaborate or seek consent; now expectations have changed (e.g., Squires et al. 2022; Thomas and Krupa 2021). For me, working with remains in the Morton Collection labeled Seminole, who are treated at length in this book, has been most instructive.

When I relocated to Florida in 2007, I came to understand that Seminole and Miccosukee tribal members generally avoided their ancestors' remains given cultural beliefs and ontological positions about the dead. Instead, they hired mostly non-Natives to oversee their Tribal Historic Preservation Offices and repatriation efforts. So soon after beginning my research, in 2011, I reached out to staff associated with the Seminole Tribe of Florida's Tribal Historic Preservation Office (STOF-THPO) and Ah-Tah-Thi-Ki Museum. I had discovered named decedents in the Morton Collection and thought staff or tribal members might shed some light on their biographies. Information was not forthcoming, however. As my work proceeded, these interactions shifted, becoming less extractive and more collaborative (Gaudry 2011). In May 2014, I met with STOF-THPO staff at the Big Cypress Reservation to seek approval, share my findings, and reiterate my openness to future collaborations. I then presented and published skeletal data in varied forums (Geller 2015, 2017, 149–54, 2020; Geller and Stojanowski 2017). These publications are cited in *Becoming Object*, though I do rework and expand earlier writings. STOF-THPO staff have never communicated to me that the skeletal data discussed in talks or publications are "sensitive tribal information," a concept outlined by the Tribal Legal Development Clinic (2020) in "The Need for Confidentiality within Tribal Cultural Resource Protection." In keeping with prior requests from the STOF, however, photographic images of skeletal materials are not included in this book.

More recently, the STOF has revised its position on developing research and publication. In spring 2023, STOF-THPO staff communicated to me and colleagues, during a consultation unrelated to the Morton Collection, that the tribe is not consenting to new studies of human remains or associated grave materials. Nor are researchers currently undertaking analyses of Seminole remains permitted to publish the results of their finds. There has been no discussion, however, about inclusion of skeletal data from past publications. This turn of events underscores the dynamic relationship between the past and the present, as well as draws attention to an ethical gray area that invites an extended conversation.

Relationality also means that clarification about the selection of terminology is necessary. The ethnic and racial labels that appear in these pages show that some names do not time travel well given shifting sociopolitical conditions and cultural beliefs. "Naming is a pragmatic process; its truth depends on its effects," philosopher of science Isabelle Stengers (2018, 135) reminds us. Today, terms like "Caucasian," "Negroid," "Mongoloid," "Kaffir," "Indian," "negro," or "mulatto" are inappropriate or offensive. (As Judith Butler [1997] observed, names can impart social existence and inflict injury.) Here I only use these terms when directly quoting historic documents or to conjure historic figures' sentiments. To evoke a history of settler colonialism that has negatively transformed, exploited, and displaced communities, as well as political activism that seeks to ameliorate this history, I capitalize "Native" and "Indigenous" (Weeber 2020; Youngging 2018). I primarily use "American Indian" but identify the tribe when applicable. "Native American" is used in reference to legislation or governmental policy. "Black" is capitalized when referring to people who are part of the African diaspora, while "black" with a lower case is an adjective indicating a color (Appiah 2020; Tharps 2014). "White" is capitalized but for different reasons. As the American Psychological Association (2019) explains in its style guide: "We believe that it is important to call attention to White as a race as a way to understand and give voice to how Whiteness functions in our social and political institutions and our communities" (see also The Diversity Style Guide 2019). Following the International Holocaust Remembrance Alliance, I use "antisemitism." According to IHRA (2022), "Hyphenated spelling allows for the possibility of something called 'Semitism', which not only legitimizes a form of pseudo-scientific racial classification that was thoroughly discredited by association with Nazi ideology, but also divides the term, stripping it from its meaning of opposition and hatred toward Jews." These semantic shifts demonstrate how race is socially constructed; it has no biological basis but distinctions between groups may be based on perceived biological differences (e.g., skin color, skull shape), which become laden with meaning.

For terms pertaining to sex, gender, and sexuality, it is also important to distinguish derogatory or archaic descriptions from modern ones. In the case of a person who sells her or his sexual labor, I use "prostitute" given the term's historic applicability to the nineteenth century. I recognize, however, that many contemporary sex workers regard "prostitute" as a pejorative; it serves to stigmatize, oversimplifies complex life stories, and connotes a lack of agency (Smith 2013).

Additionally, terms related to two-spiritedness require exposition. Historically, writers, from sixteenth-century chroniclers up to twentieth-century ethnographers, used the term *berdache*, which translates as a kept boy, male prostitute, or catamite (Angelino and Shedd, 1955, 121). The concept suggests passivity, is reductive in its emphasis on homosexuality, and decontextualizes despite cultural differences (or rather, as a colonial category, it presumes that Western beliefs about sex, gender, and sexuality are universal). Many critiques—from queer and Indigenous (and queer Indigenous) writers—have followed in time (e.g., Driskill et al. 2011; Herdt 1997; Jacobs et al. 1997a; Medicine 2002; Thomas and Jacobs 1999). To encapsulate lives that disentangle individuals' biology from their social identities from their erotic preferences, linguistic designators used by an Indigenous community are most appropriate. For instance, Shoshoni speakers use *tainna wa'ippe*, which translates as "man-woman" (Lang 1997, 103). If Indigenous linguistic designators are unknown, I use "Two-Spirit." This term is not interchangeable with "third gender," which is too narrow a descriptor of socio-sexual variance in Indigenous communities. And while I do raise the issue of transgender as connected to two-spiritedness in chapter 6's consideration of contemporary decolonial work, I emphasize that it is tied to sociopolitical processes that are recent in historic date and germane to Western society.

Rather than use the phrase "gender variance," one that circulates in literature about Two-Spirits (e.g., Jacobs et al. 1997a), I have also opted for "socio-sexual variance." I use "socio-sexual" as a heuristic rather than regard it as historically accurate. That is, this term did not circulate in the nineteenth century but is useful for explaining differences between and within groups. Moreover, the lived experiences discussed in this book are not just informed by gender. For this reason, socio-sexual aims to capture the interrelatedness but not the interchangeability of sex, gender, and sexuality (Geller 2017). The term also refers to social identities as intersectional—complex, contingent, and crosscut by multiple variables (i.e., gender, sexuality, age, race/ethnicity, class, etc.).

At the scale of the individual, to name can christen at a life's outset or mourn at its conclusion. I oscillated about whether to use first names or surnames in these pages. Traditionally, biographic writing maintains that surnames are most appropriate. But I depart from orthodoxy and use first names in a few instances. In the case of Samuel Morton, I do so for several reasons. Pragmatically, I do not wish to confuse him with other individuals who shared his surname. To name Samuel also emphasizes the sociopolitical distance between him and the "specimens" in his collection, the majority of whom go unnamed. Anonymization is a facet of necropolitics that makes it easier to erase lives perceived to be disposable or ungrievable (through killing, forced relocation, enslavement, incarceration), to collect their remains, to rechristen them with neutral-seeming descriptors (e.g., "specimen"), and to conduct scientific investigations. Silences are powerful because they signal these nefarious processes of becoming object. But I also realize that in using Samuel's first name, I run the risk of further dehumanizing the collection's decedents. To avoid doing so, I name these individuals when possible. Their identification counters the intentional forgetting and invisibility that are constitutive of longstanding necropolitical processes. As we have seen more recently, such naming can also catalyze political resistance as one comes to represent the many who have suffered.

ACKNOWLEDGMENTS

My study of the Samuel George Morton Cranial Collection was conducted primarily at the University of Pennsylvania and was facilitated by Stacey Espenlaub, Lucy Fowler Williams, and Janet Monge. I am especially grateful to Stacey for her extensive knowledge of repatriation, unflagging support for this project, and long friendship.

Thank you to the staff at the various archives where I have conducted research: the Academy of Natural Sciences of Philadelphia (Clare Flemming, Megan Gibes); Ah-Tah-Thi-Ki Museum (Anne McCudden, Jonathan McMahon, Mary Beth Rosebrough); American Philosophical Society (Charles Greifenstein); Bowdoin College Library's George J. Mitchell Department of Special Collections + Archives (Marieke Van Der Steenhoven); College of Physicians of Philadelphia and Mütter Museum (Annie Brogan, Anna Dhody, Sofie Sereda); Historical Society of Pennsylvania; Germantown Historical Society (Alex Bartlett); Library Company of Philadelphia (Connie King, Sarah Weatherwax); Medical University of South Carolina's Waring Historical Library (Brooke Fox, Susan Hoffius); National Archives in Washington, DC; National Library of Medicine (Stephen Greenberg); Penn Museum (Alex Pezzati); University of Miami's Special Collections at Richter Library; and Wistar Institute (Nina Long). And a special thanks to Kristen Ramirez for her research assistance.

This research was supported by the University of Miami's Provost Research Award (2013 and 2014). I was also able to write a sizeable chunk of this book as a 2021–2022 Faculty Fellow at the University of Miami's Center for the Humanities. The center's director Hugh Thomas and my fellow fellows—Susanna Allés-Torrent, Ager Gondra, Marina Magloire, Chrissy Arce, Henry Green, and Cae Joseph-Masséna—offered valuable feedback on a draft of chapter 3. I am especially grateful to Miranda Suri, Shannon Novak, Sabrina Agarwal, and Alanna Warner-Smith for reading chapter drafts, providing thoughtful and constructive feedback, recommending readings, and/or engaging in conversations about the function of a footnote. Extended discussions about the bioethos of dead bodies with Thomas Champney, with whom I have the privilege of sitting on the University of Miami's Anatomical Advisory Committee, have also been invaluable.

I would also like to thank those members of Native and descendant communities who have deepened my understanding of the sensitive issues discussed in this book, whether in the context of repatriation visits or through their writings. Staff from the Seminole Tribe of Florida's Tribal Historic Preservation Office, especially Paul Backhouse, Annette Snapp, and Domonique deBeaubien, were also generous with their time when I visited the Big Cypress Reservation in May 2014.

Over the years, I have given many keynotes and invited talks about Samuel Morton and his cranial collection. They provided wonderful opportunities to think out loud, as well as to engage with students and colleagues. Invitations proffered came from: Boston University's Department of Archaeology for the 11th Biennial Graduate Student Forum; the British Association for Biological Anthropology and Osteoarchaeology (BABAO) Annual Conference 2014; the 10th Annual Kolb Senior Scholars Colloquium and the 2021 Settler Colonialism, Slavery, and the Problem of Decolonizing Museums Conference, both at Penn Museum; and Departments of Anthropology at University of California–Berkeley; Florida Atlantic University; Queens College–CUNY; Cornell University; and Syracuse University.

Earlier portions of *Becoming Object*, the skeletal data specifically, appear in the following places: "Hybrid Lives, Violent Deaths: Seminole Indians and the Samuel G. Morton Collection," in *Disturbing Bodies: Perspectives on Forensic Anthropology* (2017), edited by Zoë Crossland and Rosemary Joyce (Santa Fe, NM: SAR Press, 137–56); "The Vanishing Black Indian: Revisiting Craniometry and Historic Collections" (coauthored with Chris Stojanowski), in *American Journal of Physical Anthropology* 162, no. 2 (2017): 267–84; "Labor Codes," in *Bioarchaeology of Socio-Sexual Lives* (2017; New York: Springer); and "Building Nation, Becoming Object: The Biopolitics of the Samuel G. Morton Crania Collection," in *Historical Archaeology* 54, no. 1 (2020): 52–70. The ideas presented in these early publications are much expanded in chapters 3, 4, and 5.

Thank you to the three anonymous reviewers who provided thoughtful and constructive feedback on an earlier draft of this book. While any errors or omissions are on me, their comments were much appreciated. I am also quite grateful to Mary Puckett, my editor at the University of Florida Press, for shepherding this project along with patience and grace.

This book is dedicated to my parents Sidney and Barbara Geller. While they may have migrated south more recently, I know that in their heart of hearts they remain Philadelphians (Fly, Eagles Fly!). And, as always, the gratitude I have for my dearest Teddy Bear is immeasurable. You were in utero when I began the research for this book and my work on it has tracked up to your teen years. Thank you for loving me despite my sometimes-inadequate attempts to balance the rigors of scholarship and parenting. You are the BBE.

ABBREVIATIONS

ANS	Academy of Natural Sciences
APS	American Philosophical Society
Catalogue	*The Catalogue of Skulls of Man, and the Inferior Animals, in the Collection of Samuel George Morton, M.D.*
Corps	US Army Corps of Topographical Engineers
HSP	Historical Society of Pennsylvania
MAI	Museum of the American Indian, Heye Foundation, of New York City
Morton Collection	Samuel George Morton Cranial Collection
NAGPRA	Native American Graves Protection and Repatriation Act
Penn	University of Pennsylvania
Penn Museum	University of Pennsylvania Museum of Archaeology and Anthropology
STOF	Seminole Tribe of Florida
THPO	Tribal Historic Preservation Office

Introduction

The librarian leaned over my laptop. "Legend has it," she said, "John James Audubon really collected the skulls Morton claimed as *his* own." Her voice was lowered so as not to disturb the other researchers in the hushed archive at the Academy of Natural Sciences (ANS).[1]

For the past few weeks, the ANS had provided a quiet and cool-ish reprieve from the humid stickiness of Philadelphia. The city is a hot mess in July. On that summer day, the heat had percolated into the old building—its sputtering air condition no deterrent—and infiltrated my single-minded concentration. I was having difficulty transcribing the chicken-scratch scrawl of old letters. The librarian's whispered comment came as a welcome interruption. It was not that she presented me with a new twist in the history of the Samuel George Morton Cranial Collection (hereafter shortened to the Morton Collection). Audubon had collected human skulls, several of which he then passed on to Samuel Morton (b. 1799, d. 1851), a physician, natural historian, and one of the forefathers of American anthropology (figure I.1). But ornithology remained Audubon's passion. Rather, reflecting on the librarian's offhanded comment, I was reminded of how controversy[2] and confusion have long surrounded Samuel[3] and the skulls he amassed. While this book aims to clear up confusion, it is doubtful that my account will ameliorate controversy.

A Man of His Times

Shortly after Samuel's death, the ANS purchased the Morton Collection from his widow, Rebecca Grellet Pearsall Morton. There it continued to grow under the curation of Dr. James Aitken Meigs. In 1966, the ANS loaned the Morton Collection to Penn Museum and granted formal ownership in 1997. Today, the Morton Collection is comprised of roughly 1,300 skulls (or crania, which lack mandibles). The total number continues to

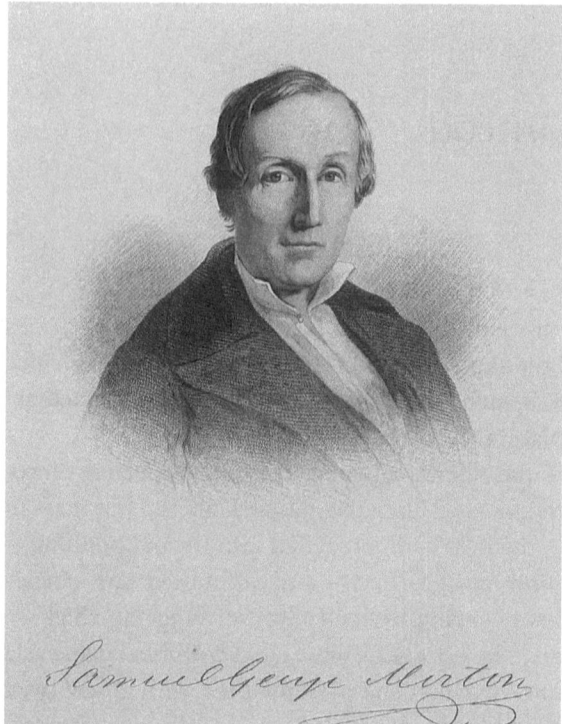

Figure I.1. An illustrated portrait of Samuel George Morton included among the personal correspondences and family photographs compiled by Elizabeth Pearsall Smith; these letters and photographs were then interspersed throughout *Recollections of John Jay Smith*. Image courtesy of the Library Company of Philadelphia.

decrease, however, as descendants reclaim the remains of their ancestors, transforming object back to vital and potent subject.[4]

Over the years, many writers have cited Samuel's study of the skulls he procured as evidence of his scientific racism. Others have sought to explain this fact away by characterizing the physician as a *man of his times*. Whether to condemn or apologize, I find both takes on Samuel to be reductive; they represent him as a caricature, his conclusions as foregone. "Nothing is more misleading," Pierre Bourdieu (1990, 55) reminds us, "than the illusion created by hindsight in which all the traces of a life, such as the works of an artist or the events at a biography, appear as the realization of an essence that seems to preexist them."

To avoid narrating Samuel's biography as an inevitable outcome, I attend to the interesting and complicated times in which he lived—an interlude between the nation's cohesion following revolution and its civil unraveling. This historical span was defined by enslavement of Black people, seizure of Natives' land, and denial of suffrage to all who were not White and male. Exclusion was baked into the body politic from the nation's constitution. While men like Samuel were responsible for necropolitical nation-building, to see him only as a villain (or hero as his contemporaries maintained) is too simplistic a summation.

During the course of my research, I found that as a man of his times Samuel held myriad roles. Scientific racist, definitely. On this aspect of his biography, many writers have expounded (e.g., Blakey 1987; Fabian 2010; Gould 1981; Redman 2016; Thomas 2000). But he was also a son, brother, husband, father, friend, Christian, professor, Philadelphian, and American. And, above all, an opportunist who sought financial gain and professional recognition. "Dr. Morton was ambitious of usefulness and fame," his brother-in-law John Jay Smith (1892, 145) recounted decades after Samuel died. A carved panel on the monument adjacent to his gravestone attests to his professional successes; "Physician, Naturalist, and Ethnologist" it reads. Samuel's sizeable cranial collection became the means that helped him to realize these ends. As Ann Fabian (2010) has discussed in her treatment of nineteenth-century skull collecting, Samuel, while not a singular example, was one of the more voracious and esteemed seekers. Beyond the idiosyncrasies of an individual life, however, Samuel's biography reveals how the intellectual histories of fields such as medicine and anthropology are not "objective" but shaped by the lives and times of their practitioners.

If not for likeminded colleagues, Samuel could never have amassed the great number of skulls that he did. As my research took me down an archival rabbit hole, to institutions located elsewhere in Philadelphia and beyond, skepticism expressed by the ANS librarian—that Samuel alone was responsible for the collection's assemblage—proved perceptive. The professional network he fostered over a lifetime, I found, was tentacular and far-reaching. After Samuel's death, his colleague Dr. William Ruschenberger reflected: "Of the whole number, 690 were presented to him by 138 donors, a fact which shows the number of friends Dr. Morton interested actively in his favorite branch of natural science. This collection is one among the striking monuments of his industry, and of the kindness of his numerous friends in every quarter of the globe" (1852, 31–32). (Surely this number of donors would be greater were we to account for circuitous routes traveled by skulls and the numerous hands through which they passed before arriving in Philadelphia.) Who were his donors? Correspondences indicate they were friends and Friends (of the Quaker sort), physicians, gentleman planters, enslavers, committed naturalists, amateur paleontologists, foreign diplomats, and military officers. Occupational differences aside, they were mostly White, Christian men of some financial means. The replies they inked in letters to Samuel often concluded with "Your Obedient Servant." We may read this common valediction two ways: as an expression of nineteenth-century social propriety *and* compliance (or complicity) with institutional authorities.[5] As evidence of the latter, skulls and correspondences testify to these men's involvement in settler colonialism and imperialism during the nineteenth century.

In the United States, especially, there were professional opportunities to be had for men with ambition and an ability to rationalize suffering. But not for all men; that is, one's skin color, national origins, and class status did matter. From others' misfortune, physicians, naturalists, and ethnologists developed clinical practices, authoritative ideas about bodies, and pedagogical norms. Through medical and scientific studies of racial and sexual differences, Samuel and these men played an active part in shaping their complicated and interesting times. They materialized beliefs about national citizenship, character, and borders that valued Whiteness, Christianity, and heroic masculinity. Their complicity in the necropolitics of American nation-building is undeniable though little explored. "Studying up," as outlined by Laura Nader (1972, 286), is one way to reveal how "major institutions and organizations that affect everyday lives" exercise power. In this book, I examine institutions and individuals connected to medicine, science, the military, and governance.

But, as Nader stressed, it is insufficient to only study up. One must study down and sideways, too. To this end, we may turn to the individuals whose skulls make up the Morton Collection. Documenting how men of medicine and science transformed subjects into objects is a lesson in the process of forgetting and distortion. To narrate the latter's stories, or the stubborn silences that thwart such an effort, offers ingress into the heterogeneous lives excluded or erased from the American body politic.

Studying up and down, then, has the potential to atone for the sins of disciplinary forefathers. We may also help to dismantle contemporary White supremacy while advancing decolonial projects. That these contradictory phenomena exist today speaks to the persistence of ideas from Samuel's times *and* the reparative, ethical logic of our own. For anthropology, more specifically, I see the Morton Collection as a barometer of the discipline's embrace of colonialism and the racist and xenophobic illogic that underpins it. A historic analysis allows us to gauge changes in anthropology's representations of the Other. We may track mythmaking about practitioners, from eulogization to vilification (or vice versa). Or we can chart the sociopolitical conditions that morphed methodology, a shift from purportedly objective, categorical analysis to research that has sought out collaboration and consent of participants and/or descendants. We can hope that from deliberation about culpability and flexible morality in the past, fairer weather ahead entails more ethical practices that consolidate into a new ethos.

Nineteenth-Century Biopower

This story begins in Philadelphia. The city was a hub of medicine and politics in the late eighteenth century. Local physicians established the first medical school in the American colonies, the University of Pennsylvania's Medical Department, in 1765. Samuel and many of his colleagues would go on to earn their medical degrees from that esteemed institution. Though the nation's capital moved to Washington, DC, in 1800, Philadelphia remained at the forefront of medicine for the better part of the nineteenth century. The nation desperately needed properly trained medical practitioners capable of treating myriad infectious diseases. Yellow fever, scarlet fever, whooping cough, cholera, typhus, smallpox, consumption, and more flourished, taking on epidemic proportions in urban environs. They were all cause for public health concern.

At the time of Samuel's birth, physicians had produced disease classifications for diagnostic purposes—a "form of experience was being institutionalized," per Michel Foucault (1978, 25). Yet, effective treatments remained elusive. Take the case of yellow fever, the virus that killed Samuel's father, George, in 1799. As documented by the Philadelphia physician Benjamin Rush (1809), yellow fever outbreaks occurred with frightening regularity and resulted in high mortality rates—in 1793, 1794, 1797, 1798, 1799, 1802, 1803, and 1805. Yellow fever's spread was variously attributed to the heat of the sun, cool or impure air (miasma), fatigue, intemperance in eating or drinking, fear, grief, sleep, and immoderate evacuations of blood or excreta. (Germs had yet to be proposed as a mechanism of contagion.) Recognizing that the public's health was in jeopardy, Rush advocated for bloodletting and purging to treat the disease's ill effects. Symptoms included (though were not limited to) fever, jaw pain, headaches, an erratic or slowed pulse, swelling in the limbs, hemorrhaging, and vomiting (Rush 1794, 1809). Suffice to say that yellow fever was not something you wanted to contract, and simply being alive seemed to up your chances of doing so (although certain risk factors like age or health status made one more susceptible). Other physicians then cross-referenced Rush's observations in their own studies, thereby setting a foundation for American medicine.

As a physician, anatomy professor, and natural historian in Philadelphia, Samuel's professional activities worked to normalize these medical practices and physicians' control over bodies. He traveled from hospital wards to dissecting tables to lecture halls to museums—spaces that produced "one or more truth discourses about the 'vital' character of living human beings, and an array of authorities considered competent to speak that truth" (Rabinow and Rose 2006, 197). His work in these interconnected institutions contributed to the emergence of *biopower* as the fundamental mechanism used by the state to exercise control over the people living within its borders, whether citizen or noncitizen.

Foucault's writings on "bio-power"[6] were seminal and have proven influential. Prior to the eighteenth century, he argued, sovereign power had exercised "the right to *take* life or *let* live" (1978, 138). But, at "the threshold of our modernity" (Foucault 1978, 148), the mechanisms of political power transformed. Techniques emerged to control bodies and safeguard life—"a power to *foster* life or *disallow* it to the point of death" in the words of Foucault (1978, 138). He described two interrelated forms of biopower, a disciplining of the individual body (*anatomo-politics*) and regulation or "massifying" of a population (*bio-politics*). The latter, he explained, "focused on the species body, the body imbued with the mechanics of life and serving as the basis of the biological processes: propagation, births and mortality, the level of health, life expectancy and longevity, with all the conditions that can cause these to vary. Their supervision was effected through an entire series of interventions and *regulatory controls: a bio-politics of the population*" (1978, 139). In his historic analysis, Foucault made transparent the intricacies of biopower's operation in myriad institutional settings—in the school, barracks, prison, factory, and clinic. Medicine played an especially pivotal role; in teaching hospitals and anatomical theaters, its practitioners generated beliefs about bodies. Categorically speaking, bodies were either normal or pathological, a framing that he adapted from his teacher Georges Canguilhem (1951). As the nineteenth century unfolded, with the proliferation of medical institutions, students, and specialist publications, these beliefs consolidated and became hegemonic.

Ideas about biopower help to contextualize Samuel in the development of biomedicine; he was a key player. The concept also clarifies a crucial aspect of this intellectual history—that Samuel's work and legacy advanced American nation-building. Samuel was instrumental in catalyzing biomedical interventions, public health initiatives, and scientific standards—in fostering life—during the first half of the nineteenth century. He and colleagues treated a variety of diseases and human failings. In the process, they disregarded or honed regulatory interventions introduced by earlier physicians like Rush. To document their activities is to retrace "the history of humans' involvement in the making of scientific facts and the sciences' involvement in the making of human history" (Latour 1999, 10).

For these men of science, only certain lives were worth enhancing, proliferating, and prolonging. The darker side of biopower, "letting die" (Foucault 2003), involved the transformation of certain populations into biological and cultural threats. There are aspects of Samuel's medical practice that testify to his production of these "ungrievable lives" (sensu Butler 2009). His work in the medical department of the Philadelphia Almshouse comes to mind, as do his writings about pulmonary consumption (Morton 1834), both of which are discussed in chapter 2. But his cranial collection is the most compelling. Initially, he acquired skulls to train medical students, but, in short order, he did so to satisfy his interest in natural history. Medicine and natural history in the nineteenth century were not discordant fields; both contributed to reifying ideas about national character. Without a Hippocratic oath to hold practitioners accountable, however, natural historians were less likely to see "letting die" as an ethical violation of disciplinary norms.

The nationalist rhetoric of the day drew a clear distinction between ideal citizens and expendable noncitizens. Medical treatises referred to the mentally ill as "the uncontrollable mad," "incurable lunatics," and "the idiotic and insane." News sources and pamphlets described Blacks as dangerous and untrustworthy; they "revolted" and "rebelled" against their enslavement. In military correspondences, government officials deemed Natives "hostile," "savage," "restless," or "uncivilized," thereby justifying seizure of their land. Those amenable to removal, or at the very least compliant, were "friendly."

A eugenic strategy was needed to combat the threat that these groups posed to racial degeneracy. Persons afflicted by mental illness, poverty, promiscuity—most inmates in urban almshouses—were subject to confinement or incarceration. For Others, physical elimination or social death was justifiable to safeguard the state and improve the species. "In a normalizing society, race or racism is the precondition that makes killing acceptable," Foucault (2003, 256) argued. Warfare, he continued, acted as one eugenic strategy by which state powers realized racial purity. Physicians and natural historians like Samuel were also instrumental. From the battlefield to the anatomy classroom or hospital dissecting table, racism made race, a creation of categorical and unequal difference.

To understand how a politics that fosters life can also justify making die and manipulating dead bodies, contradictory positions held by Samuel and his colleagues, Achille Mbembe's (2003, 2019) writings on *necropolitics* provide a powerful frame.[7] With biopower as a reference point, he defines necropolitics as the destruction of human bodies and targeted populations by sovereign powers. Necropower refers directly to the techniques, both discursive and material, used to realize these ends. Rhetorical strategies advanced the racial distinctions between us and them in the name of American nineteenth-century nation-building. As for the more tangible, technological interventions (e.g., muskets, shotguns) made die, as did spatial segregations (e.g., reservations, slave quarters, prisons, asylums, those "repressed topographies of cruelty" in Mbembe's words [2019, 92]). There are also bodies—traumatized, slain, and violated during warfare.

Mbembe (2019, 66) asks, "When politics is considered a form of war, the question needs to be asked about the place that is given to life, death, and the human body (in particular when it is wounded or slain)?" He continues, "How are these aspects inscribed in the order of power?" In answer, he recognizes that necropolitics often, if not always, has involved bodily violation intended to terrorize and/or annihilate those perceived to be Other. "In the case of massacres, in particular, lifeless bodies are quickly reduced to the status of simple skeletons. Their morphology henceforth inscribes them in the register of undifferentiated generality: simple relics of an unburied pain; empty, meaningless corporealities; strange deposits plunged into cruel stupor" (Mbembe 2019, 87). Human remains—in fragments or left exposed or secreted within graves or unceremoniously disinterred—testify, albeit silently, to "states of injury," structural violence, and mass killings. Certainly, the skulls making up Samuel's collection do; he was the beneficiary of expansionist policies and violent martial conflicts that revised national borders and, in so doing, made certain lives precarious.

Samuel never served in the military. His upbringing in the Society of Friends may have influenced this decision. Pacifism was an important aspect of Quaker religious doctrine in theory if not in practice. When Friends felt the cause was just, for instance, they made autonomous decisions to serve in the military or pay war-related taxes (Valentine 2013). Samuel's disownment from the Society of Friends in the 1820s indicated his dissatisfaction with many core tenets of Quakerism. Conscientious objection may have been one he found difficult to sustain. Regardless of his stance on armed conflict, Samuel did benefit from the wars that US forces waged against American Indians and their Black allies. Using craniometric methods he then created a racialized and gendered hierarchy, which legitimated emergent ideas about American citizenship and contributed to "creeping" genocide (Levene 1999).

There is a striking parallel between the involvement of White physicians in nineteenth-century American nation-building and the anatomical science and medical experimentation during Germany's Third Reich. Of the latter, Sabine Hildebrandt (2016) has tracked how the corpses of murdered Holocaust victims were dissected in anatomy labs and medical classrooms throughout Germany and Austria. Opportunism then led to outright ethical transgression when physicians' needs dictated executions. "Clinicians, who traditionally worked exclusively with living human beings started to include the planned death of their research subjects in their study designs, and anatomists and pathologists crossed the boundary from work with the dead to work with the 'future dead,'" writes Hildebrandt (2016, 249). Such research yielded pedagogical specimens, dissertations, and publications, among other things. The text often referred to as "Pernkopf's Atlas," for instance, was created by an ardent Nazi anatomist who based its detailed illustrations on prisoners executed in death camps. It is still a source of information for physicians, though one that has raised ethical consideration more recently (Atlas 2001; Yee et al. 2019).[8] For this reason, I extend theorizing about necropolitics to examine how medico-scientific practitioners like Samuel *made future dead*, a concept borrowed from Hildebrandt. This process involved *becoming-object*, an idea of Mbembe's that I expand upon (though do not hyphenate) in subsequent chapters, and *maintaining object*, which I introduce to address the posthumous treatment of human remains.

Yehonatan Alsheh reminds us that corpses generated by mass violence and genocide—these "simple relics" in Mbembe's analysis—are not only evidence of murders perpetrated or lives eradicated. There is a "remarkable capacity of corpses to resist attempts to reduce them to a mere illustration of a theoretical principle," Alsheh observes (2014, 13). Here we can read against the grain of necropolitical agendas. Human remains can bear witness—sometimes years after their violation. They can offer incontrovertible proof of diverse and complex life histories, different ways to be human in the past that require attention to the intersection of race, ethnicity, gender, sexuality, age, and more. Courts of law, scientific analyses, and descendants' mourning rituals shape meaning and engagement in profound ways. And for those descendant communities who assign agency to ancestors, human remains possess posthumous vitality—a politicized relevance and an emotional resonance. This recognition is also a facet of nation-building, one that seeks to make reparations for historic violences, present the heterogeneity of a body politic, and advance a decolonial project.

A Biohistorical Approach

To investigate how human remains can simultaneously be "simple relics" born from necropolitical conditions *and* past individuals with politicized afterlives, a biohistorical approach offers a valuable conceptual framework and methodology.

In "The Birth of Social Medicine," Foucault defined *biohistory* as "the effect of medical intervention at the biological level, the imprint left on human history, one may assume, by the strong medical intervention that began in the eighteenth century" (2000, 134). Modernity, he believed, left so indelible a mark on the body that it shifted what it means to be human. As to how that change occurs, Foucault looked to biopower. In *The History of Sexuality*, Foucault linked the two concepts: "If one can apply the term *bio-history* to the pressures through which the movements of life and the processes of history interfere with one another, one would have to speak of *bio-power* to designate what brought life and its mechanisms into the realm of explicit calculations and made knowledge-power an agent of transformation of human life" (1978, 143; emphasis in original). Physicians were instrumental in the transformation of humans' existence. They did so by catalyzing and solidifying hegemonic approaches to bodies—hegemonic in the sense that they became dominant and commonsensical. Increasingly medicalized beliefs about bodies circulated in physicians' specialized publications, learned societies, and private correspondences, while their treatment of bodies at hospitals, on autopsy or dissecting tables, and in classrooms or anatomical theaters made for normative practices.

What resulted was a *biomedical bodyscape*. Elsewhere I have outlined the attributes of this bodyscape (Geller 2009). In brief, bodies are broken down, or fragmented, into parts that are laden with cultural meaning. In a biomedical bodyscape, these meanings are reductive (difference is strictly dichotomous not complex or heterogeneous) and deterministic (biology equals social destiny). Reiteration of approaches by physicians and the physicians they then train (and so on and so on) serves to idealize certain bodies and stigmatize others. Take the skull, for instance. As I make clear in the chapters to come, it was an object often fetishized by White physicians and natural historians. They studied it to gain insight into race, gender, and class. Institutional powers then used information gleaned from skulls to distinguish the human from the less than or nonhuman. Necropolitical interventions effectively disenfranchised or eradicated the latter. Samuel's part in this biohistorical shift was pivotal—he was initially celebrated, later forgotten, and eventually vilified when resurrected. A biomedical bodyscape, however, departs markedly from bodyscapes maintained by cultures that venerate ancestors and regard human remains as social actors. For them, a skull's vitality is undeniable.

Foucault's understanding of biohistory is certainly germane in this book, but it is also lacking. His primary concern was the analysis of discursive practices as they played out in institutional settings. Granted he has an implicit understanding that bodies are biocultural phenomena, but their actual corpo-reality, that is, biophysical or biochemical information, was not an empirical starting point for him. For a more holistic biohistorical approach—one that brings together the discursive and material—we can turn to methodology formalized by biological anthropologists.

Among forensic anthropologists and bioarchaeologists, biohistory scales from the individual to the population. For William Duncan and Christopher Stojanowski, it is a method that makes use of "forensic techniques to examine individuals whose connection to public imagination or historical consciousness initiated the analysis" (2016, 264; see also Andrews et al. 2004; Komar and Buikstra 2008; Paradise and Andrews 2007; Stojanowski and Duncan, eds. 2017). In their framing, Stojanowski and Duncan (2017, 3–4) are careful to distinguish biohistory from osteobiography. While both approaches use biophysical and biochemical data to help narrate the mundane and significant aspects of an individual's life, archaeological context and anthropological concerns generally underpin osteobiography. Differences aside, both methods' attention to individual bodies invites consideration of the anatomo-politics that Foucault regarded as a facet of biopower.

Other researchers have applied a biohistorical approach at the population level to document biological changes produced by social, political, and economic interventions. Many case studies focus on peoples enslaved or violated during settler colonialism. Lesley Rankin-Hill, for instance, has conducted biohistorical work to document "the adaptations of humans of

African origins to biological, environmental, and sociocultural stresses of involuntary migration and resettlement in the New World" (1997, 11; see also Blakey 2001; Edgar 2009; Watkins 2012). Diaspora and enslavement came to mark the health, fertility, morbidity, and mortality of Black Americans in profound ways. Turning to the southeastern United States, Larsen and colleagues (2002) have conducted a biohistorical study to document the declining health of Native peoples in the wake of Spanish colonialism. These biohistorical studies identify biological traces—markers of disease and trauma—that link up to biopolitics, those interventions designed to massify a population. But rather than fostering life, we recognize how necropolitical experiences became sedimented over time or had intergenerational effects.

In addition to studying in vivo changes, a biohistorical approach extends understanding of the connection between medico-scientific interventions and dead bodies. This framing is implicit in the work of several scholars though they may not evoke the term biohistory (e.g., de la Cova 2019, 2021; Novak 2017; Novak and Warner-Smith 2020; Nystrom 2014; Watkins 2018; Watkins and Muller 2015). From their studies, we learn about the violent processes and technologies of power that have affected the management of dead bodies, as well as the knowledge that researchers have produced from their analyses. We can also learn how the composition of legacy collections are far more arbitrary and curated than representative because of the circumstances that lead to their formation.

In the nineteenth century, Samuel's interventions set important precedents for the fields of medicine and anthropology. Like many of his colleagues, he saw human skulls as natural historic specimens equivalent to taxidermized birds, fossilized shells, insects, and geological minerals. Assemblage en masse to assess variation within a single species made a collection. But the decedents comprising the Morton Collection diverged from nonhuman specimens in important ways. "All the people in the collection had in common . . . their or their community's disempowerment," notes Ann Kakaliouras (2021), during a precarious moment of US nation-building. Settler colonialism, military campaigns, and brutal industrialization impelled collection. The management of human "specimens," unlike those nonhuman ones, also entailed the erasure of individuality. To morph subjects into objects, men of medicine and science needed to be indifferent to structural and interpersonal violences, as well as adept at cataloguing, categorizing, measuring, and labeling.

When Samuel died in 1851, he had amassed well over 900 specimens.[9] For the more than 170 years that have followed, individuals and institutions have sold, lost, traded, fragmented, loaned, relocated, rehoused, repatriated, and reburied skulls in the Morton Collection. This changing state of affairs is informative about the dynamic process of maintaining object, as well as the malleability of Samuel's legacy. In the chapters that follow, I address both concerns in greater detail.

Cranial and archival materials have traveled confusing but separate paths. The further decontextualization and dehumanization of decedents who make up the Morton Collection has been one outcome. Details about individuals' biographies and origins have disappeared, as have specifics about the routes (and hands) through which skulls traveled prior to arriving in Samuel's office. The movement of archival materials reflects the whims of benefactors and historic shifts in Philadelphia's intellectual institutions. For example, Venia Phillips, librarian at the Academy of Natural Sciences, wrote to George Stuart in 1952 about four boxes of letters that had "come from the descendants of Dr. Morton's wife." As of 1943, they were housed at the Ridgway Library on Broad and Christian Streets. But, in the 1960s, all holdings at Ridgway Library were moved to the Library Company of Philadelphia at 1314 Locust Street.[10] (Samuel and Rebecca's brother-in-law John Jay Smith served as librarian [1829–1851] and treasurer [1840–1857] at the latter institution [Abbot 1913, 28, 29]). Today, to complicate matters, the letters are on deposit at the Historical Society of Pennsylvania (HSP), which is directly adjacent to the Library Company, at 13th and Locust Streets.

Becoming Object is the result of years researching Samuel and the Morton Collection. This work involved combing through archives and libraries throughout Philadelphia for pertinent written, illustrated, and photographic sources, as well as analysis of skulls at Penn Museum. Because of the dynamic histories of the collections, embarking on this research has sometimes felt like reassembling a jigsaw puzzle with several key pieces lost and gathering dust behind the bookcase. Joining the biological and historical together—another pragmatic aspect of a biohistorical approach—has been invaluable for circumventing some of the methodological challenges.

At Penn Museum, I conducted forensic and craniometric studies to document age, sex, pathology, and trauma.[11] My analysis concentrated on the skulls of individuals affiliated with the so-called Five Civilized Tribes[12] of the southeastern United States (n=41). In this region, with passage of the

Indian Removal Act of 1830, we can see manifest destiny in the making. Violent pacification and assimilation of Native peoples in the American West was preceded by the US Army's actions in the Southeast. But admittedly, there is much more that can be said about settler colonialism as it played out in other regions of the United States. And while not the focus of this book, seeing that Samuel also acquired skulls from locations around the world, the collection begs deeper discussion about US imperialism, more broadly.

I also recognize that my biohistorical analysis relies on a legacy set in motion by Samuel and his medical colleagues. That is, his training as a physician (and his training of student physicians who went on to educate subsequent cohorts, and so on and so on) established methods and a shared discourse—for example, terms and descriptions like specimen; cranial regions like glabella and parietal; pathology like cribra orbitalia—that aimed to transmute living subjects into scientific objects. Does my inclusion of forensic information about decedents in the Morton Collection, which I see as a means to humanize those long regarded as specimens, instead maintain object by replicating the very violence that I aim to undermine? The tricky challenge for contemporary researchers who claim no ancestral connection to the past lives they study is to signal analytical proficiency while not whitewashing the negative effects of the discipline's colonial legacy. For my part, expository parentheses and the ironic use of scare quotes (e.g., "specimen," "hostile") go a long way, as does the narration of decedents' osteobiographies, those life histories that draw from osteological data. Granted these stories may be quite difficult to sketch out, as I discuss shortly, but they are an important complement to death histories, those postmortem changes and meanings attached to a decedent by actors with varied intentions (e.g., kin, scientists, teachers, nonspecialists) (Geller 2012).

In addition to osteological analysis, I conducted traditional (in-person) archival research at ten institutions.[13] Personal letters, diaries, photographs, original research notes, and book marginalia were examined. On one especially exciting day in the archive, I encountered Samuel's will among the genealogical papers housed at the HSP. During archival work, I prioritized the following information pertaining to Samuel: personal life; kin and their biographies; and relationship to original collectors (e.g., professional, personal). I also compiled biographical information about the men who acquired skulls for Samuel, as well as how they did so (e.g., by looting graves, roaming battlefields, after dissecting cadavers). As far as the decedents whose skulls were collected, I sought information about the following: cultural affiliation; physical description; scientific analysis; social identities (e.g., warrior); and names when given for an individual. Finally, I documented the shifting proveniences of skulls, trying to track movements from their places of origins to the institutional locations they were sent. I quote often from primary source materials so that the reader might gain a somewhat unfiltered sense of past individuals' sentiments.

This said, I realize of course that inclusion of some archival writings and images may lead one down a slippery slope. I am reminded of the photographs in Saidiya Hartman's *Wayward Lives* (2019). One stands out: that of a young Black girl posing nude for the artist Thomas Eakins (he, too, makes an appearance in chapter 1 of this book). Hartman recounts uncertainty about the image's classification—"Art? Science? Pornography?" (2019, 27). Yet she is sure that it is a defilement of the unnamed child, a reification of Black women's commodification and hypersexuality that tracks back to enslavement. "The odalisque is a forensic image that details the violence to which the black female body can be subjected," she writes (2019, 27). Yet, while compelling and affective, is the image's inclusion in her book—now viewable for a modern readership—a further violation of the child? This is a question that Hartman does not ask herself. (Or is this question precluded by her positionality, seeing that she is personally and politically invested in a Black feminist historical project?)[14]

The photograph raises a host of other questions, as well—about the circumstances that led to its creation, the life of this anonymous child, and the experiences of young Black women at the turn of the century, more generally. But for Hartman, archives have often proven unresponsive, an issue with which other scholars have also struggled (e.g., King 2019; Moss and Thomas 2021; Thomas et al. 2017; Trouillot 1995). To narrate the gaps and unknowns has required her "to speculate, listen intently, read between the lines, attend to the disorder and mess of the archive, and to honour silence" (Hartman, 2019, 34). (The origins of this method, her practice of *critical fabulation* [Hartman 2008], is one to which I return.) Additionally, Michel-Rolph Trouillot's (1995) *Silencing the Past* has been methodologically instructive for navigating the forgotten or distorted. Of history's production, he reminded us that "power is constitutive of the story," for this reason "the production of traces is also the creation of silences" (1995, 28, 29). Recognizing that the silences I encountered while researching Samuel and the Morton Collection were not neutral, what then did they signify?

The Significance of Silence

At the outset of my research, some silences struck me as deliberate, others accidental. But overall, they seemed insignificant. In the case of missing information about skulls, I simply chalked it up to their mobility coupled with institutions' inconsistent or incompatible recordkeeping. As for Samuel's papers, it was not surprising that his and kin's selections sought to craft a legacy that haloed the physician in a flattering light. They did not aim to be comprehensive. As my research progressed, however, my position shifted on archival silences. I began to think less about absence and more about process, the ways by which certain "facts" of life became authoritative and others were made negligible.

Some silences were suggestive of agentive choices. Take Sarah Mapps Douglass, who I discuss in chapter 1. Among other things, Sarah was a Quaker, abolitionist, educator, and prominent Black Philadelphian. For reasons that go unspecified, in her will she instructed kin to destroy all her private correspondences, as well as her "lectures on Anatomy and Natural History to Mothers" (Winch 1999; see also Bacon 2001, 28). For information about Sarah's life, one must seek out materials contained within the archives of her family and friends (for instance, the Grimké sisters, Sarah and Angelina, counted among her close contacts). Often, however, silencing was directly tied to the nefarious exercise of power. The necropolitical conditions that facilitated Samuel's work created "disposable lives" in Hartman's (2008, 11) words, as did the subsequent use of his studies to justify exclusion from the body politic. For these reasons, the archives I visited revealed little about the decedents composing the Morton Collection or omitted altogether narratives about lives that defied easy categorization (e.g., Black Indians, Two-Spirits).

To access silenced lives though not necessarily to speak for them, Hartman proposes critical fabulation. "The intent of this practice," she writes, "is not to *give voice* to the slave, but rather to imagine what cannot be verified, a realm of experience which is situated between two zones of death—social and corporeal death—and to reckon with the precarious lives which are visible only in the moment of their disappearance" (2008, 12). But Hartman also realizes that historians (or biohistorians), unlike fiction writers, must not stray too far from the evidentiary boundaries set by the archives. An inability to tell certain stories because of silent sources—about the violence of enslavement, disenfranchisement, dehumanization—is no less a tragedy. But it can disrupt official History and national mythologizing. Vocalization may not be possible, but visibility occurs that offers compelling, tangible evidence of lives perceived to be disposable.

As Trouillot also recognized, there is a *materiality* to history. "History begins with bodies and artifacts: living brains, fossils, texts, buildings" (Trouillot 1995, 29). Whereas he emphasized the sway of the monumental—"mass graves and pyramids bring history closer while they make us feel small," he wrote (1995, 29)—it is arguable that scale is irrelevant. A skull is no less powerful despite having a more negligible material mass. (In fact, given its humanity, one may argue that a skull is more powerful.) As aforementioned and elicited in the chapters to come, the skull's meanings are multiple. It has been a collectible, a fetish, an existential reminder, a pedagogical tool, a body of evidence, a tragedy, an ancestor. In the case of the Morton Collection, skulls also functioned as textual surfaces (or embodied texts, depending on your perspective). For this reason, I felt it necessary to approach them as alternative archival sources.

Skulls procured by Samuel's colleagues are inked, notated, and labeled. The physician's own hand is identifiable, as are those of the many men who did his bidding. Jottings about proveniences sometimes appear on cranial bones, as do ages and sexes.[15] Even rarer, a name is written. Labels with tribal affiliations are affixed to foreheads. Anatomical information testifies to physicians' training. From notations on teaching specimens—"Os Parietal," "Squamous Suture," and so forth—these men learned the proper names and locations of cranial elements and features. Writing also confirmed that skulls were used for research. Penned on many left temporal bones, presumably by Samuel, is metric information; for example, the individual labeled 1105 bore "F.A. 75°" to designate the cranium's facial angle and "I.C. 82" for internal capacity. The mobility of the Morton Collection is also indicated by multiple accession numbers. When the ANS loaned the collection to Penn Museum in 1966, a registrar inked the catalogue number L-606 to supplement Samuel's original numbering system. This cataloguing was followed by the addition of 97–606 when the ANS's formal transfer of ownership occurred in 1997. So specimen 1105 became L-606-1105 and then 97-606-1105.

To regard skulls as textual surfaces also makes visible the shared experience of *precarity*. The concept is related to but should not be confused with precariousness. "Lives are by definition precarious," Judith Butler (2009, 25) notes. "Their persistence is in no sense guaranteed." Given the state of medical care in the nineteenth century—prior to the introduction of anesthesia, antiseptic, and antibiotic agents—infectious diseases made all lives precarious. And physicians like Samuel were aware of their failings. The omnipresence of death loosely unified nineteenth-century Americans irrespective of race, gender, religion, or regional location. Hence, biopolitical interventions. Facets of nation-building like enslavement, Indian removal, and scientific racialization, however, require us to recognize the extent to which precarity structured the lives and deaths of certain groups. Butler (2009, 25–26) explains: "Precarity designates that politically induced condition in which certain populations suffer from failing social and economic networks of support and become differentially exposed to injury, violence, and death. Such populations are at heightened risk of disease, poverty, starvation, displacement, and of exposure to violence without protection." Precarity impresses itself on bodies in very real, observable ways (though this concern was less explored by Butler). Trauma signals the violence and fatal intent wrought by a bullet, musket ball, or bayonet. In the case of the Morton Collection, these marks have included fractures and gunshot wounds. Structural violence is also discernable by identifying the marks of longstanding malnourishment, impoverishment, and deprivation or stress. More specifically, as bioarchaeologists have documented, pathological evidence like porotic hyperostosis and cribra orbitalia can signal chronic infections that exacerbate a group's precarity (e.g., Klaus 2012, Tremblay and Reedy 2020; Walker et al. 2009).[16] Granted, the Morton Collection—comprised of only cranial remains, few in number, and specially selected in some cases—does not a robust sample make. But when such pathology is coupled with copious archival and historic documentation the presence of disposable lives becomes undeniable.

How to narrate these silences is a question with which I have also grappled.[17] This concern is as much about content as it is about structure (or writing style). Because this book is told in a loosely chronological fashion, I have prioritized its flow. To this end, I use endnotes unsparingly. To clarify, my intent is not to trivialize or relegate certain lives and/or information to the margins. Notes do not indicate lesser but an alternative, to borrow from Katherine McKittrick. "I believe," she (2021, 18) writes, "that bibliographies and endnotes and references and sources are alternative stories that can, in the most generous sense, centralize the practice of sharing ideas about liberation and resistance and writing against racial and sexual violence." (For McKittrick there is overlap between foot/endnotes and citational sources because, dissimilar from anthropologists, scholars in the humanities include the latter in the former.) Her use of footnotes throughout *Dear Science and Other Stories*—as the traditional location for citations and as an alternative one for "a lesson that cannot be contained within the main text" (2021, 19)—offers a provocative way to rethink their function and to dismantle a hierarchy of information.

But, dissimilar from McKittrick's book, *Becoming Object* does relate a linear narrative about Samuel's life and histories of violences. For this reason, I realize that endnotes may be insufficient alone in a work seeking to advance a decolonial project. It is also necessary to disrupt that story with lives historically (and literally) pushed to the margins given their race, gender, or class. (To riff on Nader, one must write down and up and on the sides.) So, as I revised *Becoming Object*, some migration from endnotes to main text occurred. Despite my best attempts to finesse the transitions, at certain junctures, I acknowledge that their integration does more important work as an interruption and complication to the linearity of *Becoming Object*'s story.

Organization of the Book

Becoming Object begins with an overview of Samuel's formative years in Philadelphia. His family's experiences with immigration, employment, infectious disease, and urban dwelling were representative of White, American citizens at the start of the nineteenth century. Samuel's enmeshment in the Society of Friends presents an important contradiction in his upbringing, however. As I discuss in chapter 1, "The Friend," his childhood involved immersive schooling in Quakerism. To what extent did these spiritual and moral positions make an impression on him? Progressive lessons learned about abolitionism, gender equality, and pacifism are hard to square with his later medico-scientific work, which promoted ideas about the inferiority of women and certain races and benefited from violent military incursions. Time spent at the University of Edinburgh's medical school is where Samuel seems to have dispensed with his Quaker beliefs. In Europe, he cultivated personal and professional relationships with men who became quite (in)famous (e.g., Thomas Hodgkin, Robert Knox, George Combe). His European education complete and medical degree in hand—"a licence [*sic*] to kill and cure all over the world," a friend joked in a letter (Chaloner 1823)—he returned to Philadelphia in 1823.

Back home, curiosity and analytical devotion contributed to Samuel's professional successes, but we cannot discount his opportunism, ambition, and privilege. As a respected member of the city's medical community, he played an important role in formalizing, or normalizing, biomedicine. He and colleagues developed biologically deterministic beliefs about class, race, and gender, which then legitimized nascent sociopolitical inequalities and worsened disparities in health care. During this juncture in his life, he also began to collect skulls in earnest, initially to train medical students but soon in the interest of natural history. Chapter 2 documents his daily travels through the halls of medicine and science. His activities in these institutions fostered certain lives and let others die.

Although Samuel's stint as a medical school lecturer spurred his desire to acquire skulls, natural history increasingly came to occupy his professional efforts. Several factors may account for the shift, not least of which was his inability to effectively treat patients who fell victim to various epidemics. The cholera epidemic of 1832, which spread from Europe to Canada and then swept down the United States' eastern seaboard, greatly impacted the almshouse residents in Samuel's care. But more devastating for him was the loss of his young niece Gulielma to scarlet fever. In the aftermath, his brother-in-law and sister-in-law, John Jay and Rachel Smith, questioned Samuel's abilities as a physician. In contrast, the skulls he collected—skeletonized and belonging to the disenfranchised, subjugated, or ancient—did little to remind him of decomposition's mess and odor, decedents' identity, or kin's grief. No one demanded that he explain or apologize for his craniometric work.

Rather, Samuel's ethnological studies garnered him international attention. As his ideas about human races developed, some friendships flourished, and others fizzled. Samuel and the phrenologist George Combe cultivated a mutually beneficial relationship and shared concern for national character. But his hardening position on the plurality of origins for distinct, human races, or polygenism, alienated old friends like James Cowles Prichard and Thomas Hodgkin. Both men were active in the Aborigines' Protection Society and offered pointed criticism of the wars waged by the US government against American Indians.

Conversely, Samuel found opportunity in the Indian removal policies enacted by President Andrew Jackson. By 1830, as necropolitical events unfolded, Samuel largely abandoned Quaker lessons learned in his youth about the immorality of Indian land dispossession. Or, at the very least, the advancement of science provided sufficient rationalization for the research he conducted. Samuel rarely if ever acquired skulls himself, however. Rather, he relied on an extensive network of colleagues. In chapter 3, I consider members of the US military who procured skulls for him; in closing their correspondences, they often penned the expression "Your Obedient Servant." Many of these individuals were medical staff. As physicians, they had been tasked with a Hippocratic duty to do no harm. But benevolent aims were often difficult to reconcile with the exercise of biopower. With passage of the Indian Removal Act in 1830, medical officers became deeply enmeshed in the necropolitics of US nation-building. They chronicled diseases but mostly remained indifferent to the waves of sickness that decimated Native groups. Physicians normalized the precarity that American Indians experienced. This response attests to their complicity in letting die.

Once landscapes had become depopulated of Native inhabitants, it was all the easier to disinter bones from their burial mounds and cemeteries. As military officers, medical men were also involved directly in violent confrontations. A more nefarious collection method, one that signals their making of the future dead, found them taking heads directly from battlefields. To demonstrate necropolitics in action during this tumultuous period, I relate the experiences of several medical officers who campaigned in the southern United States. While I chronicle the specifics of their stories, their interactions with American Indians set important precedents for future campaigns of conquest, assimilation, and collection. These men's activities and biographies also offer a pointed contrast to the dearth of information about the individuals comprising the Morton Collection.

In the manifesting of the US nation-state—in establishing and maintaining the body politic—White Americans were validated as citizens and received proper burials when they died, usually in cemeteries not far from their homes. Such was not the case for the "hostile" Indians and "rebellious slaves" (as described in official accounts) with whom they clashed. Their bodies and fragmented parts were transported far from ancestral lands and final resting places. It was only after death that these Others acquired a sort of social worth through disinterment, fragmentation, examination, and incorporation in collections like the one compiled by Samuel. This process of becoming object erased the complexities of individuals' identities and the historic entanglements of all peoples living in America. Instrumental in this process was boundary making.

In chapter 4, "Border Making, Border Crossing," I discuss how boundary making as a necropolitical strategy defined rhetoric, (re)shaped landscapes, and informed studies of bodies. Central in this process was the US Army Corps of Topographical Engineers. The corps was, in the words of historian William Goetzmann (1959, 4), "a central institution of Manifest Destiny." Like chapter 3's medical officers, the topographical engineers discussed here had a heavy hand in orchestrating Indian removal, as evidenced by the maps they drew and the human skulls they sent along to Samuel. To justify expansion of the United States' borders, military officers' rhetoric painted American Indians as either "friendly" or "hostile." Their distinction did build on the logic of earlier European colonizers. But this rhetoric increasingly became politicized and popularized (or weaponized) with the US government's forced relocation of American Indians. Friendly Indians were amenable to moving beyond state borders or willing to stay within them and assimilate. Indians deemed hostile resisted colonial encroachment, demarcated boundaries, and negotiated relocations. Characterizing these responses as hostility was necessary because it allowed White settlers and soldiers to perform heroism. Their violent deeds, carried out in the name of nation, became cause for celebration among many US citizens, a point brought home by the exploits of Captain Justin Dimick during the Second Seminole War.

Men like Dimick were often the original purveyors of skulls in Samuel's collection. The physician, in turn, studied them for quantifiable information about racial differences. His craniometric inquiries functioned as another type of boundary making. One that represented race as natural, bounded, simplistically categorical, and hierarchical. These intellectual efforts contributed to an exclusionary body politic, an understanding of national citizenship underpinned by heroic masculinity and Whiteness. Processes of racialization effaced the complexities of identities and specifics about named decedents in the Morton Collection. Though not entirely. Traces remain, as evidenced by the skull Samuel labeled 707. "EOKLO-EMATHLA" was inked in bold letters across the frontal bone but stricken from official texts. What might we learn from this individual's life, his "livingness" as conceived by McKittrick (2021), despite efforts, subtle and violent, that acted to erase him from the annals of History?

Silences, I believe, also call attention to the effacement of past lives that defied the racial categories established by Samuel and colleagues. To this end, in chapter 4 I think through the multiple meanings of hybridity. Samuel deliberated extensively about the concept, arguing that miscegenation decreased a pure race's fertility rate and was worthy of juridical punishment. While there were many who pointed out the deficiency of his ideas, Charles Darwin being one notable critic, they nevertheless became prime fodder for advocates of slavery and anti-miscegenation policies.

Few today (outside of White supremacists) would find value in Samuel's take on hybridity as contamination. Though shorn of its biological essentialism, the concept has continued to generate intellectual debate with political implications. Come the end of the twentieth century, scholars began to explore hybridity's capacity to subvert or transgress power dynamics—an in-between identity claimed or a boundary strategically navigated (e.g., feminist studies [Anzaldúa 1987; Haraway 1991]; postcolonial studies [Bhabha 1985, 1994; Hall 1990]). More recently, assessments of hybridity have found its "redemptive features," to quote Stephan Palmié (2013, 464), lacking or at least in need of critical attention. To this end, archaeologists who study colonial encounters have held forth: Card (2013), Liebmann (2008, 2015), Loren (2013), Silliman (2013, 2015), Tronchetti and van Dommelen (2005), and van Dommelen (2005), among others. Their criticisms are numerous, but rather than rehash them, I instead draw attention to what I find valuable about hybridity. That is, it provides an entry point for exploring process over form. "It is not *what* is a hybrid but *when*," proposes Palmié (2013, 472; emphasis added). As a compelling example, I consider the possibility of a Black Seminole included among the decedents of the Morton Collection (the *what*, or rather *who*). In the southeastern United States during the nineteenth century, complicated, historic relations between Blacks and American Indians were the outcomes of individuals' choices, albeit ones constrained by dire conditions (the *when*). These alliances were evidence of strategic resilience, as well as resistance to the state's necropolitical interventions. The hybrid identities and ancestries that ensued, despite legislators' and medico-scientists' best efforts to simplify differences and manage bodies, confirmed the fallacy of purity and the longstanding reality of entangled lives.

During this time, biopolitical regulation of bodies was not limited to racial minorities. Chapter 5, "The Beloved Woman," examines the role that physicians and ethnologists had in stifling women's political and economic involvement in American society. This period saw the demise of midwifery and growing legitimacy of obstetrics and gynecology. The disease model that underpinned physicians' perspectives designated women's bodies dangerous and pathological. Pregnancy was an especially risky endeavor, they maintained, and so required medical intervention. As further evidence of women's inadequacies, scientists cited the smaller size of their skulls. They embraced Samuel's craniometric studies, which equated lower cranial capacity with arrested physiological development and inferior intelligence.

Bodily differences were then used to explain the lowly place of women in cultural evolutionary schemas, as well as to justify their second-class status in the body politic. Biology was social destiny. And social destiny had a spatial arrangement. A partitioning of men and women into appropriate spheres, contingent on class, age, race, and religion. As a woman of her interesting times, Rebecca Grellet Pearsall Morton, the wife of Samuel, reproduced the day's traditional framing of "true womanhood." She was a White, middle-class, Christian wife, mother, and homemaker. Archival sources represent Rebecca as beloved, while their stubborn silences hint at her deference and passivity.

As a counterpoint to Rebecca, this chapter also identifies deviations from true womanhood—the radical, the fallen, the subversive. Lucretia Mott (Quaker, suffragette, abolitionist, and social reformer), a Philadelphia acquaintance of Samuel's, is discussed. Also orbiting his sphere, were unbeloved women, those prostitutes and impoverished inmates incarcerated at the Philadelphia Almshouse. As for the subversive, I bring to the fore individuals whose socio-sexual variance transgressed heteronorms altogether. Native "Beloved" women—a title bestowed on certain female-bodied individuals active in warfare and political life—are illustrative. These persons, like Black Indians discussed in the previous chapter, were evocative of hybridity, denied citizenship, and expunged from official histories. A biohistorical analysis of the Morton Collection reveals their traces. This type of socio-sexual variance was not homogeneous across tribal groups, I argue. In some cases, Native Beloved women were a longstanding category of personhood; they predated European conquest but became stigmatized during colonialism and Christianization. For other tribes, sociopolitical circumstances connected to US nation-building prompted Native peoples' responses. Rather than a social norm, such persons are survival strategies incarnate in the face of necropolitical nation-building.

After his death, eulogies portrayed Samuel as much beloved by his kin and colleagues. But, with the passing years, this sentiment did not stick. In *Becoming Object*'s final chapter, I track Samuel's shifting legacy. Memorialization first turned to indifference and, much later, aversion. Twentieth-century sociopolitics had their part to play as did anthropology's reckoning with its historic ties to colonialism. Nevertheless, facets of Samuel's study of dead bodies, which forged normative practices established by nineteenth-century physicians, became disciplinary common sense. Consent from the deceased or next of kin was unnecessary, and a utilitarian position—that is, science served the greater good—provided ethical justification. With the Morton Collection as an important precedent, such an ethos guided the creation of most legacy collections, hence their fraught significance today.

As the twentieth century ended, the controversial nature of the Morton Collection became clear. Passage of the Native Graves Protection and Repatriation Act (NAGPRA) of 1990 impelled researchers to check their own positionality and privileges. It certainly did for me, as I describe in chapter 6. The federal law also recalibrated institutions' relations with descendant communities. In the case of the Morton Collection, repatriation has advanced a decolonial project in two ways: it brought researchers and descendant communities into collaboration, and independent tribal nations have exercised autonomy over their ancestors. Yet, because of the law's limitations and institutional inertia, NAGPRA is not an end unto itself. For my part, and with Hartman's critical fabulation as a provocation, I return to the disruptive narratives of Black Indians and Two-Spirits. In previous chapters, these individuals served as reminders of the cruelties of colonialism and the complexities of past lives. In chapter 6, I evoke them as cautionary tales. As Indigenous scholars have pointed out, when Native communities soft-pedal historic enslavement, disenroll Black Indians, or reiterate homophobic and heteronormative beliefs, they may inadvertently derail a decolonial project (e.g., Byrd 2011; Driskill 2004, 2016; Micco 2006; TallBear 2003, 2013).

In tracking this book up to the sociopolitical present, we come to our own interesting times. In the wake of a national reckoning with racial injustice, attention has turned to the skulls of Black decedents in the Morton Collection. They have generated much media attention and a conscientious response from Penn Museum. At the writing of this book, repatriation of these decedents was scheduled for early February 2024, as are additional reparations. Critics continue to express their discontent, however. They would like to see the Morton Collection returned in its entirety. While expedient, I do not see this as feasible in all cases. I discuss the skulls acquired from Egypt and Cuba, whose inclusion in the collection was a consequence of imperialism. Their international repatriation is not without challenges, though I do offer some suggestions for how to move forward ethically and compassionately. Recognizing that this book will hardly be the last word on Samuel or the Morton Collection, I end the chapter with a coda that also functions as a prelude.

1

The Friend

Were it not for an aborted mutiny at sea, Samuel George Morton's birth in a new nation might never have occurred. In the summer of 1773, his father, George, left Clonmel, Ireland. He and older brother John were Philadelphia-bound. In Waterford, they boarded the *Charlotte*, a ship captained by Richard Curtis (Jordan 1911, 1714). George was all of 17 years old, his brother 19. Given their youth, they may have regarded the mutiny as part of the transatlantic adventure. From Ireland, their father, Thomas, expressed relief and derision:

> we Can't be thankfull Enough for your preservation, not only from the Boisterous Seas, but from them Abandoned Villains who Sought your distruction for A Short & Ill purchased liberty by which they would have buried in the deep near 80 Souls, but providence Enterposed and discoverd their dark design, Nothing apears too desperate for some of our Wicked Country men to Attempt, no Wonder they should be held in Derision in America as the greatest part that goes is the Very Scroff of the Nation.[1] (Jordan 1911, 1714)

George and John traveled to America as free passengers. Many of their Irish compatriots, however, were indentured servants, their passage paid in promised labor (Grubb 1988). Regardless, whether one was free or contracted, economic opportunity in a society not defined by strict social stratification beckoned from across the ocean. Philadelphia promised to fulfill many European immigrants' nascent American dreams. In the late eighteenth century, the city's inhabitants were multicultural, and its port was well-connected to global markets (Miller 1985, 138–39). Into the latter, the *Charlotte* docked on July 4. The date had yet to acquire its symbolic weightiness, but in retrospect seems providential given the contributions that George's son Samuel would make to the US nationalist project.

As George disembarked, the American colonies were moving toward open rebellion. In May of 1773, British Parliament had passed the Tea Act.

Seven months later, colonists responded by dumping several boatloads of British East India Company tea into Boston Harbor. They did so in the guise of American Indians; war paint and ferocious whoops added to the theatrics. The result was a stereotypical representation of Indianness that sustained through the centuries—Indigenous but disobedient and therefore dangerous (Deloria 1998). In the decades to come, the US government evoked these reductive descriptions to justify violent expansionism, land usurpation, and forced assimilation. Medical inquiries about disease and scientific study of skulls, as I discuss in later chapters, reified this cultural evolutionary logic.

As a recent arrival from Ireland, George may have found these depictions of American Indians familiar. England justified its colonization and subjugation of Ireland by deeming its Gaelic inhabitants inferior, pagan, barbaric, and degenerate (Canny 1973). "We find the colonists in the New World," historian Nicholas Canny (1973, 596) has remarked, "using the same pretexts for the extermination of the Indians as their counterparts had used in the 1560s and 1570s for the slaughter of numbers of the Irish."

This history allows us to situate Thomas's comment about the "Very Scroff of the Nation." The Morton family was descended from English who colonized Ireland in the sixteenth century (Jordan 1911, 1712). Thomas wished to distinguish his familial stock from "scroff," those Irish of Gaelic or Catholic background who sought cultural or religious refuge in America. As for his sons, George and John's emigration was impelled by the promise of economic prosperity. Even prior to disembarking on American shores, their family ties and Protestant birth lent them an advantage. A family relative, Samuel Neale, penned an introductory letter to Israel Pemberton, a prominent Quaker in Philadelphia (Thayer 1943). He emphasized the boys' enterprising nature and homegrown challenges:

> Thy interposing on their behalf will be an additional favour conferred on me & may yield a prospect of prosperity to these youths, who gave up freely to leave their parents to endeavor to seek a distant land a living by industry and labour which has often succeeded to establish a settlement for life amongst a people much less tainted by luxury & vice than in this Island where corruption & licinticusness [sic] runs like a torrent & I fear will bring upon us a national scourge. (Neale 1773)

The letter was effective. John secured a position with Pemberton, and George found employment in the firm of Levi Hollingsworth, a successful

Quaker merchant whose commodities included flour, grains, and whiskey (G. Morton 1774).

John's time in the American colonies was short-lived, however. Eight months after his arrival, he fell ill and died (Jordan 1911, 1714). Benjamin Booth, a friend of the brothers who attended the dying John, identified his sickness as consumption (Booth 1774). George conveyed the sad news to his parents. In a reply, his father Thomas expressed grief tempered by pragmatism: "Such is the uncertainty of this life, that them that put their trust in it, will surely be disappointed" (T. Morton 1774).

Birth in a Nation

George, like the new nation he now called home, moved forward with cautious optimism. During the American Revolution, he served as an assistant commissary of issues in Philadelphia for the Continental Army (Waldenmaier 1944, 26). Postwar, George's business ventures vacillated. His decision to take a bride suggested that he had found a modicum of fiscal stability by 1784. Jane Cummings, the daughter of John and Margaret (née Hinman), came from one of Philadelphia's respectable Quaker families. George courted his "Jenny" with letters containing private jokes, snippets of romantic poetry, and terms of endearment, which grew more intimate with time.

That he also regarded marriage and business as analogous attests to his practicality. To Samuel Neale he wrote: "In my opinion there is as much nicety in chasing a Partner in Trade as there is in chasing a Wife—if there is not a similarity in their dispositions and pursuits you seldom find that such connections are permanent. Apropos—Before this reaches you I shall in all probability be engaged with a partner for Life" (G. Morton 1784b). In November, George penned a letter to Margaret asking that she consent to his and Jane's union. He assured her that the proposal was not motivated by financial gain. "I can declare with the greatest Sincerity that the high opinion I have of the Dear Girl & her attachment to me, would be a sufficient inducement for me to make this proposal if you had not one shilling in the world" (G. Morton, 1784a).

George and Jane married on 23 February 1785 in Philadelphia's St. Peter's Church. Reverend Robert Blackwell officiated. The bride wore a white dress of satin brocade. Over a century later, her great-granddaughter Helen Kirkbride Morton retained a portion of the garment, though she herself never married.

From Ireland, George's father Thomas sent hearty congratulations (T. Morton 1785). He was pleased that his son had chosen a young woman of "agreeable accomplishments" and laudable "family connections."[2] Her Quaker upbringing posed no problem for her new in-laws. The Society of Friends, however, did not reciprocate the warm feelings. Within months of the marriage, members of the Philadelphia Monthly Meeting on Arch Street moved for Jane's disownment—"By which conduct she has disunited herself from us, until she becomes truly sensible of her errors and condemns the same to the satisfaction of this Meeting; which we desire for her."[3] Jane's desires, however, clearly lay elsewhere. A year after their marriage, George waxed romantic while on a business trip: "I hope and ardenly [sic] wish the end of this week will be spent in your Arms" (G. Morton 1787).

In due time, Jane gave birth to a total of nine children. Six of the babies did not survive infancy. The deaths were mourned, but they were not unexpected. In late eighteenth-century Philadelphia, infant mortality rates averaged 187 deaths per 1,000 live births (Graff 1995, 28). These rates did drop with time but only slightly; by the 1820s, there were 182 deaths per 1,000 births (Klepp 2004, 64). One's race, class, religious affiliation, and geographic location (i.e., urban vs. rural) were significant determinants of survivorship (Klepp 2004). Unskilled laborers—a group often beset by poverty and composed disproportionately of people of color—had the most dismal mortality rates with 254 infants per 1,000. Infants born into the Society of Friends were situated at the other end of the spectrum with 146 infants dying per 1,000 (Graff 1995, 28). Their survival may have benefited from access to health care, crude though it was at the time; Quaker men often pursued careers in medicine.

Of the three Morton children to survive, Samuel George was the youngest. He was born on 26 January 1799 during a winter of extended duration and abundant snow (Darlington 1891, 118). The summer season in Philadelphia proved equally as challenging. Reports of yellow fever began to circulate in mid-June. By the end of the month, the College of Physicians confirmed its presence with trepidation. Many had witnessed firsthand yellow fever's lethal effects in 1793, 1797, and 1798; death tolls during each of these epidemics had ranged between 5 and 10 percent of the urban population (Shannon and Cromley 1982, 357). (At the end of the eighteenth century, about 41,000 people called the city home, and an additional 20,000 residents lived in the Northern Liberties and Southwark areas.) While physicians had grown adept at describing yellow fever's symptoms, they remained uncertain about the etiology and best course of treatment. The college did recommend that the Board of Health enforce certain regulations to curtail its spread (Currie 1800, 9–16). The affected should be removed to the country and their residences cleaned deeply, the physicians suggested. But the Board of Health demurred, and the number of cases continued to increase. It was during this exchange that George took ill with yellow fever. He succumbed on 27 July 1799 and was buried at Gloria Dei Church.[4] The Morton family was not alone in their grief; George was one of approximately 1,000 Philadelphians who fell victim to the yellow fever epidemic of 1799.

Though he retained no memory of his father, Samuel worked to fill the gap left by his death. Family members, specifically stepfather Thomas Rogers and uncle James Morton, were supportive, as were physicians who mentored Samuel during the early stages of his medical training. Years later, when he was middle aged and a father himself many times over, Samuel inquired about George. In answer, uncle James (1838) wrote: "You desire to know if there was any likeness between your Uncle Samuel + your Father. I never saw your Father after the year 1784.... They both had round faces and nearly the same coloured eyes + hair but your Father was paler + a better limbed man, certainly more like my Brother Sam than myself." The physical description may have been sufficient for Samuel, whose correspondences seldom betrayed any exuberant affection. His Quaker upbringing had schooled him well in emotional stoicism.

Growing Up Quaker

The rapidity with which infectious diseases spread in Philadelphia's populous, urban environs made death seem as if it was omnipresent and ever lurking. Outbreaks of yellow fever, cholera, scarlet fever, whooping cough, typhus, croup, and smallpox recurred throughout the nineteenth century. Resignation rather than romanticization characterized most people's responses. When medicine failed to comfort those in need—and it failed often during this period—religion filled the void. For Jane, the death of George compelled her to reconnect with Friends in Philadelphia's Quaker community. In 1800, she was officially brought back into their socioreligious fold, as were Samuel and his sister, Anna.

As for Jane's oldest son, James, her father-in-law Thomas suggested that she send him to Ireland. There George's brother, who was also named James, could care for, educate, and eventually adopt him. The solution seemed sound enough; George had died in debt, Jane's compromised financial situation left few options, and uncle James was childless. Within the year, the 11-year-old boy had arrived safely in Clonmel. Thomas, with words that rang bittersweet, noted how James bore a likeness to his dearly departed George (T. Morton 1800). In subsequent correspondences to Jane, he sent updates about James's health and activities, as well as assurances of his sustained financial support.

But his letter on 1 November 1803 began with an ominous tone. "The lord giveth and the lord taketh away. Blessed be his holy name. It's a hard task on me to be the bearer of intelligence that I fear will strike deeply in your bosom; our dearly beloved James is no more!" (T. Morton 1803). He had contracted croup. Physicians' standard treatments—an emetic to induce vomiting and blistering—proved inadequate. The letter concluded on a more pragmatic note. Thomas now needed to alter his will. The Irish Mortons would support Samuel in future educational and professional endeavors.

Jane bore the news of her son's death with "resignation to the will of providence" (T. Morton 1804). The response was befitting a Friend. Quakerism maintained that the death of kin, even after a long and drawn-out illness, should be met with grace and tranquility (Gould 1830). Mourning offered an opportunity to reflect on one's mortality, but it was an internalized and subdued affair.

At the time of James's death, Jane, Samuel, and Anna were living at West Farms in Westchester, New York (Jordan 1911, 1715; Meigs 1851, 10). They had relocated shortly after George had died. Jane's sister Ann Cheesman resided in Westchester, and the Society of Friends was well established in the region. In the spring of 1801, Jane requested a certificate of membership to the Purchase Monthly Meeting.[5] So that her children received a proper education in all things Quaker, Jane enrolled them in a Friends' boarding school. Matriculation into these coeducational institutions was quite common in the nineteenth century. "By 1800 American Friends had become convinced that the school should completely take over educational responsibilities from the family for a large part of the youth's formative years" (James 1962, 102). In addition to reading, writing, and arithmetic, Samuel would have been well schooled in dress, morality, and spirituality (O'Donnell 2013, 410). Boarding schools also functioned to foster solidarity and sustain the Society over generations. Girls and boys would meet there, marry when they came of age, and cultivate Quakerism in their own children (Haviland 2006, 20). The coeducational composition of boarding schools hints at the Quaker community's high regard for women. Femi-

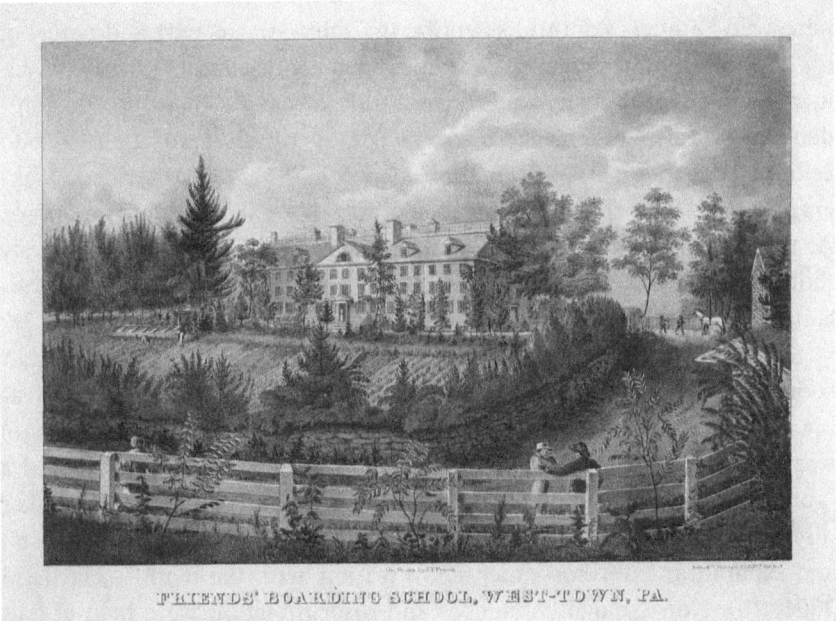

Figure 1.1. *Friends' boarding school, West-town, PA*, by John Taylor French, ca. 1848. Image courtesy of the Library Company of Philadelphia.

ninity was not seen as an impediment to one's intelligence or leadership abilities. This lesson was likely not lost on Samuel, whose mother went on to become a minister.

The paths of Friends living in scattered regions of the tri-state area—New York, Pennsylvania, and New Jersey—would cross repeatedly in boarding schools' classrooms, public places of worship, commercial settings, and private residences. Everyone seemed to know or be related to everyone else. It is in one of these spaces that Jane met her second husband, Thomas Rogers. Like Jane, Rogers was acquainted with the pain of familial loss. His first wife Anne (née Dawson) gave birth to two stillborn babies. Four months later she followed them to the grave. And, like Jane, after their deaths, Rogers found comfort among his Quaker brethren. He and Jane married on 13 December 1811.[6] Two months later, Jane requested a certificate of removal from the Purchase Monthly Meeting to join Rogers, who was living in Philadelphia.[7]

By all accounts, Rogers left quite the impression on his new stepson (Patterson 1854, xxii; Wood 1853, 5). He and Samuel bonded over geology, among other topics in natural history. Devoutly religious, Rogers may have perceived Samuel's youthful scientific investigations as part and parcel of his commitment to Quakerism. In his seventeenth-century writings, William Penn advocated strongly for the study of nature, insisting "that students should use their senses to appreciate the physical world and also to acknowledge that it is God's creation" (Cantor 2013, 523). American Quakers perceived their spirituality and scientific empiricism as complementary. As the nineteenth century unfolded, however, science grew progressively more secularized, and Samuel came to place more faith in it than Quakerism, as evidenced by his eventual disavowal of the Society (see chapter 2).

Samuel did not remain under Jane and Rogers's roof long. His mother soon enrolled him at the Westtown School in Chester County, Pennsylvania (Jordan 1911, 1715). Established in 1799, this Quaker boarding school was a day's ride from the city (figure 1.1). Its rural isolation facilitated a "guarded education"—one that was "imbued with a right sense of Quaker discipline, Christian faith, the testimonies of simplicity, integrity, pacifism, and separation from 'too much conversation' with the world" (Haviland 2006, 20). Non-Quaker influences and discrimination were held at bay, as were infectious diseases like croup, whooping cough, and scarlet fever. Similar to other Quaker boarding schools, Westtown was a coeducational institution. While Samuel's future wife Rebecca Grellet Pearsall did not attend the school, both of his brothers-in-law—John Jay Smith and Robert Pearsall Jr.—were alumni, as were several of their children (Smith 1892). (Years later, his Smith nieces and nephews would pen letters to their parents expressing great dissatisfaction with the school's rules and discipline.)

While many Friends favored gender integration in education, bringing non-White races into schools like Westtown was another matter entirely. The position points to a contradiction at work in the Quaker community. Alleviation of human suffering was a core religious tenet, one learned by adherents at an early age. The Society also maintained a longstanding and public denouncement of slavery and support for manumission (Philadelphia Yearly Meeting of the Religious Society of Friends 1797, 91–98). But, as Quaker scholar Elizabeth Cazden (2013) has pointed out, the reality was much more complicated.

Despite an egalitarian ethos, the Society of Friends was exclusionary in its approach to membership. Black Quakers were few in number. One example of such discrimination comes from the pen of Sarah Mapps Douglass (b. 1806, d. 1882). Douglass's ancestry encapsulates the intersectional complexities, the hybridity, of birth in the new nation (Bacon 2001; Dunbar 2008, 84). On her mother Grace's side (née Bustill), Sarah's grandfather was Black, and her grandmother was of mixed race, born of a White Englishman and Delaware Indian woman. But even the family's education and middle-class status did not safeguard them from racism. Sarah described her experiences with segregation at Philadelphia's Arch Street Meeting. "Even when a child," she reflected, "my soul was made sad with hearing five or six times during the course of one meeting this language of remonstrance addressed to those who were willing to sit by us. 'This bench is for the black people.'... And oftentimes I wept, at other times I felt indignant" (Lerner 1971, 512). (Perhaps these experiences are the reason Sarah instead came to frequent the Ninth and Spruce Meeting. Lucretia Mott, who is discussed further in chapter 5, counted among the attendants, and the two women became well acquainted [Smith 1925, 643].)

Racist attitudes extended from the meetinghouse to the counting house. For many Quakers, commercial opportunities often trumped anti-slavery activism. Some Friends continued to rely on the labor of enslaved Africans, while others found it difficult to avoid trading in goods procured from plantations in the southern colonies and Caribbean islands (Cazden 2013, 355).

These contradictions also played out in scholastic settings. There was widespread support for the education of men and women of color. As described in 1791 by Clement Biddle, a Quaker and early chronicler of Philadelphia: "It ought not be omitted, that there is a school for the Africans of every shade or colour, kept under the care and at the expense of the Quakers, into which are admitted gratis, slaves as well as free persons of whatever age of both sexes, and taught reading, writing, arithmetic, knitting, sewing and other useful female accomplishments" (as quoted in Smith 1995, 19). But Biddle's statement also testifies to the education of enslaved and freed Blacks in spheres separate from Quakers of white skin and European ancestry. Again, Sarah Mapps Douglass's life is demonstrative.

According to the historian Margaret Hope Bacon (2001), as a youth, Sarah attended a school for Black children run by Arthur Donaldson, a White Quaker, before switching to one established by her mother. She herself, for several decades, went on to teach Black boys and girls, first briefly in New York City and then Philadelphia. When Sarah sought to study physiology and anatomy, however, her educational options were decidedly limited. For the 1852–1853 session, she took courses at the Female Medical College of Pennsylvania (Lindhorst 1995, 174).[8] Established in 1850, this Quaker-backed institution was one of the first in the nation to train women in medicine (Lucretia Mott's husband James served on the original board of trustees [Lindhorst 1995, 173]), and Sarah was the first Black woman to enroll. The college's founders modeled the space and curriculum after Penn's medical school. At the former, according to Susan Wells (2001, 212), female students conducted dissections using the same textbooks and procedures as their male counterparts. But, she argues, their scientific work often necessitated strategic, creative, and transgressive gender performances (a topic to which I return in chapter 5). Sarah, for instance, regarded physiology as instructive for helping "poor women gain some control over their own reproductive lives" (Bacon 2001, 30). And while she may have learned about skulls' racialized dimensions, it is unlikely that Sarah gave much credence to ideas about Black inferiority.

Perhaps the hypocrisy of the Society's (and society's) stance on segregated education was not lost on Samuel. But given the dominant ideas circulating about racial difference during his youth, it is unlikely that he saw people of color as equal. And even if he regarded them as equal, and there is nothing in his later writings to suggest that he did as we will see in subsequent chapters, he would have still seen them as separate. While he may have found sex-segregated schooling less logical in his early years, the older he got, the more he found himself in public spaces accessible only to men.

In the fall of 1814, Samuel transferred from Westtown to a Quaker boarding school for boys in Burlington, New Jersey. The Gummere Academy was newly opened by brothers John and Samuel Gummere. John, who was later elected to the Academy of Natural Sciences (ANS) and American Philosophical Society (APS), gave instruction in natural philosophy and mathematics while his brother lectured on chemistry (Hallowell 1883, 38). Samuel came to regard his six months there as the highpoint of his early education (Meigs 1851; Patterson 1854; Wood 1853). Of course, nostalgia may have softened his memories of any pedagogical challenges faced at the boarding school. In his eulogy, Charles Meigs (1851, 12) remarked that Samuel "did not even there acquire any strong bias or affection for mathematics."

The Apprentice Doctor

During his formative years, time spent at various Quaker boarding schools likely informed Samuel's beliefs about race and gender. But, as he moved beyond the insular world of his youth, each new life experience seemed to loosen the hold of his early education.

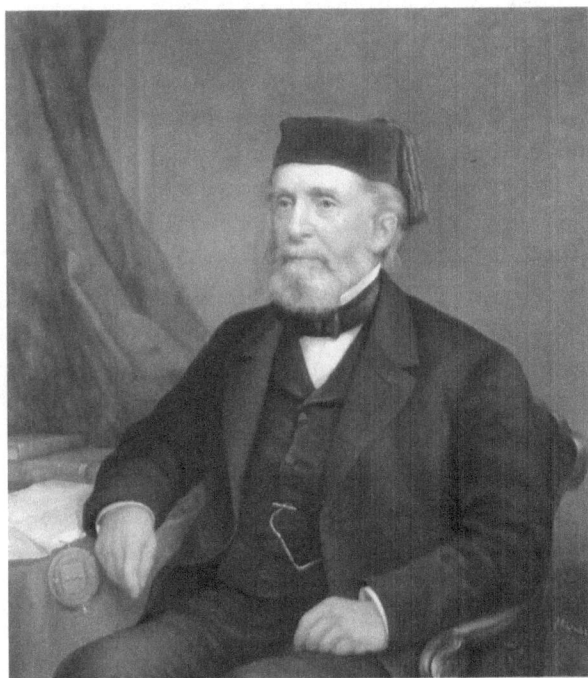

Figure 1.2. John Jay Smith, portrait by James Reid Lambdin, ca. 1880, oil on canvas; 42 × 34 inches. Image courtesy of the Library Company of Philadelphia.

Indecision about a proper career path made for some starts and stops. Initially, Samuel began an apprenticeship with Philadelphia hardware merchant and Friend Benjamin H. Yarnall (Smith 1892, 69). His mother approved. Commerce granted a young man ongoing access to respectable social circles, the "better sort" of people in the city's class hierarchy (Smith 1995, 11). As Samuel began to pursue other intellectual interests, however, he grew dissatisfied with mercantilism. To remedy some of the deficiencies in his schooling, he attended a course of lectures on natural philosophy at the University of Pennsylvania. There he met one of his future brothers-in-law, John Jay Smith (figure 1.2).

Of their budding friendship, John Jay (Smith 1892, 62) would later write: "I now made the acquaintance of my long-tried friend, and subsequent brother-in-law, Samuel George Morton, then residing in Front Street near Market, with his mother, a preacher of the Society of Friends, his stepfather, Thomas Rogers, and his sister Anna. Both Sam and I had a turn for reading, and he especially for study. We united in studying Hebrew together, at the drug-store of evenings." In addition to Hebrew, the two had much in common. Both were raised Quaker. Both attended Westtown, though at different times. Both were unhappy in their then current professional positions (John Jay was an uninspired apprentice to a druggist). Both had a youthful wanderlust. One summer, John Jay, Samuel, Anna Morton, and two unnamed ladies ventured by steamboat to various destinations in New York. Another of their adventures involved an informal geological expedition along the Delaware River. They were in search of a change in scenery, a limestone cavern called the "Devil's Hole," and rock crystals for Samuel's mineral collection. The day was deemed a success despite the near death of the horse they had hired as transportation (Smith 1892, 69).

Averting a fiscal crisis—dead horses are costly to reimburse—solidified the young men's relationship. From their friendship, family ties were then woven. John Jay introduced his sister-in-law Rebecca to Samuel, and the two were married in 1827 (see chapter 5). Until his death in 1851, Samuel's family lived just a few city blocks from the Smith residence, ensuring that cousins grew close with the passing years. The brothers-in-law also achieved and celebrated each other's professional successes, Samuel as a man of science and John Jay as one of letters. Robert Pearsall Jr., brother to Rebecca and John Jay's wife Rachel, filled out their triumvirate as a man of commerce. But, in 1816, they were all still on the verge of manhood—just about to make those crucial decisions that would shape their futures. For Samuel, his mother's death on December 5 provided a catalyst.

There was a silver lining to be found in the dark cloud of Jane's passing. Those physicians who oversaw her care—Drs. Caspar Wistar, Joseph Parrish, and Joseph Hartshorne—set Samuel down a respectable career path (Wood 1853, 6). While not as lucrative as commerce, physicians were perceived to be society's better sort of citizens (Smith 1995, 8). Parrish, by all accounts a pious Quaker doctor and dedicated abolitionist, took Samuel under his wing. His decision to mentor Samuel may have been motivated by something more than his interest in medicine, perhaps a kindness extended to a grieving, lost young man or a sense of community obligation. Like many things in Samuel's life, timing and personal connections, more so than his "intelligence and studious tendencies" (Wood 1853, 6) or "spark of scientific talent" (Fabian 2010, 18–19), proved advantageous. Regardless, Samuel soon abandoned his mercantile position and began medical training as a private pupil of Parrish. Later, he expressed much gratitude for his mentor's tutelage, as evidenced by dedications in not one but two publications (e.g., Morton 1823, 1834).

Knowledge gained as a medical apprentice was contingent on a mentor's predilections and personality (Bell 1943, 4). In Parrish's case, his amicable nature was quite popular among young men in Philadelphia. The eager and attentive convened in his office twice weekly. There the physician held forth on his experiences with surgery and medical practice (Wood 1840, 26–27). In the early nineteenth century, the meetings were a necessary first step for men who aspired to undertake formalized medical training. Apprenticeships, which usually lasted three years, provided practical knowledge while institutions schooled medical students in the theoretical (Baer 2001, 7; Rothstein 1987, 15). Parrish himself had undertaken private study with the estimable Wistar before graduating in 1805 from the Medical Department at the University of Pennsylvania.

The first of its kind in the American colonies, Penn's medical school can trace its founding to 1765 (Medical Faculty of the University of Pennsylvania 1839, 89).[9] It was one of the leading medical schools in the United States for much of the nineteenth century (and arguably remains so today). In its earliest version, the institution was a medical department grafted on to the College of Philadelphia. Founding faculty members had modeled it after their alma maters in Europe—in London, Paris, Leiden, and above all Edinburgh. Prior to the school's establishment, physicians and clergymen were often regarded as one and the same. Akin to medical missionaries, they catered to individuals ailing in spirit and body (Carson 1869, 20–22). But the creation of a formal institution designed to train medical practitioners signaled a clear distinction between the two professions, as well as a transforming conception of the body's relation to the soul.

While faculty members may have distanced themselves from theology, they were more tolerant of natural history (Carson 1869, 24). By the time Samuel matriculated, Penn had established professorships in botany, natural history, natural philosophy, and comparative anatomy under the aegis of the faculty of natural sciences (Carson 1869, 134). These subjects may have satisfied the curiosity of a physician in training, but they were not mandatory. Courses that counted toward curricular requirements included: anatomy; chemistry; midwifery (just wrested from the hands of women who were deemed "ignorant" and "conceited"); institutes, practice, and clinical medicine; materia medica (a precursor to pharmacology); and surgery (which was unavoidably painful and often fatal prior to the mid-nineteenth-century introduction of anesthesia and antiseptic agents) (Carson 1869, 98). Students were also tasked with writing a thesis. And, most important for their hands-on training, they completed a clinical session at Pennsylvania Hospital. (The Hospital of the University of Pennsylvania, the nation's first teaching hospital, was not established until 1874 [Bynum

1994, 51].) Of this required work, anatomy with its training in the theatrics of dissection, engenders additional reflection for what it has to say about the development of biomedicine in general and Samuel's research interests specifically.

Anatomy and Dissection

For the budding anatomist, dissection granted unprecedented access to the body's depths and inner workings. In Philadelphia, Dr. Thomas Cadwalader was among the first to conduct public dissections in 1731, some of the earliest in the American colonies (Middleton 1941, 101–2). He had trained in England and France, and colleagues urged him to share his teachings. In attendance was Dr. William Shippen Jr. Inspired by Cadwalader's initial efforts, Shippen in turn performed his own series of dissections. He took an advertisement out in the *Pennsylvania Gazette* on 25 November 1762: "Dr. Shippen's Anatomical Lectures will begin to-morrow evening at six o'clock, at his father's house in Fourth Street. Tickets for the course to be had of the Doctor, at five Pistoles each, and any gentlemen who incline to see the subject prepared for the lectures and learn the art of Dissecting, Injections, &c., are to pay five Pistoles more" (as quoted in Carson 1869, 40). Dissection may have served to educate physicians. But it was also spectacle—a performance accessible to any White male who could afford the price of admission (or tuition). Women, people of color (whether enslaved or freed), and paupers were only permitted entry as cadavers (Sappol 2002). By the nineteenth century, dissections had moved from rented rooms into institutional spaces.

Historically, medical schools' faculty and student bodies were overwhelmingly White, male, and of some financial means. In Penn's case, an institution with ties to Quaker abolitionists and their suffragist spouses, such homogeneity signaled the contradictions of lived reality. (And it continued to do so for many decades thereafter. The first Black man, Nathan Francis Mossell, graduated from the medical school in 1882 [Mossell 1941, 14–18]. The first White women, Gladys Girardeau and Alberta Peltz, did not receive doctorates in medicine until 1918 [Anonymous 1919, 565]. The double bind that racism and sexism weave is evidenced by the fact that Penn's School of Medicine did not graduate a Black woman, Arlene Bennett, until 1964 [Epps et al. 1993, 635].)

At Penn, Samuel received his primary instruction in anatomy from the aptly named Dr. Philip Syng Physick, a forefather of modern surgery and

Friend. Physick had stepped into the Penn position after Wistar's death in 1818; he was assisted by Dr. William Edmonds Horner (Carson 1869, 183). The lecture room used for practical anatomy was designed with demonstration in mind. Able to accommodate 600 men, it was described in the following way: "Sixty feet square with the seats circularly arranged about a central area, in which the demonstrations are made, and which is lighted from the roof immediately above it. The seats rise by a paraboloid ascent, so graduated as to allow the students in each row to see over the heads of those in the row beneath" (Medical Faculty of the University of Pennsylvania 1839, 102). The spatial layout of the anatomical classroom allowed students to gaze upon, or rather into, dissected bodies—to disassemble parts from the whole, distinguish the pathological from the normal, and deepen analysis in general. Although Jefferson Medical College is featured (Penn's local rival), the artist Thomas Eakins depicted this space so realistically in his paintings *The Gross Clinic* (1875) and *The Agnew Clinic* (1889). His renderings call to mind concerns raised by Foucault about the medical gaze in clinical settings: "But to look in order to know, to show in order to teach, is not this a tacit form of violence, all the more abusive for its silence, upon a sick body that demands to be comforted, not displayed?" (1973, 84).[10]

Given his upbringing in the Society of Friends, Samuel may have meditated at the onset of medical training about the extent to which his religious beliefs and anatomical studies were compatible. Quaker doctrine held that life was fragile, death ubiquitous, and the body corruptible. As the preacher Elias Hicks sermonized, "The body should serve only as a tabernacle for the soul during its probation. . . . We may be gay, strong, and nimble to-day, and to-morrow a lifeless corpse" (transcribed in Gould 1830, 38–39). Such a view may explain why Quaker men gravitated to medicine as a profession.

As for dissection specifically, Samuel was ambivalent. Genealogical documents recollect his distaste: "Dr. Morton's abhorrence + detestation of vivisection—Once called by duty to be present at an execution of a criminal—he sickened at the spectacle, and was rendered ill for a week" (Anonymous n.d. a, 272).[11] Yet, his later anatomy lectures stressed the importance of dissection. "Anatomy is on all hands acknowledged to be indispensable to the healing art," Samuel stated in his introduction to the course (Morton 1831, 7). He continued, "Human anatomy can only be learned by dissecting the human body" (1831, 11). The sentiment paraphrased earlier lessons from his French instructor René-Théophile-Hyacinthe Laënnec. About disease and its transformation of organs, Laënnec had written: "The opening up of corpses is the means of acquiring this knowledge" (as cited in Foucault 1973, 166). Practical experience, however, was not always easy to gain.

In the nineteenth century, the number of anatomical students burgeoned, and the supply of cadavers dwindled. Generally, doctors sourced bodies from the almshouses, prisons, and potter's fields (Halperin 2007; Richardson 1987; Sappol 2002). Samuel was no different, and when he served as medical staff at the Philadelphia Almshouse's infirmary, from 1827 to 1835, he, too, saw opportunity in his charges' deaths (see chapter 2). In death and decomposition, those at the margins—the poor, the prostitute, the criminal, the enslaved Black, the Native—found (or, rather, were granted) social worth (a facet of becoming object to which I return in chapter 4). A spirit of utilitarianism prevailed among physicians—one that insisted on the repayment of social debts and the development of science for society's greater good.

When the supply of cadavers proved insufficient, medical practitioners turned to grave robbers, or resurrectionists. Such activities generated legislative action and mob violence. The year Samuel entered medical school, for instance, New York's legislators criminalized grave robbing (Novak and Willoughby 2010). But as historian Michael Sappol (2002, 112) points out, such measures had little impact on anatomists who could easily feign ignorance about cadavers' origins and thus go unpunished. A greater deterrent to physicians were riots. These events destroyed medical facilities and threatened the safety of instructors and students. Between the years 1785 and 1855, at least 17 anatomy riots occurred at institutions of medicine (Sappol 2002, 3).

Engendering less public controversy was the pedagogical use of anatomical and pathological specimens. When the widow of Dr. Caspar Wistar, a former professor of anatomy at Penn, gifted her husband's personal collection to the medical school on 2 June 1818 (Dorsey 1818), she established an important precedent. Students could now extend their training by referencing specimens in an institution's Anatomical Museum or Pathological Cabinet, as these collections came to be called. For Samuel, they would prove instructive when he began to amass skulls. As institutional collections grew, medical schools and hospitals created curatorships. For example, Samuel's son Thomas George served as a curator from 1860 to 1864 for the Pathological Cabinet housed at Pennsylvania Hospital. Initially acquired and bestowed by Samuel's mentor Joseph Parrish (T. G. Morton 1864), the collection became a more formalized Pathological Museum under the guidance of Thomas George (Anonymous n.d. a, 309). For his part, he diligently identified, prepared, catalogued, and exhibited everything from the intestines of cholera patients to enlarged prostate glands to "schirruses" of the testicle.

Nor did the public react violently to the surgical procedures and postmortem examinations that generated the specimens in collections. Dissimilar to dissection, which violated corpses and erased decedents' identities, these practices required consent from the patient or next of kin, took place in private venues away from the gazes of medical students, minimized corporeal disfigurement, and proceeded in a timely fashion (Crossland 2009, 109–10; Sappol 2002, 103). Samuel's autopsy provides a case in point. After his death in 1851, six doctors assessed his body, focusing on select body parts (heart, brain, lungs, liver, and spleen). The inspection occurred prior to his formal burial though after the requisite 24-hour waiting period (Philadelphia Medical Examiner 1851). Furthermore, none of Samuel's organs appear to have ended up in anatomical museums or pathological cabinets.

A mainstay of every medical school curriculum, an anatomy course shocked, familiarized, and inevitably desensitized students. The medical gaze was certainly instrumental in this process, but the experience also assaulted one's senses of smell, sound, and touch. Some students found dissection exciting, while others like Samuel did not. Regardless, those who successfully completed a course's lab practicum and lecture series had their view of the human body altered profoundly. Dissection broke down physical boundaries but erected conceptual ones. For anatomists coming into their own, it reiterated the difference between subject and object, doctor and patient, decedent and specimen, soul and body. The impact of anatomical museums on physicians' psyches was more subtle. Fragmentation and decontextualization of body parts further obfuscated the identities of the decedents to whom they had once belonged. In the case of skeletal materials, this depersonalization and objectification proceeded with even greater ease. Yet, dissimilar from the normalization of dissection in medical training, the pathological cabinet has morphed from pedagogical tool into morbid spectacle.[12]

When Samuel's course and clinical work came to an end, he next tackled a written thesis about the "Popliteal Aneurism." It is possible that his anatomy professor Dr. Physick influenced the decision. The popliteal artery runs behind the knee joint and continues into the femoral artery. A widening or bulging of this vessel can cause a blood clot or prevent blood flow altogether. When it did, physicians often amputated the sufferer's leg. But, in 1785, British surgeon John Hunter developed a procedure to treat the condition, which involved the ligation, or tying up, of the femoral artery (Ellis 2001, 66–67). Physick was one of the first surgeons in the United States to successfully apply Hunterian ligation; in 1803, he used animal ligatures to tie up the femoral artery of a 35-year-old patient identified as H.B. (Morton and Hunt 1880, 46). Subsequent physicians, Samuel being one, continued to expand on the causes of and resolutions for popliteal aneurysms. Once his thesis was written, however, he had little if anything to say publicly on this medical subject and its treatment.

Having completed the final logistical hurdles of medical school—the proper formatting of his thesis and payment, that is—Samuel earned the initials M.D. in March of 1820. (Even then, the university powers that be had very specific formatting requirements: "The Essay must be in the candidate's own hand-writing, and must be written uniformly on paper of the same size, the alternate pages being left blank" [Medical Faculty of the University of Pennsylvania 1839, 104].) Within a month he was elected to the ANS, indicating that he was as much a man of natural history as he was of medicine.

Rather than set up a medical practice in Philadelphia, Samuel opted to continue his training in Europe. He did so at his Uncle James's urging and with his full financial support. But, before leaving, he did two things. First, Samuel solicited his mentor for a letter of recommendation. As historian Whitfield Bell (1943, 5) relates, the request was a typical one: "When his American education was completed, therefore, his resolve taken to go abroad, and his passage booked, the medical student turned to his Philadelphia instructors for letters of introduction to the great and near-great of the medical and scientific worlds of Britain and the Continent which he was about to enter." In confirmation of his former student's abilities, Parrish (1820) provided a glowing recommendation:

> Samuel George Morton M.D. commenced and completed his medical education under my direction. His diligence as a student, superadded to excellent natural talents, has rendered his attainments highly respectable—and after passing an honorable examination, before the Medical Faculty in the University of Pennsylvania, he received the degree of Doctor of Medicine—Altho' the connection of Preceptor and Pupil is now dissolv'd—yet I regard him as a younger brother in

the Profession, in whose welfare I feel an affectionate interest, and trust the friendship formed between us, will strengthen with years, and only terminate with Life—

The second thing Samuel did in preparation for his time abroad was to attend a meeting of Philadelphia's Society of Friends. Like many a traveling Quaker physician before him (Bell 1943, 6), he petitioned for a certificate of transfer. His request was recorded in the minutes on 22 March 1820: "Samuel George Morton expecting to embark in a short time for Ireland and to visit some other places in Europe requested an [sic] certificate to Clonmell [sic] Monthly Meeting."[13] He would remain in Europe for more than four years. His time there proved transformative. As several authors have discussed, Samuel encountered ideas and individuals that shaped his perceptions of human differences and offered the scaffolding on which anthropology was erected (Bieder 1986; Desmond and Moore 2009; Fabian 2010; Spencer 1983). Courses and clinical work in Edinburgh and Paris also extended his medical knowledge. But, ironically, Samuel's development as a natural historian and physician occurred at the expense of his spiritual relationship with the Society of Friends.

"Transatlantic Semibarbarian"

Samuel sailed from New York to Liverpool in May 1820 (Meigs 1851, 14). Letters from this period indicate that he was warmly received by his extended family in Clonmel. For his Irish relatives, Samuel filled a void left by the death of his older, ill-fated brother James. Connecting with George's kin was also fulfilling for Samuel—emotionally, intellectually, and financially. His uncle James encouraged Samuel to enroll at the University of Edinburgh's medical school (Meigs 1851, 15; Wood 1853, 7). A friend from Clonmel later jested about Samuel's decision as an American to attend a Scottish university: "They in their national arrogance, would look on you as a transatlantic semibarbarian and taking pity on your ignorance" (Fitzgerald 1823). Samuel, however, found little to deter him from the adventure, not even poor health. (An "affection of the liver" assailed him upon arrival to Ireland and seems to have compromised his immune system thereafter [Wood 1853, 7, 18].) Despite the setback, Samuel was adamant that a degree from Edinburgh would benefit an American man's medical practice. Earlier generations of physicians had proven so—Benjamin Rush, William Shippen, Caspar Wistar, Philip Syng Physick, among others (Bell 1943). Further enticement for Quaker students was the university's position on religious affiliation. Unlike many other institutions in Europe, Edinburgh was under secular control and did not require a religious test on entry (Cantor 2005, 64). The university may have permitted Quakers to enroll, but women and people of color still could not matriculate. Though interestingly, Edinburgh's medical school accepted Jewish men as students (Cantor 2005). It appears that a categorical distinction between the Semitic and Caucasian races, a notion Samuel later "supported" with empirical evidence, had yet to gain ground at the university.

Seeing that the University of Edinburgh served as a model for the founders of Penn's medical school, its regulations and requirements were familiar to Samuel. Like Penn, students could pursue course work in medicine and natural history. To expand his knowledge about the latter, Samuel enrolled in geology with Robert Jameson (Patterson 1854, xxiv). Of Jameson's lectures, Charles Darwin—who attended Edinburgh shortly after Samuel, from 1825 to 1827—did not mince words: "The sole effect they produced on me was the determination never as long as I lived to read a book on Geology, or in any way to study the science" (Darwin [1887] 2010, 24). If subsequent publications about geology are any indication, Samuel did not find Jameson's lectures as off-putting (e.g., Wetherill et al. 1826). He and Darwin did have a similar ambivalence about dissection, however. "It has proved one of the greatest evils in my life that I was not urged to practice dissection," Darwin ([1887] 2010, 19) wrote years later, "for I should soon have got over my disgust; and the practice would have been invaluable for all my future work." Both men also found it difficult to reconcile their spirituality and worldviews. As a consequence of much personal turmoil, Darwin's renunciation of Christianity came later in his life (Desmond and Moore 2009; Lander 2010; Pleins 2013), whereas Samuel's forsaking of his Quaker birthright occurred while studying in Europe.

Initially, Samuel's membership in the Society of Friends opened doors for him in Edinburgh. Thomas Hodgkin, a pious Quaker and English medical student who later lent his name to lymphoma, was one of Samuel's first friends in the city (figure 1.3). A month after the two met, Hodgkin described his impressions of the Philadelphian in an 1820 letter to his brother John. Samuel was "particularly fond of mineralogy & Geology & has had considerable opportunities for cultivating them whilst travelling over a great part of the United States.... His sentiments with regard to the Indians & his confirmation of some of my ideas respecting them rendered

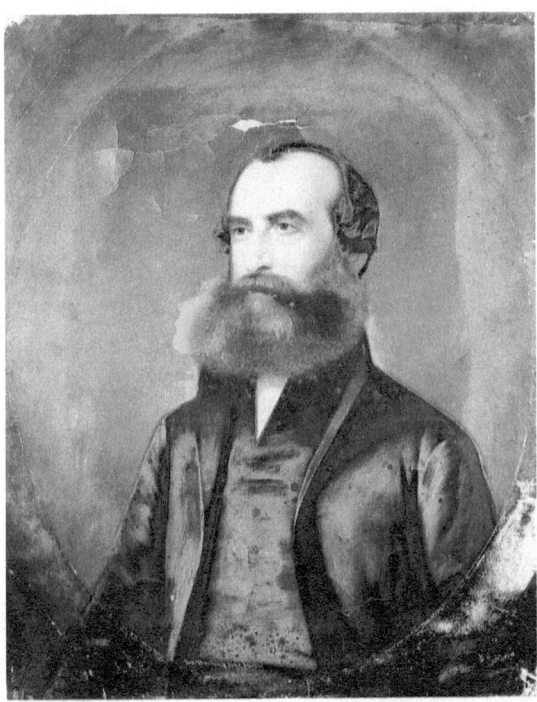

Figure 1.3. Thomas Hodgkin (1798–1866), physician and social reformer. Oil painting by John Burton and Sons. Wellcome Collection. Retrieved from https://wellcomecollection.org/works/fgr2re5y/images?id=ahtpbay9. Attribution 4.0 International (CC BY 4.0).

him very interesting to me" (Kass and Kass 1988, 71). As he alludes to in his letter, Hodgkin was particularly sensitive to the plight of American Indians and quite critical of European colonizers and Christian proselytizers. In "Essay on the Promotion of Civilization," which he penned a year prior to meeting Samuel, Hodgkin stressed that White men had "done far more to degrade, corrupt and exterminate their uncivilized fellow creatures than all the heathen world, since the creation of man" (as quoted in Kass and Kass 1988, 39). He would also vocally oppose the US government's forced relocation of the Cherokee, which President Andrew Jackson's Indian Removal Act of 1830 had set in motion. These positions were decidedly at odds with the sociopolitical ideology, the necropolitics, undergirding Samuel's later scientific work, as I discuss in chapter 3. Over the course of a long friendship, it is difficult to say how the two men squared their contradictory stances on nation, humans' origins and differences, and colonialism. Correspondences continued for more than twenty years, but do not reveal if the relationship sustained due to heartfelt collegiality or passive aggression.[14]

Perhaps Samuel was more obliging at the outset of their friendship. Hodgkin had an extensive network of acquaintances. He counted among the guests of the Millers, a wealthy family at the social center of Edinburgh's Quaker community (Cantor 2005, 65; Kass and Kass 1988, 76). William Miller, an engraver, and his wife, Jane, often played host to those Friends studying at the university (Bell 1943, 12–13; Cantor 2005, 65). An obituary for Jane paid homage to the couple's social skills: "For nearly forty years their delightful home at Hope Park was famous for its free and gracious hospitality; while their kindly greetings, and their cultured social intercourse were helpful and cheering to many who had gone to reside in Edinburgh as students at the University or at the Ladies' College" (Anonymous 1908, 88). Given Samuel's membership in the Society, relationship with Hodgkin, and the Millers' sociability, it is probable that the family invited him into their home at some juncture during his time in Scotland.

There is, however, nothing to suggest that Samuel formalized his connection with Edinburgh's Society of Friends. Indeed, the opposite seems to have occurred. Samuel did petition to transfer from the Philadelphia to the Clonmel Monthly Meeting, out of deference to his stepfather. But there is no evidence that he actively requested a certificate of admittance to the Edinburgh Quaker Meeting. In explanation, many nonlocal Quaker students found that they did not welcome "the prospect of having their lives scrutinized by Edinburgh Friends . . . [and] many took advantage of the situation to loosen their links with their parents' religion" (Cantor 2005, 68). By the time Samuel returned to Philadelphia in 1824, his name disappeared from the Society's records. And, when he married Rebecca, as we will see in chapter 5, she was censured by Philadelphia Friends for taking a husband outside of the religious order. The temporary removal he sought prior to his trip became permanent. Samuel died a practicing Episcopalian. Like many things in his life, the decision to change religious denominations suggests an opportunity seized rather than a spiritual connection felt.

As his Quakerism waned, Samuel's circle of friends expanded. Common interests, acquaintances, and circumstances suggest that he and the Scottish anatomist Robert Knox were familiar with one another. After graduating from Edinburgh's medical school in 1814, Knox served as an assistant surgeon in the British Army (Lonsdale 1870, 10). He was stationed at South Africa's Cape of Good Hope. According to a nineteenth-century biographer, his military service included time spent collecting zoological specimens, noting environmental conditions, and dissecting local Natives

(Lonsdale 1870, 9–13). His adventures offered provocative and illustrative examples in the anatomy classes he taught years later. "Gentlemen," he expounded to his students,

> I hold in my hand the cranium of a Caffrarian chief, whom I saw on the hostile field, leading his undisciplined but brave tribes forth against British infantry; and for a time he maintained his position against fearful odds. His dauntless spirit, that could bear no curb, brought him within close range of our troops, and of course he fell under a rattling fire. I was fortunate enough to secure his body, and to bring this ethnological specimen home to England. Look at the development of this cranium, and compare it with the known Europeans presented in such numbers to your observation. (Lonsdale 1870, 149)

Delivered no doubt for dramatic effect, Knox's account underscores the facility with which men involved in violent colonial expansionism, especially military physicians, obtained Native peoples' skulls. His statement, with its use of "Caffrarian," also demonstrates how men of science used language to strip decedents of their humanity. Derived from the Arabic *kafir*, or infidel, the term is a variation on "Kaffir." European colonizers first applied it in the early seventeenth century to the Xhosa-speaking peoples of South Africa's Eastern Cape Colony (Hughes 2006, 31, 280). By the nineteenth century, British writers evoked Kaffir as shorthand for savagery and inferiority, a dismissal of the native Blacks against whom they waged war. With time, it became a highly offensive ethnic (or racial) slur. Today, its usage is taboo and punishable by law in South Africa (Hughes 2006, 281–82).

In fall of 1820, Knox left South Africa, landing in Edinburgh by the start of the new year (Lonsdale 1870, 16). At the time, Samuel and Hodgkin were midway through their first term in medical school. But Knox's stay in the city was an abbreviated one. By October, he had moved to Paris (Lonsdale 1870, 18). Coincidently (or not), Samuel and Hodgkin arrived in France's capital that same month (Kass and Kass 1988, 86; Meigs 1851, 15). French lessons counted among the young men's activities. Knox had also invited Hodgkin to share a private dissecting room at l'Hôpital de la Pitié, one of two institutions in Paris that was "well supplied with bodies for students' use" (Bates 2010, 48–49; see also Kass and Kass 1988, 92). Though Samuel does not appear to have joined them, he and Knox did have overlapping interests, suggesting that their paths crossed more than once. Both men harbored an affinity for skulls, polygenism, and scientific racism. As I discuss in chapter 3, the extracurricular activities of military physicians were often the source of skulls in Samuel's collection. His comparative anatomical study of them benefited from and perpetuated violent Euro-American colonialism. Yet, Knox's experiences—in contrast to Samuel who remained safely ensconced in his Philadelphia study—were firsthand ones.

Paris provided Samuel with a break from the moral strictures of Quakerism. "He had endeavored so to combine study with amusement as not to become weary of either," a memoirist remarked (Meigs 1851, 16). But for Samuel, medical studies were a priority. Throughout that winter, he and Hodgkin attended clinical lectures given by René-Théophile-Hyacinthe Laënnec (b. 1781, d. 1826) (Morton 1834, viii; Wood 1853, 11). Laënnec was the professor and royal lecturer at the Collège de France. The invention of the stethoscope counted among his many contributions to medicine. With the instrument, he listened for internal abnormalities in the thorax, which ultimately yielded a greater understanding of pulmonary tuberculosis (Daniel 2000, 43–45). In his discussion of the clinic's birth, Michel Foucault (1973, 135) discussed this practice of listening in relation to the medical gaze, a prelude to "the opening up of corpses" (in Laënnec's words) where knowledge came from looking. Hodgkin went on to effectively apply Laënnec's technical lessons in stethoscopy (Bynum 1994, 47). Samuel, for his part, extended his professor's notions about tuberculosis in an illustrated treatise about "pulmonary consumption" (Bynum 1994, 51), a topic to which I return in the next chapter.

Previous scholars have also suggested that, while in Europe, Samuel first met the phrenologist George Combe (Bieder 1986, 71). The same year Samuel arrived in Edinburgh, in 1820, George and his brother Andrew established the city's Phrenological Society (Shapin 1975). A point of pride for the society's members was its museum. There an extensive skull collection, inspired by the pathological cabinets amassed by physicians, was prominently displayed. Donations were always welcomed as were visitors (though only on Saturdays) (Combe 1824, xv–xvi, 55). Had Samuel paid the price of admission, he would have been able to view the skulls of executed criminals and the mentally impaired, as well as those identified as Hindoo, Chinese, and Sandwich Islander. While there is no direct evidence that he interacted with George until years later in Philadelphia (Spencer 1983, 324), as discussed in the next chapter, it is difficult to imagine that his curiosity about phrenology was not at least roused during his time in Edinburgh.

Samuel's thesis, a meditation on bodily pain titled *Tentamen Inaugurale de Corporis Dolore, etc.* also alluded to phrenological ideas (Spencer 1983). "There is no doubt," he wrote, "that the origin of all the varieties of character are congenital, and those differences for a greater part must be ascribed to the structure of the brain" (Morton 1823, 32–33).[15] Of course, Samuel may have also gleaned ideas about brain structure and its connection to character from his teachers. The line between medicine and phrenology during this period was a fine one. Ideas often floated about like so many clouds—drifting, amorphous, sometimes substantive—without a nod to their sources. For example, in the case of James Gregory, Samuel's professor of practical medicine at Edinburgh, phrenologists cited his writings to argue that the brain was the seat of the mind and intelligence (e.g., Combe 1830, 3; Smith 1838, 26). Additionally, Dr. Phillip Syng Physick, to whom Samuel dedicated his Edinburgh thesis, helped found Philadelphia's Central Phrenological Society in February 1822.[16] As stated in the society's constitution, its object was "the study of the manifestations of mind as depending upon the proportionate development of the Brain."[17] Such work necessitated a background in "comparative anatomy" and "natural history," two subjects that had long piqued Samuel's interest.

In August of 1823, Samuel received his medical degree from the University of Edinburgh. Over the next ten months, he traveled between France, Italy, Ireland, and England. During his extended stay, he had lost his spiritual connection to the Society of Friends, while his understanding of human differences—anatomical, mental, cultural—deepened. In June 1824, Samuel boarded a ship in Liverpool, and on the 28th of that month he disembarked at the port of New York. Curiously, the ship was named the *James Cropper*. Its eponym was a wealthy Quaker merchant who, even as Samuel traversed the Atlantic, was actively working to end the slave trade (Davis 1986). The name may have rung a bell. Hodgkin and Cropper were acquaintances, united against slavery and critical of Europeans' subjugation of Native peoples. According to Hodgkin, the Quaker merchant was a Liverpudlian point of contact for newly arrived American Indian youths (Hodgkin 1824). Cropper then directed them to Hodgkin, who oversaw their European education. Such patronage was an important dimension of the "considerate" colonialism that Hodgkin promoted and, according to him, Samuel supported at one point in his life (Hodgkin 1824).

The passenger list for Samuel's voyage was composed entirely of European immigrants.[18] Some aboard the *James Cropper* were new to the United

States. Others, like Samuel, regarded their arrival on American shores as a homecoming. Secure in his citizenship and professional training, he returned to Philadelphia, his "native" city, with plans to resume his medical practice. He did so during a pivotal period in medicine. Starting in the early 1820s, as I discuss in the next chapter, there was a dawning realization among medical practitioners that treating ailing patients and educating aspiring physicians could generate symbolic and financial capital.

2

"Licence to Kill and Cure"

When Samuel graduated from Edinburgh, his friend John Chaloner (1823) sent cheeky congratulations: "You are now as great a man as Prince High and Low, having obtained a licence [sic] to kill and cure all over the world." Though off the cuff, the remark proved prescient. Samuel's professional career was as much defined by the doctoring he did (or tried to do effectively) as it was by his study of skulls. When he returned to Philadelphia in 1824, Samuel settled at 411 Mulberry Street[1] and set about making a name for himself as a physician. Extensive training from two prestigious institutions should have given him an edge in the medical marketplace. Success was neither immediate nor easy to come by, however.

Biomedicine's beginnings in the nineteenth century may have yielded a proliferation of institutions, practitioners, and information. But the field's advances were undercut by competing doctrines and invalidated by patients' high mortality rates. This chapter chronicles Samuel's ambition, as he navigated a nascent, competitive, and changing medical field. He traveled daily between the city's institutions of medicine and science. In these spaces, his work to foster life contributed to the emergence of biopower (I refer the reader back to the introduction for an overview). Samuel's activities at the Philadelphia Almshouse, which proved pivotal for his development as a physician, illustrate just how the state came to exercise authority over the life and death of its citizens. There he ministered to the city's disenfranchised residents, including those devastated by the cholera epidemic of 1832. But Samuel also found opportunity in the suffering of almshouse inmates. The socioeconomic distance between himself and his patients made it all the easier to justify medico-scientific study of their ailing or dead bodies. In hospital wards, he collected clinical information, while organs and skeletal elements were sourced from dissecting tables. These activities—biopolitical techniques that helped with the "administration of bodies and the calculated management of life" (Foucault 1978, 140)—were the springboard for subsequent ethnological work that came to involve colleagues located well beyond Philadelphia.

During this juncture in his life, he began to collect skulls in earnest, initially to train medical students but soon in the interest of natural history. Medicine and natural history in the nineteenth century were not discordant fields; both contributed to reifying ideas about national character—an ideological foundation for the body politic that deemed some ideal and Others expendable. To advance these efforts, Samuel conducted craniometric analysis. With time, and for varied personal and professional reasons, natural history came to occupy his intellectual efforts. In this shift, we can see an increasing embrace of, or an inurement to, letting die.

The Philadelphia Almshouse

Doctors were in demand during the first half of the nineteenth century due in large part to an expanding middle class, which had the financial means to access physicians more easily (Sappol 2002, 63). Concomitantly, the number of men with medical aspirations grew. From 1792 to 1839, graduates of Penn's Medical Department increased more than twenty-two-fold—from 7 to 158 (Medical Faculty of the University of Pennsylvania 1839, 96, 99). The promise of prestige and profit drove students' interest in the business of medicine as much as intellectual curiosity and altruism. As a result, competition among physicians became fierce (Fabian 2010, 26; Wood 1853, 8–9). As listed in the *Philadelphia Directory and Stranger's Guide, for 1825*, for instance, Samuel was one of 169 practicing physicians in the city and its suburbs (Wilson 1825).

To stave off inconstant employment, he strategized. First Samuel turned to friends in the Philadelphia community. As historian Ann Fabian has noted, he found a mentor in Richard Harlan (2010, 19–21). Or, perhaps, since Harlan was three years his senior, it is more appropriate to characterize him as an elder brother figure. While the two men had much in common, a subtle sibling-like rivalry long simmered beneath the surface of their relationship, eventually boiling over. Like Samuel, Harlan came from a respected Quaker family. He apprenticed under Joseph Parrish, acting as his anatomy assistant during Samuel's stint as a private pupil. When Parrish's tutelage came to an end, Harlan enrolled in the Medical Department at Penn. He graduated in 1818, just one year prior to Samuel's acceptance (Medical Faculty of the University of Pennsylvania 1839, 35). And, importantly, human skulls held a special fascination for both physicians. Accordingly, Harlan introduced him to the members of the Academy of Natural Sciences (ANS) of Philadelphia (Patterson 1854, xxiii).

ANS began as a casual conferral among friends with shared interests and soon formalized into an institution that set the nation's scientific research agenda (Peck and Stroud 2012). Pennsylvania's legislature officially incorporated the ANS on 25 April 1817 (Necker 1818, 385). Like American medical schools' emulation of Old World institutions (e.g., University of Edinburgh), the founders of the ANS also looked to European examples—the Royal Academies in Paris, Stockholm, Lisbon, and Berlin—for inspiration. Harlan counted among the ANS's seminal members, having joined in 1815 (Academy of Natural Sciences of Philadelphia 1877, 8, 11).[2] Samuel's nomination and election followed in five years' time, and from the beginning he was committed to making the ANS a vibrant intellectual institution of national renown. Over the years, Samuel held several administrative positions: recording secretary (1825–1829), corresponding secretary (1831–1840), vice president (1840–1849), and president (1849–1851). It is also likely that Harlan supported his friend's election to the venerable American Philosophical Society (APS) in 1828; he had been a member since 1822.

Whereas Harlan and Samuel's interests in natural history fostered collegiality (or at least a healthy competition), their work as physicians generated friction. Naturalists took their scientific research seriously, but their medical practices paid the bills (Fabian 2010, 27). For Harlan, a medical staff appointment at the Philadelphia Almshouse, also known as the Bettering House, ensured fiscal stability; he was hired in 1822 and soon transitioned into a surgical position (Agnew et al. 1890, 14–15; Lawrence 1905, 393–94). Samuel was brought on in 1827 and remained on staff for eight years (Lawrence 1905, 394).[3]

As historian Charles Rosenberg (1982, 124) has related, "the almshouse-hospital was always a last resort" for its residents. Their misfortune took myriad forms—abandoned wives, abused servants, orphans, crippled or aged laborers, sufferers of syphilis and consumption, "filles de joie" (a euphemism for prostitutes), impoverished widows, drunkards, pregnant women (many of whom were unmarried), vagrants, and the deranged (Smith and Shelton 1985a, 1985b). Segregation, by race and sex, also added to some inmates' misery (Clement 1985, 86–88; Rosenberg 1982, 121–22). The least desirable locations (e.g., attic) were reserved for Black men, for instance. Their numbers at the almshouse were disproportionate to the city's larger populace. From 1812 to 1813, for instance, Blacks counted for 8–9 percent of the city's population but were 15 percent of the people admitted to the almshouse (Clement 1985, 32, 198n14). "Most of them were not in bondage," Priscilla Ferguson Clement (1985, 32–33) clarifies, "because the gradual abolition of slavery in Pennsylvania had begun in 1780." Nevertheless, their lives were defined by extreme poverty and racial discrimination, both of which impeded employment and good health.

For ambitious physicians like Harlan and Samuel, however, the almshouse was rife with professional opportunity. In his *History of the Philadelphia Almshouses and Hospitals*, Charles Lawrence (1905, 57), a superintendent at the almshouse from 1891 to 1900, enumerated the ways. Medical staff positions were stepping stones to more prominent professorships. Rush, Wistar, Parrish, and Physick had all served at the Philadelphia Almshouse prior to accepting positions at the University of Pennsylvania. Almshouse wards also functioned as living classrooms where physicians' students could receive free clinical instruction (Rosenberg 1982, 141). Physicians were able to hone medical treatments, as well as collect information about varied diseases. Indeed, Samuel's own study of pulmonary consumption, *Illustrations of Pulmonary Consumption* (1834), benefited from his clinical interactions with almshouse inmates. While the treatise garnered accolades from medical colleagues, the beauty of the 12 colored plates belied the grim origins of the fragmented body parts. As disclosed by Samuel for Case 9: "S. D., a black labourer, aged thirty-eight years, was admitted to the Philadelphia Alms-house hospital, January 3, 1833, with confirmed consumption. He is a tall, athletic man, with a remarkably broad, expanded chest, and other external appearances of a once robust frame" (1834, 57–58). Thirty hours after the man's death, Samuel and colleagues dissected his heart and lungs. A figure of funicular abscesses, sectioned from the inmate's left lung and then drawn by artist Alexander Rider, appeared among the plates (plate IV, figure 2) in Samuel's book.

As a member of the almshouse's medical staff, one also had easy access to the unclaimed corpses of recently deceased inmates. The distance from patient ward to dissecting table and graveyard was a short one (Lawrence 1905, 160–62), and Samuel regarded this fact as a boon. It was unimaginable to him that certain societies stigmatized the practice. "Some of the most enlightened nations of Europe deny even tacit acquiescence in the dissection of paupers, who have been a burthen [sic] to the community during their lives, and who have none to mourn over them in death," he lectured to his students (Morton 1831, 6). For Samuel, dissection provided his (inmate) charges in the almshouse with a way to seek redemption and his (student) charges at the medical school with an important pedagogical tool. A win-win, as he saw it.

Ever an opportunist, Samuel personally acquired some of the first skulls in his collection from the almshouse's "Insane Department." For those confined to the ward's cells, insanity was a generic diagnosis, attributable to "idiocy," "mania" (of a religious nature or induced by excessive alcoholic drink, i.e., *mania à potu*[4]), "dementia" (caused by masturbation in men but not women who, instead, were said to suffer from "moral insanity"), and "melancholia" (D'Antonio 2006). Conditions in the ward were deplorable in the early nineteenth century (which likely exacerbated inmates' vulnerability). As Lawrence (1905, 57) described:

> They were placed in dark, close and damp cells in the eastern wing, and the medical gentlemen did not seem to trouble themselves very much about them. They appeared to think that insanity was incurable, and even the mildest cases were in cages like wild beasts, and exposed to the gaze and jeers of heartless visitors, who laughed at them and treated them as though they were monkeys or other animals on exhibition in a zoological garden.

Very little had improved by the time Samuel became medical staff at the almshouse. Such treatment suggests that the occupants deemed "insane" were regarded as less than human, a qualification that made it easier to lay claim to their bodies after they died. In total, Samuel acquired at least 14 of these inmates' skulls; they are listed in the various editions of *The Catalogue of Skulls of Man, and the Inferior Animals, in the Collection of Samuel George Morton, M.D.* (hereafter *Catalogue*). One entry in the *Catalogue*'s published version reads "14. ANGLO AMERICAN Female. *Died insane, 1830. S. G. M.*" (1840a, 4).[5] But a handwritten annotation in the *Catalogue* is more expansive: "Skull of the celebrated Mrs. Fortesque, who was in succession seduced, thrown upon the town + abandoned. She became melancholy, entered the Almshouse + died insane in one of the cells of that institution in the 30th year of this age. She was of respectable family + had been remarkably beautiful. A.D. 1830" (Morton 1840b). Interestingly, this biographical information did not find its way into the revised version of the *Catalogue* (a third edition published in 1849). Whether out of deference to Mrs. Fortesque's kin or a mistake in copy editing, the reason for its omission remains unknown. Other annotations were formalized in publication, however. For "45. ANGLO-AMERICAN. Lunatic. *S. G. M.*," Samuel's handwritten note states, "45. For several years confined in the cells of the

Philad. Almshouse" (Morton 1840a, 1840b). The annotation for "63. NEGRO Lunatic. S. G. M." also reads "63. Died in Philad. Almshouse A.D. 1832, aged 65 years." Both handwritten notes appeared in the *Catalogue*'s third edition. Perhaps Samuel had no issue (or felt no shame in) offering additional information about the circumstances of these decedents' deaths. As for the 11 other "lunatics" and "idiots" in the *Catalogue*, there are no annotations, but presumably their skulls were acquired in a similar manner.[6] Skulls in the Morton Collection labeled either "lunatic" or "idiot" are, for the most part, the only ones that Samuel collected himself.

The tracking of this subtle information—the inclusion, omission, or erasure in various editions and archival sources—suggests just how the identities of individuals whose skulls make up the Morton Collection were transformed. I discuss this process of *becoming object* more fully in chapter 3. The change from human being to scientific specimen is obvious in the colonial interventions of medical officers and military men to whom Samuel outsourced collecting. They were dispersed throughout the United States' expanding boundaries, which allowed Samuel to move beyond his own backyard. After this time, around 1833, he instead began to foster a concern with racialized differences; relatively few "lunatics" or "idiots" are listed in the *Catalogue* thereafter.

Almshouse inmates found the claims staked on their bodies disquieting. "To impoverished Philadelphians in the almshouse . . . their bodies were often virtually all that they owned and thus the primary means whereby they might achieve some measure of control over their own lives," writes historian Simon Newman (2003, 17). Resistance to regulation while alive was feasible to an extent but quite impossible after death. At issue here was consent of any kind (e.g., broad, informed, implied, passive). Dissection often, if not always, occurred in its absence. Coercion and medical paternalism informed patient-physician interactions, while the advancement of medicine and science was evoked as sufficient justification for dissection of inmates' cadavers and culling of anatomical or pathological specimens from them (Sappol 2002, 125, 277). In contrast, autopsies occurred with the consent of individuals (prior to death) or their next of kin. Historian Michael Sappol (2002, 103) has recounted additional ways in which they were different from dissections: they occurred in private rooms without the spectacle of the anatomical theaters; they were reserved for the privileged members of a community; they did not signal shame, stigma, or punishment; they targeted specific areas of the body to discern cause of death.[7]

Despite inmates' remonstrations and the theoretical requirement that paupers' bodies be buried, their dissection continued for several decades with a wink and nod. In the wake of the Burke and Hare scandal of 1829, it was far less suspect than purchasing cadavers from resurrectionists.[8] Though, importantly, not all physicians affiliated with the almshouse endorsed dissection of inmates' cadavers. In 1845, a decade after Samuel had ended his tenure, six members of the hospital's board issued a public statement, characterizing such opportunism as un-Christian and cruel (Lawrence 1905, 160–61). Supplying medical schools with paupers' cadavers, regardless of the reason for their misfortune, was far too high a price to pay, they wrote. While the protest engendered discussion, there was no real change in policy for fear that grave robbing would occur at the city's cemeteries. Thereafter the public referred to physicians' activities as "Buzzard practices" (Lawrence 1905, 270–71). On 13 June 1883, the Pennsylvania legislature officially sanctioned physicians' dissection of paupers' bodies, providing a patina of legitimacy.[9] As directed in the Anatomy Act, kin, friends, and charitable organizations had 36 hours after death to claim a decedent's body. The bodies of unclaimed individuals, who were buried at the public expense, were to first "be used within the State for the advancement of medical science."[10] A utilitarian argument continued to hold weight.

As the dispute over dissection of almshouse inmates demonstrates, medical staff squabbled with each other and administrators. Harlan and Samuel were of like mind, however; neither man took issue with dissection of their impoverished wards given the benefits to anatomical science (e.g., Harlan 1835; Harlan in Gannal 1840, 211; Morton 1831). Their early correspondences also communicated a mutual respect. A letter from Harlan dated 3 August 1827 is effusive and filled with intimate details about his trip to Baltimore:

> I am sincerely indebted to you for the trouble I have exposed you to. Indeed when I think how often my demands have been repeated, and the cheerful alacrity with which they have been performed on your part, I fear I have much to fulfill ere I shall be able to strike a balance. Nor do I forget that friendship essentially consists in a *mutual* interchange of kind offices. I am sure however, that when the occasion offers, my *will* to serve you will never fall short of the *power*.

Harlan slyly noted in the same letter that, had more time afforded itself, he might have been "seduced from celibacy" by the "elegant and accomplished" ladies whose acquaintances he was pleased to meet. Two days later, he penned a follow-up, informing Samuel he had been delayed. Feminine wiles and a repressed libido were not the cause. Rather, a job opportunity had presented itself. The chair of anatomy at the University of Baltimore unexpectedly opened and was rumored to pay $3,000 a year. Harlan requested secrecy and assistance with scheduled patients. "P.S. Two surgical patients were to call at my office on Monday at 9 oclock—Mr. Cuffman and Mr. ____. If possible will you see them at that hour." The postscript was jotted down as an afterthought and not posed as a question.

In the months that followed, Harlan championed Samuel's admittance to the venerable APS.[11] The two men also shared a predilection for human skulls. Harlan's collection rivaled Samuel's own until a fire destroyed it in 1839—the same year that *Crania Americana* was published (Fabian 2010, 20). But their relationship soured with time. Samuel's increasing commitments may have made him less obliging or his ambition more tenacious. As a physician at the almshouse, he grew confident in his medical abilities (Anonymous n.d. a, 272).[12] Come January 1830, Samuel joined with other notable physicians to form the Philadelphia Association for Medical Instruction, a "proprietary" medical school. (I elaborate on this particular type of medical education later in the chapter.) Of the founders' eminence, Dr. Alfred Stillé (1846, 7) made the following remarks in a closing address to students:

> But it is no easy task to emulate the intellectual and moral worth of such men as the benevolent and judicious Parrish, and of Doctors [Franklin] Bache, [George] Wood, J[ohn]. Rhea Barton, [Charles] Meigs, [Jacob] Randolph, Morton and [W. W.] Gerhard. The gentlemen . . . had still their reputation to achieve when first they entered upon their career as public teachers; but now that their fame is sacred and familiar as household words, who can doubt that they nobly fulfilled their object, and gave to their classes a full remuneration for their time and money.

In the meantime, Harlan's bid for the Baltimore job proved unsuccessful, and so he remained on medical staff at the Philadelphia Almshouse. Collegiality became strained. A strongly worded correspondence dated 9 December 1831 indicates a falling out between the two men. Samuel's visit to the private home of a paying patient had stoked Harlan's ire. "Sir," it began (he forsook the "Dear"):

> You can not be ignorant that I have long since lost all confidence in your probity as a man and talents as a physician; notwithstanding

which you visited a patient of mine yesterday, and prescribed in a manner totally different from my views of the nature of the case—on being made acquainted with this transaction, I found it out of my power to assume any further responsibility for the patient, who did not long survive.

This is not the first time, sir, that your illegitimate and ungentlemanly interference has deprived me of patients, by what you are in the habit of denominating "acts of friendship or of kindness" but you may rest assured that I am perfectly well acquainted with the full import of such phraseology, and I warn you for the future to abstain in every case from any interference of a similar nature, or you will force me to appeal to measures to maintain my past rights, very disagreeable at least to you, if not totally destructive to your reputation. (Harlan 1831)

It is not clear whether Samuel penned a response to explain the circumstances of the patient's demise or to counter the defamatory comments. But he did take the outburst in stride. After all, Harlan was quick to anger and known to alienate friends (Fabian, 2010, 19–21). Samuel saved the correspondence (it was included among his letters housed at the APS). He also amended it with an equanimous allegory at the bottom: "Apologue. A citizen of Athens, while walking by the Ilissus, met a vulgar fellow who pelted him with mud. 'Spare thy dirt,' said the Athenian, 'a thing so easily washed off can do me no injury.'" After this exchange, the two men continued to serve as acting attending physicians at the almshouse. But their friendly correspondences ceased.

The Cholera Epidemic of 1832

If Harlan's waspish comments did not have Samuel rethink his effectiveness as a physician, the outbreak of cholera in 1832 made clear the limits of his (and all practitioners') medical ability to foster patients' lives.[13] "I trust none of your family or friends have fallen victims to the horrible new disease which I find by the papers has at length visited your city," a concerned Gideon Algernon Mantell (1832) wrote to Samuel from Lewes, England. It was 27 September 1832, and, as Mantell explained, for weeks, 100 Londoners had been dying daily. He continued, "Like all new diseases the laws which govern it being unknown it has set theory and practice at naught, and our best practitioners candidly confess they are as much at a loss now as they were at first to lay down any general plan of treatment!" Mantell was in no danger of contracting the "Pest," as he referred to it, however. The obstetrician and amateur paleontologist was safely ensconced in the countryside caring for patients and collecting fossils. The same could not be said of Harlan or Samuel who found themselves in the thick of the epidemic.

Originating in South Asia and seasonal in its recurrence, cholera had long been endemic to India. But, in the early nineteenth century, its westward spread resulted in epidemics (followed by pandemics), first in Europe and then the Americas (Clemens et al., 2017).[14] The news of its advance preceded actual outbreaks, generating fearful anticipation among physicians, politicians, and the public. The disease was novel, and there were many unknowns—about its etiology, treatment, and lethality.

In early June 1832, its presence was first reported in Grosse Île, Canada. As recommended by the Quebec Medical Board, this island port was set up as a quarantine station for European immigrants (Bilson 1980, 8–12). But the measures implemented at Grosse Île proved ineffective against the transmission of cholera. It traveled uninvited and often undetected among ships' passengers and then continued unabated down the eastern seaboard (Pyle 1969; Rosenberg 1962; Sanitary Board 1832; Whooley 2013, 31–37). In the United States, the epidemic eventually extended up and down the Atlantic coast, into the Midwest, and as far south as New Orleans. Cholera came to trump yellow fever and smallpox as national concerns.

In his analysis of the 1832 epidemic, Rosenberg (1962) has argued that medical providers grappled ineffectively with cholera for several reasons. A revolution in trade and transportation fostered global connections that facilitated its spread. Increasing urbanization meant overcrowding and squalid living conditions for the less fortunate. Governmental concern for public health was nascent; indeed, multiple cholera epidemics throughout the nineteenth century were what jumpstarted efforts.

That the 1832 cholera epidemic would eventually reach Philadelphia was not in question. But how best to ameliorate its deadly toll? Fortunately, prior waves of sickness had imparted some valuable lessons about appropriate sociopolitical responses during a public health crisis. An extant municipal Board of Health, which the Pennsylvania legislature established in the wake of the tragic yellow fever outbreak of 1793 (College of Physicians of Philadelphia 1799), had the wherewithal to commission an emergency sanitary board. They selected Samuel's colleagues—Richard Harlan, Samuel Jackson, and Charles Meigs—to survey the situation in Canada and identify feasible methods of treatment. The Board of Health also created biopolitical guidelines (i.e., quarantine protocols) and implemented public policies (e.g., street cleanings; isolation hospitals) (Osborne 2008; Watson 2009). These efforts indicate how local governance and physicians ardently worked to foster life. But the cholera epidemic also offers lessons in precarity. Marginalized groups—on account of their occupancy in the almshouse, incarcerated status, or racialized identity—were at the greatest risk of succumbing to cholera. And while physicians did not actively facilitate these deaths, the impact that the infectious disease had on these communities came as no surprise.

The first case of cholera was reported in Philadelphia on 5 July 1832 (Pyle 1969, 62). Those wealthy enough fled for more rural environs. An estimated 161,980 remained in the city (Scharf and Westcott 1884, 1726). Inmates of the almshouse counted among the Philadelphians unable to leave. How best to prevent the disease from impacting them, Samuel and colleagues deliberated. They convened a special meeting of the almshouse's Board of Physicians and Surgeons within days of cholera's arrival.[15] Acting in the capacity of secretary, Samuel recorded the group's resolutions:

"*Resolved*, That the Medical Board recommend to the Board of Managers the propriety of prohibiting the introduction into this house of any case of cholera.

"*Resolved*, That it also be recommended to the Managers to make provision for such cases of cholera as may occur within the limits of their administration, and that said accommodations be located as near as practicable to this infirmary." (Lawrence 1905, 117)

In line with the Board of Health's policies, a separate hospital was established for Almshouse patients who contracted cholera. Samuel counted among the acting attending physicians (Pennsylvania Senate 1832–1833, 233). Admirably, these men who cared for patients did so voluntarily and without compensation. Though Samuel did reap some benefit; at least two of the skulls in his collection were from inmates who died during the cholera epidemic. Both had been people of color and confined to the Lunatic Asylum. In Samuel's (1840a) *Catalogue*, for "63. NEGRO Lunatic. *S. G. M.*" the handwritten annotation reads "63. Died in Philad. Almshouse A.D. 1832, aged 65 years." For "64. MULATTO Lunatic, female. *S. G. M.*" handwritten on the adjacent page is "64. Died of the Cholera, 1832, aged

18 years." In total, and despite the proactive stance taken by physicians at the almshouse's hospital, 134 individuals developed cholera and at least 61 individuals succumbed to the infectious disease (Osborne 2008, 37).

The incarcerated did not fare much better than paupers. Like the inmates of the almshouse, men imprisoned at Arch Street Prison also represented a population at risk. Indeed, many shuttled back and forth between the two institutions (O'Brassill-Kulfan 2019). Conditions at the prison were quite appalling; to discourage recidivism, cells were crowded while food and bedding were scant. When cholera arrived in Philadelphia, dissimilar from other cities, local governance did not immediately release prisoners, a decision that exacerbated the epidemic's negative impact (Rosenberg 1962). Harlan described vividly events unfolding at Arch Street Prison in a letter he penned to John James Audubon.

> The Cholera has raged dreadfully in some localities here—I was engaged on Monday superintending the removal of the sick prisoners from the jail in arch St. at the request of the City authorities—I was there three times during the day—60 were sick at one time, the suffering, and agony of the dying wretches, was an awful sight to witness, 26 died there that day, and about as many more who were removed to the various local Hospitals—I have treated altogether up to present date 35—of whom 18 from prison. 16 have died—and only one remains today—my success is rather encouraging considering the habits of the poor wretches whose cases fell under my care—most of the fatal cases were in a dying state when admitted—I would not have recd. them, but for the wish to alleviate suffering and scatter the tenants of the infected rooms of the jail—The Newspapers do not give an accurate account, because numbers are cured in the early stages whose cases are never reported—the statements of deaths are more accurate—and I suppose the greatest mortality has not exceeded 100 per diem—today only 26 deaths reported, there will probably be more tomorrow. . . . My term of duty as Surgeon to the alms House commenced at the 1st of August—the sik [sic] for the surgical wards have also suffered, but not so much as the poor tenants of the cells, it has nearly cleaned them out—some respectable, but weakly families in the city have already suffered—My time is usefully, at least, if not profitably employed, night and day. cholera, cholera, cholera!!!! [5 August 1832 (Herrick 1917, 28–29)]

When all was said and done, about one-quarter of prisoners, 80 of 310 individuals, died at the Arch Street Prison. Though, as Harlan noted in his letter, these numbers were underreported.

Cholera also offers an early example of the racialization of disease and suffering. From the epidemic's outset, physicians made observations about its disproportionate impact on ethnic or racial groups (Rosenberg 1962, 60). While in Canada on Sanitary Board business, Harlan described its effects on Caughnawaga, a community of 1,000 "Christian Indians" located 11 miles west of Montreal (Sanitary Board 1832, 8). This group suffered terrible losses; 137 of its members contracted cholera and 70 died. Among the takeaways summarized in the Sanitary Board's report: "The native Indian population appeared to be strongly predisposed to the disease, which afflicted them with a dreadful mortality" (Sanitary Board 1832, 17).

In Philadelphia, where physicians' interactions with American Indians were few and far between, they determined that cholera disproportionately impacted the city's Black occupants. Racial discrimination and impoverishment made for lives defined by precarity. As reported in the weekly *Cholera Gazette*: "The ravages of the disease were more extensive in the coloured than in the white portion of the population, in proportion to numbers" (Jackson 1832, 250). Part of this impact may have had to do with the disproportionate number of Black men—nearly half of all prisoners arrested for vagrancy—who made up the inmates at the Arch Street Prison (O'Brassill-Kulfan 2019, 257). For physicians, those racial groups most at risk for contracting cholera, Native and Black communities, offered further evidence of their physical, social, and moral fallibility.

Though interestingly (and inversely), during the city's yellow fever epidemic of 1793, physicians cited the purportedly low mortality and morbidity rate of Blacks as evidence of their immunity to the disease (Hogarth 2019). Years later, Samuel reiterated the idea in an introductory lecture titled "The Diversities of the Human Species." Native Africans, he told medical school students, might be intellectually and morally inferior, but they were physically hardier in the face of "destroying epidemics which infest the rice plantations and other marshy districts of the southern states" (1842, 10). These "differences among the several races of men" were "primeval" (Morton 1842, 6). Observations about these epidemics' unequal effects became key evidentiary support for his ideas about the plurality of humans' origin, a topic to which I return later in this chapter.

By September, the cholera epidemic had run its course in Philadelphia. At least 935 residents had died among a city population of about 160,000 (Jackson 1832, 246; Scharf and Westcott 1884, 1726). In comparison to other cities, the loss of life was low. New York, for instance, had 2,782 deaths among its approximately 140,000 inhabitants. For medical services rendered during the cholera epidemic, the city honored 13 physicians—"the physicians in chief of the Cholera Hospitals of the city proper" (Anonymous 1833, 204–6). They each received a silver pitcher as a token of gratitude. Harlan was one of those 13; Samuel was not.[16] The oversight, an opportunity missed for advancing his professional reputation, may have irked Samuel given his response at the Philadelphia Almshouse and the expenses accrued from his increasing familial obligations.

"Husband, Father, Friend, Physician, Lecturer"

Samuel seems to have approached affairs of the heart with the same ambition and pragmatism he did his medical practice. "It is reasonable to suppose that his professional business was increased by his marriage," George Wood (1853, 11) eulogized after his death. On 23 October 1827, Samuel wed Rebecca Grellet Pearsall (in chapter 5, I discuss Rebecca in far greater depth). Joseph Watson, the mayor of Philadelphia, officiated. There are hints that the conjugal relationship was more practical than passionate. Archival materials do not include any letters, intimate or otherwise, from Samuel to Rebecca. Or vice versa, for her formative years in Quaker boarding schools had ensured she too was literate and well read. Seeing that Samuel was an avid letter writer—the number of correspondences he penned over his lifetime was perhaps comparable to the quantity of skulls he amassed—the lack of them between husband and wife is odd. Preservation may be one reason. Intentional and careful production of a certain image for posterity may be another. Yet, included among genealogical materials compiled by their son Thomas George were love notes written by a besotted George Morton to Jane Cummings (I encourage the reader to revisit the previous chapter). And a sizeable assortment is contained within the papers of brother-in-law John Jay Smith, who would also gush about his wife Rachel (née Pearsall) Smith on the occasion of their golden wedding (Smith 1892). That is to say, proximity did not preclude the writing of love letters nor were they a genre omitted from the family's archives. In the case of Samuel and Rebecca, then, the silence may speak volumes about the nature of their relationship.

That the couple was intimate, however, was evident by the nine offspring they produced over some twenty-four years of marriage. Samuel and Rebecca named the children for various living and deceased family members: James St. Clair, Robert Pearsall, George, Thomas George, Anna, William Henry Harrison, Mary Elizabeth, Algernon, and Charles Mortimer. Given his medical and scientific pursuits, the mind boggles that he had any time for parenting responsibilities. Indeed, his friend Thomas Hodgkin often gently chastised Samuel for his delay in replying to previous correspondences. "Husband, father, friend, Physician, Lecturer, perpetual secretary of the ANS, Natural Historian, Poet, draft man, et cetera," Hodgkin (1830) jested in a letter about his friend's numerous commitments. The growing size of Samuel's brood might have accounted for some of his financial worries and grasping ambition. He turned to "proprietary" medical education as a possible solution for his economic insecurities.

Starting in the early 1800s, American medical societies chartered proprietary medical colleges. The success of these schools was predicated on the profits they generated.[17] Some were disbanded. Others were folded into or formed the foundation for larger educational institutions. One early example was the College of Medicine of Maryland. Chartered by the Medical and Chirurgical Faculty in December of 1807, this proprietary medical college later came under the aegis of the University of Maryland (Waite 1935). A third type of medical school was founded by a small group of individuals, which they ran independent of a medical society or large-scale educational institution. These schools were usually in rural locations and may or may not have had charters approved by the state legislature (Waite 1935). All offered instruction but did not necessarily confer degrees or honors. Come the early twentieth century, medical professionals denounced proprietary medical colleges, arguing that the for-profit model resulted in an inferior education (e.g., Flexner 1910). This criticism had a significant impact on Black doctors; segregationist policies denied equal access to medical education, making proprietary medical schools the only option for acquiring knowledge and clinical experience (Harley 2006).

Samuel and colleagues rode these trends. In 1830, they established the Philadelphia Association for Medical Instruction, a collective that delivered extramural lectures to private pupils (Stillé 1846, 5; Wood 1853, 12). Classes extended over the summer months when the city's heat and humidity tested even the most committed student. Samuel delivered lectures on anatomy at the school until its dissolution in 1836 (Anonymous 1904, 282). In 1839, he joined George McClellan, Samuel Colhoun, and William Rush in their efforts to open another medical school, one that could compete with Jefferson Medical College. They successfully petitioned the Pennsylvania College of Gettysburg to charter a medical department in Philadelphia (Anonymous 1904, 288). The request, known as "grafting," was common and had the potential to benefit all involved (Norwood 1970, 478). A college could enhance its reputation and extend its geographic range. Faculty members stood to profit individually, were free to make decisions without overreaching trustees, and could achieve medical reform. Requirements and regulations at the Pennsylvania Medical College were commensurate with larger institutions. Samuel and colleagues, for instance, had modeled their medical department after the one at Penn.[18] The physical layout of its two lecture rooms, a museum, reading room, chemical laboratory, and anatomical rooms for dissection were similar (Breidenbough 1882, 81).[19] The curriculum included courses on surgery, anatomy and physiology, theory and practice of medicine, materia medica and pharmacy, obstetrics and diseases of women and children, chemistry and natural philosophy, and practical anatomy. For his part, Samuel lectured on anatomy and physiology. For a time, the college was profitable. But enrollment numbers dwindled over the years. Perhaps Samuel had seen the writing on the dissecting room's wall; he resigned in 1843 amid faculty strife. Without students' fees to support the school, it closed in 1861; the outbreak of the Civil War sounded its final death knell (Breidenbough 1882, 86; Norwood 1970, 483).

During the first half of the nineteenth century, in addition to vying with each other for students, medical schools' physicians competed in the marketplace with practitioners of alternative therapies. According to medical anthropologist Hans Baer (2001, 7), therapeutic sects included "homeopathy, botanic medicine, eclecticism, hydropathy, Christian Science, osteopathy, and chiropractic." Pluralism speaks to the religious and metaphysical beliefs that continued to frame understandings of the body, as well as skepticism about nascent biomedical approaches and their technical interventions. Rush's depletion therapy, discussed in this book's introduction, was one example of the latter—influential but not without its critics. Additionally, because of the many deaths and unanswered questions spurred by the 1832 cholera epidemic, the lay public found alternative approaches to be as credible and more democratic (Whooley 2013).

Homeopathy was the most widely embraced of these healing systems. It abided by two main principles: "the law of similars," that like cures like; and "the law of infinitesimals," which maintains that a medicine's potency increases the more it is diluted (Baer 2001, 11). Physicians with medical degrees equated homeopathic medicine with pseudoscience. Financial concerns also undergirded their criticisms. "The serious economic threat posed by homeopathy's status as a professionalized heterodox medical system was one of the major factors that prompted regular physicians to establish the American Medical Association in 1847," Baer observed (2001, 4; see also Sappol 2002, 98). In line with his medical colleagues, Samuel harbored an aversion to homeopathy. When his niece Margaret fell ill, he derided his brother-in-law and sister-in-law, John Jay and Rachel Smith, for consulting a homeopathic doctor. For the Smiths, their decision to do so indicates a waning faith in medical authority set in motion with the death of their daughter Gulielma Maria. Her suffering and early demise weighed heavily on the family.

The circumstances surrounding the death of "Lady Bird" or "Guly," as Gulielma was affectionately known, were discussed in publication, private correspondences, and an unpublished manuscript (R. Smith 1835; Smith 1872, 1892). As 1835 began, she experienced excessive vomiting, weight loss, and a swelling in her neck that bled persistently. She was diagnosed with scarlet fever, and her sickness progressed with rapidity and intensity. Despite her suffering, Gulielma was a compliant patient. Samuel, with the help of two colleagues in the Philadelphia Association for Medical Instruction, Drs. John Rhea Barton and George Wood, cared for the five-year-old. According to John Jay, her uncle "attended her most faithfully and affectionately for 29 days" (Smith 1872). Her parents watched desperately at her bedside as "life ebbed fast with the discharge of blood." Treatment, affection, and religious prayers all proved ineffective. Gulielma died at the end of February. A detailed account of her final days—messy, painful, and heartbreaking—appeared in his handwritten recollections, but John Jay omitted the description from any formal publication (Smith 1892).[20] Perhaps the memory was too personal for a wider audience.

For Philadelphia's parents, the devastation wrought by scarlet fever was dreadfully familiar. European colonists introduced the infectious disease to the New World in the eighteenth century, but it was not until the late 1820s that a particularly virulent and highly contagious variant began to spread globally (Katz and Morens 1992, 299). It became the leading cause of childhood death during this period. In New York, for instance, after 1828, scarlet fever mortality rates "suddenly jumped 10-fold and remained high for long afterward" (Katz and Morens 1992, 300). As the Philadelphia physician William Potts Dewees[21] (1833, 181) explained, "It is frequent in its occurrence, extensive in its prevalence, and, at times, exceedingly fatal in its termination." While physicians agreed that scarlet fever qualified as an epidemic, the contagious nature of the disease remained up for debate. Dewees (1833, 185), for instance, argued that scarlet fever was not contagious, while *Gunn's Domestic Medicine*—the most popular home medical guide of the day—asserted that it was (Gunn 1838, 706). (We now know that this streptococcal disease is easily transmitted via respiratory droplets.)

No families were safe, even those who had already suffered and mourned the loss of a son or daughter. And should a child contract and survive a bout of scarlet fever, the likelihood of a compromised immune system was significant. To safeguard their children, the Smiths ensconced two of them, Albanus and Elizabeth, at the Westtown School (R. Smith 1835). But the ones too young to attend remained at risk in Philadelphia. After Gulielma's death, Rachel conveyed the sad news to her older siblings. In the letter, she made note of supportive kin during the emotionally fraught time. "We have had the most affectionate sympathy of a great many kind friends Aunt Rachel + Rebecca [Morton,] Uncle Robert and above all dear Grandmother + Mary have been devoted to us, to comfort and assist us." There is no mention of Samuel or his ministrations.

When John Jay and Rachel's infant daughter Margaret fell ill five years later, in 1840, they sought the opinion of a homeopathic doctor. Samuel tempered his displeasure with concern for Margaret's health (Morton 1840c).

> Dear Brother—
>
> Your note is just received, and has relieved me from some unhappy reflections; although I could not for a moment suppose that you designed to wound my feelings, or stain my professional reputation. Your communication entirely satisfies me that the kindness and confidence which have subsisted between us for five + twenty years, are not to be dissolved in an hour. I should never have opposed Dr. Singer's seeing your child, tho' I confess it would have been gratifying to have been apprised of your wishes beforehand.
>
> In treating your child for an insidious disease, I have acted to the best of my judgment; always bearing in mind the maxim of Dr. Fothergill, that in the diseases of infancy the great danger lies in doing too much.
>
> I have watched your child with extreme anxiety + solicitude, + if what has been done should unhappily prove unavailing, I shall mingle

my sorrow most unfeignedly with yours, and lament, as I have often had occasion to do before, that human judgment is so fallible—human means so uncertain.

Truly hoping that nothing may ever occur to mar our mutual regard, I remain

Very faithfully yours
S. G. Morton

I include the full correspondence here for several reasons. While Samuel assiduously saved and catalogued his incoming correspondences, his outgoing requests or replies are trickier to track down. We learn much about him from what others have said. But outside the formal strictures of his scientific publications, his voice resonates softly; it is difficult to get a sense of Samuel as a person. In this regard, his scolding of John Jay is edifying. Though the tone is softer, the letter calls to mind Richard Harlan's sharply worded reproof from 1831. Samuel displays confidence in his abilities, concern for his professional reputation, and distaste for homeopathic medicine that borders on the arrogant and insecure. What would potential patients and professional colleagues make of his in-laws' adherence to medical heresy over Samuel's learned opinion? And if an increasing number of patients sought out homeopathic practitioners, how would their decision effect the business of more traditionally trained physicians?

Additionally, the emotional distance between physician and patient that Samuel normally cultivated was difficult to sustain in the cases of his ill-fated nieces (Margaret also ended up succumbing to scarlet fever). He too may have grown demoralized by his impotence in the face of dying and death. Medicine in the first half of the nineteenth century was marked by shifting beliefs about disease, treatments, and doctor-patient interactions (Baer 2001; Rosenberg 1977a, 1977b; Whooley 2013). Even the most confident of physicians harbored uncertainty, though not necessarily humility.

Ethnological Inquiry

"When it was that he began to turn his attention especially to ethnological studies I am unable to say," George Wood (1853, 13) wondered in his eulogy to Samuel. It was likely a number of factors—an existential void left by his disillusion with Quakerism (though, in time, he affiliated with the Episcopal church), interactions with specific colleagues, erratic employment, praise for his geological and zoological studies. It also seems more than coincidence that his increased attention to ethnology was concurrent with his impotence in the face of epidemics.

According to his own recollections, Samuel had something of an epiphany about his research aims during a lecture at the Philadelphia Association for Medical Instruction.

> I commenced the study of Ethnology in 1830; in which year, having occasion to deliver an introductory lecture on Anatomy, it occurred to me to illustrate the difference in the form of the skull as seen in the five great races of men. . . . When I sought the materials for my proposed lecture, I found to my surprise that they could be neither bought nor borrowed. Caucasian and Negro crania were readily procured, and two or three Indian skulls were placed at my disposal; but for the Mongolian and Malay I inquired in vain. I resolved, therefore, to supply this remarkable deficiency in an important branch of science. (Morton 1849a, iii)

Samuel's call for crania built on earlier work conducted by a number of European scientists. Johann Blumenbach proved among the most influential, and Samuel acknowledged this intellectual debt in *Crania Americana* (1839). It was the German anatomist's five-race schema to which Samuel alluded in the above quotation. Blumenbach believed skulls to reveal valuable, morphological information about racial differences, arguing that even those of infants possessed distinguishing traits (Blumenbach 1865, 238). While all "varieties"—Caucasian, Mongolian, Ethiopian, American, and Malaysian—were represented in his collection, he did not go as far to advance a racial hierarchy. Yet, implicit in the colonialism that yielded the collection were notions about European superiority and Native inferiority.

Samuel followed Blumenbach's advice about sourcing skulls. The difficulty of such an endeavor is "not insuperable when the collector shows zeal and perseverance, and can obtain the active co-operation of men who have opportunities of helping him in his object," Blumenbach (1865, 299) stated in *Contributions to Natural History*. By his own admission, colonialism also yielded opportunity for Samuel: "Yet, I need hardly add, that had it not been for the exertions of my friends in every quarter of the globe, my object would have remained unaccomplished" (Morton 1849a, iii). His call for crania coincided with passage of the Indian Removal Act in 1830, federal legislation underpinned by settler colonial ideology, as I discuss in greater depth in the next chapter.

Here it is worth noting that his intellectual interests signaled a clear separation from the Society of Friends. Quakers had long opposed removal of American Indians from their lands. As made explicit in the *Rules of Discipline and Christian Advices of the Yearly Meeting of Friends for Pennsylvania and New Jersey*:

> Friends should not purchase, or remove to settle on such Lands as have not been fairly and openly first purchased of the Indians, by those who are or may be authorized by the Government to make such purchases; and that Monthly Meetings should be careful to excite their Members to the strict observance of this advice; and where any so remove, contrary to the advice of their Brethren, that they should not give Certificates to such Persons, but persuade them to avoid the Danger to which they expose themselves, and to convince them of the inconsistency of their Conduct with our Christian Profession. (Philadelphia Yearly Meeting of the Religious Society of Friends 1797, 61)

Samuel was quite aware of this stance given his formative education, though it did little to dissuade him from actively pursuing the skulls of dispossessed American Indians. While he may not have served in the military, many of his medical colleagues did, and his pedagogy and research benefited directly from these connections, as we will see in chapter 3.

Samuel's ethnological inquiries also drew from the day's fascination with phrenology, in no small part due to its popularization by George Combe, a Scottish lawyer. His writings on the subject reached across the Atlantic. Phrenology, for Combe, connected "different mental qualities with particular portions of the brain" (1835, viii). The portions, or organs, varied contingent on the individual. By the mid-nineteenth century, however, intellectuals grew ambivalent about the scientific basis for phrenology. Proponents saw value in the systematic study of skull shape, which offered a window into the brain's morphology. Cerebral development, they argued, revealed information about personality traits and behavior. For critics, it increasingly qualified as pseudoscience.

Somewhat surprisingly (or perhaps not given that these interesting times were full of contradictions), the abolitionist Frederick Douglass fell into the former camp. He was particularly taken with Combe's *The Constitution of Man*, perhaps given its statements about the injustices of slavery and potential equality of "Negroes," as revealed by their heads (1835, 247–49). (In the same treatise, Combe was less gracious in his characterization of "Hindoos" and Native Americans, whose brains he deemed "inferior" [1835, 158].) On an 1846 trip to Edinburgh, Douglass breakfasted with Combe. Of the phrenologist and the conversation that followed, he later wrote,

> I was a listener. Mr. Combe did the most of the talking, and did it so well, that nobody felt like interposing a word, except so far as to draw him on.... He looked at all political and social questions through his peculiar mental science. His manner was remarkably quiet, and he spoke as not expecting opposition to his views. Phrenology explained everything to him, from the finite to the infinite, I look back to the morning spent with this singularly clear-headed man with much satisfaction. (Douglass 1882, 208)

If Douglass had any qualms about Combe's hierarchical categorization of "national brains," or how it may have been used to justify British imperialism in India, he never stated so aloud or in writings. But, for Samuel, it was this aspect of phrenology that seemed to be the most appealing.

Well into the 1830s, correspondences and publications attest to Samuel and Combe's collegiality, mutually beneficial relationship, and shared concern for "national character" (Bieder 1986; Fabian 2010, 95). In *A System of Phrenology*, a publication that predated *The Constitution of Man*, Combe (1825) hypothesized about the sizes of different nations' brains and what they could communicate about intelligence. European nations, Combe (1825, 618) stated with authority, "are larger than Hindoo, American Indian, and Negro heads; and this indicates a superior force of mental character." The phrenologist continued, "A scientific mode of measurement is much wanted. These measurements are taken from individual skulls, and cannot be given as an exact statement of the average of the different national crania. They are, however, an approximation to truth, and are sufficient to show the interest of the investigation" (1825, 622). Here Combe called attention to the need for a proper technique by which to measure crania, a shortcoming that he acknowledged earlier in his 1819 publication *Essays on Phrenology*. He also recognized that his current assessment was far too idiosyncratic. A larger sample size could offer sufficient empirical evidence to support a hypothesis about hierarchical ranking. In Samuel's burgeoning collection, he would find a sufficient number of skulls for such analytical purposes.

At Samuel's request, Combe conducted a phrenological study of his collection during an 1839 visit to Philadelphia (Gibbon 1878, 53). It appeared as an appendix in *Crania Americana* (Morton 1839). Economic opportunity may have spurred the inclusion of Combe's assessments (Fabian 2010, 92). His trip to North America involved a promotional tour, which promised to introduce Samuel's craniometric work to a lay public not yet disillusioned with phrenology. He may have also viewed Combe's published statements about American Indians intriguing. Of the mental qualities he assigned them, few were complimentary. "The forehead is not largely developed, while Firmness, Secretiveness, and Cautiousness, are very prominently enlarged; as is also Destructiveness," explained Combe (1825, 611). They also had a deficiency in the organ of Conscientiousness, and their natural environs had done little to improve their savage ignorance and indolence, especially when compared to the advances made by Europeans who had settled in the Americas (Combe 1825, 300, 604).

While his ties to medical officers and Combe indicate how his circle of acquaintances expanded, Samuel's ethnological inquiries likely generated friction among several old friends. For some two decades after Samuel returned from Europe, he and Thomas Hodgkin continued to stay in touch. The British physician penned long letters, his tight script making good use of a sheet's surface area. Rather than close with "Your obedient servant," he signed "Thy attached friend," a valediction suggestive of his and Samuel's warm relationship and formative connections to Quakerism (e.g., Hodgkin 1842). But, as the years went by, the two men formed quite divergent positions on Native peoples.

In 1837, Hodgkin helped found the British and Foreign Aborigines Protection Society.[22] According to George Stocking (1987, 242), protection of aborigines took two forms: collection of ethnological information and promotion of humanitarian positions. Knowledge of difference, so it went, engendered more considerate colonialism. Cultural evolution, not relativism, was an implicit ideology, as the society members pursued the "advancement of uncivilized Tribes" (Aborigines' Protection Society 1840, 3). The Aborigines' Protection Society also worked to sway public policy at home and abroad. During its third annual meeting, in a statement directed at Honorary Members living in the United States, the society addressed American Indians' dire situation.

> The official documents published by that republic have long contained accounts of the sanguinary contests which is now being carried on between that power and the Seminole Indians, and which has already been the abundant source of misery and death to both parties.

The most recent accounts have brought the distressing intelligence that in connexion with this struggle there is great reason to fear that an extensive Indian war is likely to rage against the western frontier. The members of the Aborigines' Protection Society contemplate with horror the atrocities to which such a war must give birth; and whilst they sympathize with numerous and innocent families who are likely to become the victims of savage vengeance, they also reflect that the inevitable, though probably deferred, success of American prowess and arms, must frustrate the benevolent efforts already adverted to, and those of the many American philanthropists who have labored to promote the cause of Christianity and civilization amongst the Indians, and hasten the long menaced doom of that devoted race. (Aborigines' Protection Society 1840, 24)

The Aborigines' Protection Society was also quite pointed in its criticism of the Seminole Wars. Resistance in the face of forced relocation was certainly justifiable, they stated in a remonstration to the US president and Congress (Aborigines' Protection Society 1840, 21).

This politicized position on American Indians may be one reason Samuel declined to be an honorary member when elected to the Aborigines' Protection Society in 1839. It certainly did not line up with his indirect involvement in these conflicts, as I lay out in the next chapter. It is possible that the membership was a professional courtesy reciprocated. Samuel had helped secure a correspondent position for Hodgkin in the ANS two years prior (Academy of Natural Sciences 1877, 25; Kass and Kass 1988, 331). Regardless, he seems to have eschewed involvement in the Aborigines' Protection Society; his name does not appear in any of its annual reports. His absence is notable especially in contrast to the inclusion of James Cowles Prichard's name among the list of honorary members (Aborigines Protection Society 1838, 10–11; Aborigines' Protection Society 1840, 3).[23]

Prichard was a British ethnologist, physician, lapsed Quaker, and fellow Edinburgh alumnus. Hodgkin had originally introduced him to Samuel at medical school. Like Hodgkin and most men in the Aborigines' Protection Society—its motto was *Ab uno sanguine* (Latin for "of one blood")—Prichard was a monogenist; he believed in the unity of humankind and attributed racial differences to environmental forces (Bieder 1986, 63; Cantor 2005, 133–35; Kass and Kass 1989, 538; Stocking 1987, 245–46). Though Prichard did not go as far to advance racial equality. In European colonialism, he saw the root of suffering and the means of salvation. That is, it drove Indigenous peoples to extinction *and* functioned to generate knowledge that might circumvent their extermination (Prichard 1839). (Therein lies the contradiction at the foundation of anthropology.)

Samuel, however, grew to be a staunch polygenist; human races, plural, represented distinct species, he maintained (Gould 1981). That ideological difference, however, was not fully formed when he published *Crania Americana*. Years later, Samuel reflected on his initial belief in monogenism and eventual championing of polygenism: "My first convictions were, that these diversities are not acquired, but have existed *ab origine*. Such is the opinion expressed in my *Crania Americana*; but at that period, (twelve years ago) I had not investigated Scriptural Ethnology, and was content to suppose the distinctive characteristics of the several races had been marked upon the immediate family of Adam" (Morton 1850b). His early ambivalence may explain why Samuel dedicated the English edition of *Crania Americana* to Prichard. George Combe did not approve. In publication, Prichard (1835, 464) had derided phrenology for its "plausible and specious nature." Its intellectual shelf life would be a short one, he concluded. The characterization had clearly riled Combe, and he did not mince words about his distaste for the man (nor did he see it necessary to spell his surname correctly in his letter to Samuel).

> I am not gratified by learning that your English Edition is dedicated to Dr. Pritchard [sic]. He has an excellent intellect, and a well balanced head, with one exception, a deficient organ of Conscientiousness. I speak from observing his development. In regard to Phrenology, he has shown a lamentable defect of honest + fair dealing. A man of this kind is one who is a capital friend as long as it is his interest or inclination to be a friend; but no perfect reliance can be placed on his conduct where interest or inclination (vanity, for example, or ambition) dictate one course of action + duty another. (Combe 1840a)

In a letter penned a few weeks later, Combe suggested that the dedication to Prichard had prevented Samuel from selling several copies of *Crania Americana*. "Mr. Hewett Watson intended to purchase three copies of your work at his own expense + present them to public institutions, but when he read the dedication to Dr. Pritchard [sic] he abandoned his purchase!" scolded Combe (1840b), his "I told you so" implied by the exclamation mark. Though friends he had aplenty, Samuel keenly felt the loss of even a few sales. He had published *Crania Americana* on his own dime, a risky undertaking for one not born to wealth. Indeed, its production costs and dismal sales nearly put him in debt (Fabian 2010, 88–90). A notation in genealogical documents housed at the Historical Society of Pennsylvania confirmed his financial straits: "Many copies of *Crania Americana* lost at sea in a voyage from Phil to Boston—no insurance—a loss he could ill afford to bear" (Anonymous n.d. a, 4).

Relief came in the form of death. When his Uncle James Morton passed in 1840, his fortune transferred to Samuel. Combe (1840c) sent congratulations upon hearing the news: "This is like a scene in a play, or the winding up of a novel, it is so appropriate and so pleasing. How very rarely do men of talent and devoted to science enjoy the good things of this life? Yet none are more worthy. I greatly respect your Uncle's memory for such a judicious disposal of his Estate." His newly gained wealth coupled with *Crania Americana*'s warm reception in the United States and abroad impelled Samuel to embrace his study of natural history more fully. As one eulogist reminisced after Samuel's death, "The eminent success of this work determined definitely its author's ulterior scientific career. From this time forward he devoted his powers almost exclusively to Ethnology" (Patterson 1854, xxxv). Granted his take on ethnology is one of a cacophony of voices vying to be heard—from natural historians to phrenologists to social crusaders working to protect Native peoples. Collectively, they expressed an ambivalence about the role Others should play in the body politic. Nevertheless, "it was in the less restricted paths of science that he achieved special distinction" (Anonymous n.d. a, 143).

By the end of the 1830s, Samuel's correspondences are primarily concerned with human skulls and their procurement or ANS business. The former attest to the challenges his collectors faced. The mineralogist Parker Cleaveland wrote to Samuel in 1839 about his failed acquisition of a skull: "Our friend writes me, that he would sooner undertake to *Burke* a living Indian then to disinter a dead one" (see note 7 for an explanation of "to Burke"). In Cleaveland's estimation, the murder of an Indian was far less difficult an endeavor than the defilement of Native mortuary spaces and ancestral remains. For Samuel, who patiently bided his time in Philadelphia, concerns about the pragmatics of hands-on collection were not as immediate. Yes, as a physician, he had been held accountable to those who mourned the ones they lost. But with skulls—for most he received were fully skeletonized and belonged to the disenfranchised, subjugated, or ancient—there was little to remind him of decomposition's mess and odor, decedents' identities, or kin's grief. No one required him to explain or apologize.

3

"Your Obedient Servant"

In 1829, President Andrew Jackson sketched out a solution to fractious relations between US citizens and American Indians. "Our conduct toward these people is deeply interesting to our national character," he stressed in his inaugural message to Congress (8 December 1829).[1] The government's past efforts to civilize and settle Natives, Jackson opined, were unsuccessful. The humane option was to forcibly relocate southern Indians to territories west of the Mississippi River. The proposed policy was a departure from previous administrations, which had supported relocation but drew the line at mandated removal (Portnoy 2005, 22).

Removal in the name of nation, Jackson went on to rationalize a year later (6 December 1830), would benefit White settlers, further states' economic interests, and safeguard national borders. It was also in the best interest of Indians, the president claimed. A federal policy would segregate tribes to protect their dwindling numbers and ensure their sovereignty outside of US borders. Or, should they remain situated within the limits of southern states, it might lead Indians down a path of assimilation.

> By opening the whole territory between Tennessee on the north and Louisiana on the south to the settlement of the whites it will incalculably strengthen the southwestern frontier and render the adjacent States strong enough to repel future invasions without remote aid. It will relieve the whole State of Mississippi and the western part of Alabama of Indian occupancy, and enable those States to advance rapidly in population, wealth, and power. It will separate the Indians from immediate contact with settlements of whites; free them from the power of the States; enable them to pursue happiness in their own way and under their own rude institutions; will retard the progress of decay, which is lessening their numbers, and perhaps cause them gradually, under the protection of the Government and through the influence of good counsels, to cast off their savage habits and become an interesting, civilized, and Christian community.[2]

Responses to Jackson's proposed Indian Removal Act were mixed. Despite his rhetoric, many US citizens saw the policy as neither "liberal" nor "generous." Some opponents regarded removal as a humanitarian disaster, while others took issue with Jackson's abuse of power (Cave 2003). Women activists and evangelical mission societies launched antiremoval petition campaigns in the name of Christian benevolence (Portnoy 2005). Congress was also divided on the matter. The act was especially contentious in the House of Representatives, where it received 102 yeas and 97 nays (the Senate voted 28 to 19). Dissension did not deter Jackson, however, and he signed the Indian Removal Act into law on 28 May 1830 (Perdue and Green 2001, 89–90).[3] It was the most significant piece of legislation enacted during his two-term presidency (he served from 1829 to 1837).

The act had swift and dire repercussions. Under the guise of paternalism, Jackson's final solution legitimated the government's seizure of American Indians' lands. Poverty, starvation, threat of physical harm, and ontological insecurity had preceded migrations west of the Mississippi, but precarity also took root in lands that the US government granted Native groups. Scientific studies were instrumental in realizing this nationalist agenda.

For Samuel, implementation of aggressive expansionist policies and necropolitical conditions presented a favorable juncture of circumstances. Relocation of Indians by federal troops and local militia coincided with his 1830 call for crania, discussed in the previous chapter. His willingness to forge relations with military men indicates a complete break with the Quaker religious doctrine of his formative years, a stance that advocated for pacifism and conscientious objection. Samuel then used his institutional connections and solid scientific reputation to make friends from strangers. Military men were all too willing to send him human "specimens" acquired while manifesting the nation's destiny. From plundered graves and body-strewn battlefields, they collected the skulls of ancient ancestors and the recently vanquished. The arrangement suited Samuel since he rarely left Philadelphia.

US Army surgeons were among his most generous suppliers. Many of them graduated from the Medical Department at the University of Pennsylvania. There, and elsewhere, standardized medical training became increasingly underpinned by an epistemological view of the body as partible, transportable, and in need of curation (see chapters 1 and 2). Many also shared an interest in natural history. These men were more than happy to break up the tedium of their days with collecting jaunts (or task underlings to do so). All casually fetishized the skulls of Others. Few had little difficulty reconciling the charge they were given to foster life with the practices they enacted that let die. Their collective efforts signal a colonial necropolitics born of political opportunity, operationalized through military encounter, justified as scientific advancement, and encouraged by authorities. Medical officers' actions during the removal of southeastern tribes set important precedents for future interactions with bodies of living and dead Indians.

By Way of Fort Gibson

In the preface to *Illustrations of Pulmonary Consumption*, Samuel alludes to the investigative opportunities presented by the precarity of American Indians. The decreasing prevalence of consumption, he proposed, correlated "with the progress of cultivation and civilization" (Morton 1834, xi). To address this hypothesis, additional study of Native peoples, who Samuel believed to suffer disproportionately from the disease, was encouraged. "Medical men attached to the army have great facilities for inquiries of this kind, and those who reside in the vicinity of the Indian tribes, have it in their power to communicate much valuable information" (Morton 1834, xii). The implicit notion being that tuberculosis was a disease with distinct racial attributes; susceptibility signaled inferiority and savagery. Given his footnote about Blacks, it seems he already suspected as much: "Negroes are of course left out of the calculation: their predisposition to phthisis, however, is familiar to every American physician" (Morton 1834, 41). Physicians could then invoke predisposition to absolve themselves of letting Others die.

Samuel's colleagues complied with his requests, sending him word of the diseases they encountered at their respective posts. As Indian removal ramped up, there was much to recount. Reference to Fort Gibson occurred frequently in letters. Located in Indian Territory (today Oklahoma) along the Arkansas River, Fort Gibson's original structure was erected in 1824 at the insistence of James Calhoun, the secretary of war under James Monroe. The officers and troops stationed at the garrison were tasked with Indian removal. To do so, they had to ameliorate tensions between the Osage already living in the region and the southeastern groups being forcibly displaced there by the US government (Agnew 1980; Foreman and Foreman 2015). Their efforts were made all the more challenging by the omnipresence of disease and death.

Dr. Joseph J.B. Wright, an assistant surgeon posted at Fort Gibson from 1833 to 1835, wrote about its insalubrity. "This fort, whether deservedly or not," he commented, "sustains the character of 'charnel house of the army'" (1841, 113). For soldiers and officers alike, morbidity and mortality rates were exceedingly high. Wright catalogued a litany of maladies: pneumonia, pleuritis, bronchitis, rheumatism, catarrh, phthisis pulmonalis, ophthalmia, dyspepsia, chronic dysentery, and diarrhea. Remedies to foster life were standard for the day, inclusive of bloodletting, purges, cupping, opiates, and herbal tinctures. The variety and severity of diseases, however, provided Wright with an opportunity to test the efficacy of nascent medical treatments; he successfully used quinine to alleviate fevers, for instance. Wright (1841, 116) even acknowledged Samuel's contribution to the study of pulmonary consumption: "Among the palliatives used in the management of the cases of pulmonary consumption, large doses of opium and sulphate of iron, as recommended I believe by Dr. Morton, were exhibited with a view to control the colliquative diarrhœa, and with apparent benefit." Nor was he averse to applying Indigenous knowledge, as suggested by his description of Indian hemp's diuretic benefits.

No doubt life was precarious for US Army troops traversing an expanding nation and its frontiers. Many of the enlistees sent to the Florida frontier, for instance, were urban poor or foreign-born Whites (from Ireland, Canada, France, England, Scotland, Poland, and the German states). The meager monthly income they received, six or seven dollars, to wage war in perilous environs affirmed their neediness (Denham 1991, 41). But for the 50,000 Indians removed to Indian Territory during Jackson's presidency and by way of Fort Gibson (Agnew 1980, 3), precarity destabilized normal existence and threatened ontological security. Their expedited migration and not general welfare was the military's priority. Nor did the Army require medical officers to care for anyone other than soldiers (Gillett 1987, 75). Yet medical staff accompanying troops during removal sometimes did attend to ailing Indians. Among them was Dr. Eugene Hilarian Abadie, whom the army had designated "surgeon to emigrating Indians."

Abadie emigrated from France in 1818 at the age of eight (Tepper 1986, 832). His status as an immigrant proved no obstacle to education (as a Frenchman, he was the right kind of immigrant.) He graduated from Penn's Medical Department in 1833 (Lippincott 1919, 213). Three years later, ANS granted him a correspondent membership, solidifying his status among the Philadelphia intelligentsia (Academy of Natural Sciences of Philadelphia 1877, 17). After brief though unprofitable stints in private medical practice and with the Dispensary of Philadelphia, Abadie enlisted in the US Army; its medical department appointed him assistant surgeon in 1836. In service to his adopted nation, he was to assist with removal of captured and "hostile" Creeks, one of the so-called Five Civilized Tribes of the southeastern United States. (The US government's qualification of Indians as either "hostile" or "friendly" is discussed at length in chapter 4. But, in brief here, friendly Indians were amenable to relocation and civilizing, while hostile ones resisted these efforts, meeting violence with violence.)

Voluntary emigration of Creeks (and their enslaved Blacks) living in Alabama and Georgia began as early as 1827. Despite the increasing threat of starvation and White settler encroachment, most Native communities opposed relocation (Haveman 2018). By May 1836, spurred by desperation, the Creek fought back. Violence provided President Andrew Jackson with sufficient reason to qualify these Indians as "hostile," capture them, and forcibly remove them to territories west of the Mississippi River (Haveman 2018, 179–210). In the capacity of surgeon to emigrating Indians, Abadie accompanied a shackled group of these Creek from Fort Mitchell to Fort Gibson. Along the way, he witnessed the effects of unchecked diseases and compromised health statuses (Gillett 1987, 54–55). To his superior, General George Gibson, he quantified the numbers of lives lost. "I have the honor to report the safe arrival at Fort Gibson, of the hostile party of emigrating Creek Indians to which I was attached as surgeon, on the 3rd of Sept, having employed two months in searching our destination, and during which time we had 81 deaths out of nearly 2400 souls in the party" (Abadie 1836; see also letters transcribed in Haveman 2018, 184–85, 193–94, 204–5). Abadie deemed several of these individuals' deaths accidental—a child asphyxiated, a woman broke her spinal cord after falling, a man was shot while trying to escape, another was bayoneted by a guard (though these last two sound less accidental and more punitive). Fevers, dysentery, and cholera accounted for the remainder of deaths, 77 in total. In Abadie's estimation, the low death toll was a "fortunate state of things in the removal of so large a party of Indians." He also disclaimed responsibility. The vulnerable were the greatest at risk, he confirmed. Of the 77 who died from disease, 37 "were children under 5 years of age, 13 under 10, the balance being old and infirm, and but few in the prime of life," reported Abadie (1836). As was the case for other southern tribes, high childhood morbidity and mortality was a widespread phenomenon, which medical officers normalized in their assessments of Indian removal. And Natives were wary enough of military men to seek medical care only after exhausting other options. Observed Abadie (1836), "I at first experienced much difficulty in getting them to apply to me when first taken, they would generally resort to those of their tribe to whom they had been accustomed to apply in sickness, and too often it was after an unsuccessful trial of their remedies that they came to me only in time to see them succumb to the disease." Abadie's suggestion that these deaths were ungrievable and avoidable moves the conversation from precariousness to precarity, a distinction spelled out in this book's introduction (see also Butler 2009).

Abadie did make good on Samuel's original request to document the prevalence of consumption. In a letter, he confirmed his suspicions, "I can furnish you but few data as to the prevalence of Pneumonic Diseases among the Indians, I am of opinion however that it is more frequent than it is represented, I had many cases of Severe Pneumonia among the Creeks I attended to the West" (Abadie 1838a). While he did not send Samuel the skulls of his unfortunate Creek wards, an oversight he later remedied when stationed in Florida, Natives' vulnerability did generate collecting opportunities for other medical officers.

From his post at Fort Gibson, Dr. Zina Pitcher—an assistant surgeon with the US Army who served from November 1831 to July 1834 (Novy 1908)—outlined the convenience of it all to Samuel:

> At this moment I have a Creek (Muskogee) skeleton on hand, but not prepared for sending away. He died of pneumonia under my observation + the Osage died true game having literally eaten himself to death whilst under guard of this Post, having been arrested on Suspicion of Murder. So that in regard to nationality there is no chance of our being deceived in these cases. (Pitcher 1832)

The Creek (Muskogee) to whom Pitcher refers is relabeled as Euchee in the *Catalogue of Skulls of Man, and the Inferior Animals, in the Collection of Samuel George Morton, M.D.* (hereafter *Catalogue*); he was entered as specimen number 39 (Morton 1840a, 7). Confusion over his identity is evidenced by the writing on his skull. In very faint ink on the superior right parietal is "Muscogee Creek," reiterating the notation provided by Pitcher. But on the skull's glabellar region—located between the eyebrows and above the nose—is handwritten "**EUCHEE**"; this corrected tribal affiliation appears in the *Catalogue* (figure 3.1). (When ANS loaned the Morton Collection to Penn in 1966, L-606 was placed before the original number, e.g., L-606-39. With the official transfer in 1997, that number changed to 97-606-39. This number system is applicable to all skulls in the collection, and later in the chapter, I explain the significance of these amendments).

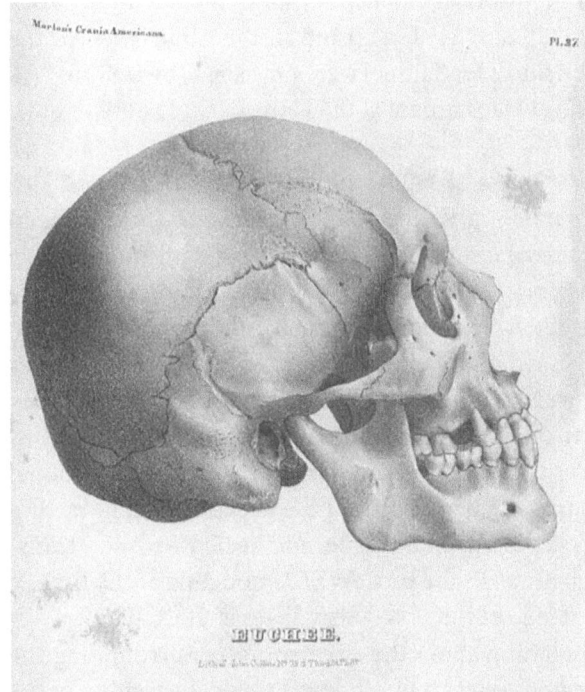

Figure 3.1. *Euchee*, a lithograph by John Collins included as plate 27 in *Crania Americana* (1839).

As for the Osage skull that Pitcher sent along, Samuel labeled this decedent's skull with the number 54. In a letter dated 4 March 1834, Pitcher expanded on his biography: "He was a young and distinguished brave who bore in his tribe the cognomen of The Buffalo tail [*sic*]. At the time he died of suicide by gourmanderie he was not as I had been told, in duress himself, but was an attaché of a war chief who had him confined for depredating upon the whites" (Pitcher 1834). The description—of an overindulgent and pillaging Indian disciplined by his own tribe—glosses over the Osage Nation's desperate circumstances and elides altogether tensions with southeastern tribes set in motion by US nation-building. The Osage cession of land to the US government began in 1808 and continued throughout the nineteenth century. In 1825, the Osage Treaty had them relinquish multiple territories to accommodate tribes removed to the west. Congenial relations were short-lived. As historian Christopher Haveman (2018, 676) relates, the Osage were facing their own tribulations as buffalo herds thinned, harsh winters prevailed, and proximity led to encroachment. The two skulls in the Morton Collection, then, signal the conflict generated between distinct American Indian groups by forced removals.

As for the Creeks in the Morton Collection, these included the specimen numbers 441, 579, 751, and 1454, as listed in the *Catalogue*. All the men who collected Creek skulls for Samuel were physicians by training. All graduated from the Medical Department at the University of Pennsylvania. See Table 3.1.

Dr. Joseph T. Pancoast (class of 1828), the secondary collector of 441, established a surgical practice in Philadelphia, offered private courses in anatomy, and served as medical staff at the Philadelphia Almshouse (Kelly 1912; Wagner 1989). His concurrent interests in natural history are indicated by membership in the ANS and the American Philosophical Society, institutions to which Samuel also belonged. Seeing that Pancoast never served in the military, just how he acquired the skull of a young Creek male from Alabama remains unclear. But the Creek decedent's identity as a warrior and markers of trauma suggest a familiarity with interpersonal violence. Blunt force trauma may have caused the depressed skull fracture on the right parietal—deep, teardrop in shape, and healed—while a transverse nasal fracture, which was in the process of remodeling at the time of death, appears on the left side of the nose (Magalhães et al. 2020).

Samuel is more forthcoming about the circumstances surrounding the acquisition of 579. In *Crania Americana*, he describes an illustration of the skull, "This plate is taken from the skull of Athlaha Ficksa, a full-blood chief of the Creek nation. He fought with great bravery in the United States service, and against the majority of his own countrymen in the present Florida war. He died in Mobile, in 1837, whence I received his cranium through the kindness of Dr. Henry S. Rennolds, of the United States Navy" (Morton 1839, 170). I discuss this decedent in greater detail in the next chapter. Here, with the objective of supporting an argument about scientific-medical practitioners' complicity in necropolitics, it is worth noting that Rennolds was class of 1831 at Penn's Medical Department (Lippincott 1919, 214). Two years after graduating, on 6 February 1833, President Andrew Jackson nominated him to serve as an assistant surgeon, and he was promoted to surgeon in 1841.

About the two other skulls, 751 and 1454, Samuel has less to say. The specimen he numbered 751 belonged to a "Creek woman from Georgia" aged 25–30 years at the time of death; the description is handwritten on her frontal bone and runs parallel to the coronal suture. Her cranium bears no traces of trauma. The collector, Dr. Joseph Walker, received his M.D. from Penn in 1836 (Lippincott 1919, 212). In due time, on 16 August 1838, he, too, was appointed US assistant army surgeon and stationed at Fort Gibson.

Table 3.1. Creek Skulls with Information

Current Catalogue #	Collector	Age	Sex	Trauma	Identity	Provenience
97-606-441	Pancoast, Dr. Joseph	20–30	M	Y	"warrior"	AL
97-606-579	Rennold, Dr. Henry S.	40–50	M	N	Athlaha Ficksa	Mobile, AL
97-606-751	Walker, Dr. Joseph	25–30	F	N		GA
97-606-1454	Woodhouse, Dr. Samuel W.	50+	F?	N		Eastern Oklahoma

Note: Creek skulls with information about the current catalogue number at Penn Museum, collector, age at time of death, sex (female, probable female, male, probable male, unknown), trauma (presence or absence), archival information about identity, and provenience.

Like Abadie, as I discuss later in this chapter, he was next posted to Florida. The Second Seminole War was coming to an end, which proved opportune for the collection of skulls.[4]

The specimen labeled 1454 did not find its way to Samuel until what would be the penultimate year of his life. Its collector, Dr. Samuel Washington Woodhouse, came from a good Philadelphia family that had originally hailed from Northumberland, England. He was a member of ANS and graduate of Penn's Medical Department (class of 1847). The Creek skull he sent Samuel was included among the natural historical specimens he acquired during the Creek and Cherokee Boundary Expeditions. These expeditions were an exercise in border creation and scientific exploration, concerns discussed in the next chapter. Colonel J. J. Abert, the chief of the US Army Corps of Topographical Engineers and another of Samuel's collectors, had ordered his men to survey and mark Creek and Cherokee lands in Indian Territory. He also asked Samuel to recommend a physician and naturalist able and willing to accompany the expeditions. Woodhouse eagerly accepted, reaching Fort Gibson, the rendezvous point, by June 1849 (Stone 1906). While Woodhouse (1992) wrote in his journals about wild, virgin landscapes, "hostile" living Indians, and assorted birds and animals, commentary about the human cranium he sent Samuel was minimal. The label still affixed to the frontal bone—at the center of the forehead—reads "1455. CREEK Indian of Western Arkansas: woman ætat. 70." Antemortem loss of maxillary (upper) teeth and significant resorption of alveolar sockets for molars, premolars, canines, and lateral incisors support this age assessment. (There was no mandible, or lower jaw, passed along to Samuel for analysis.) More likely than not this location is present-day Oklahoma, and this individual's skull was taken from one of the villages established by the Creek after they were removed to Indian Territory. Despite having survived the precarity of removal, even in death this person's ontological security was threatened by the exhumation of her body well after kin had performed mortuary rituals.

The Chain of Command

Physicians—ambitious young, White men with ties to prestigious institutions, involved in nation-building missions, and intrigued by natural history—were especially responsive to Samuel's requests for skulls. Other medical officers, like Dr. Joel Martin, were invested in "the advancement of science" but simply too busy to procure skulls themselves (Martin 1838a). So, they outsourced this work to their subordinates. Here we can see how the call for crania reverberated down the medico-military's chain of command—from medical directors to assistant surgeons to acting assistant surgeons to volunteer civilian physicians. On 16 May 1838, exactly one week prior to the military's enforcement of Cherokee removal from their ancestral lands, Martin penned a letter to Samuel. "Dear Sir" he began,

> Yours of the 9th March thro' the War Depart. did not reach me till the 30th same mo. It found me immersed in public duties and with but little time to spare for making such investigations myself as would tend to satisfy your enquiries in relation to the peculiar shapen crania which you have been informed are to be found in this country. As Medical Director to the Army etc. in the Cherokee Nation I was closely engaged in superintending, the receiving, putting up, & issuing medical supplies for some 15 to 20 Posts, in various parts of the nation, appointing and arranging citizen surgeons to each, and instructing them in their duties, etc. etc.—Among these gentlemen there is some talent & cleverness & I have invited their attention, at different points, to this interesting subject & they are beginning to forward to me their respective reports thereon.
>
> I have received from them too, several skulls, but not of the form you look for, and with me they seem strongly impressed with the opinion, that none such exist, or ever did, among the Cherokee tribe, and that if any skull has been ever seen here of that peculiar form | flat-

Table 3.2. Cherokee Skulls with Information

Current Catalogue #	Collector	Age	Sex	Trauma	Identity	Provenience
97-606-632	Martin, Dr. Joel	15 ± 6 mos.	F?	N		Cave, Springtown, Polk Co., NC
97-606-633	Martin, Dr. Joel	12 ± 6 mos.	?	N		Cave, Springtown, Polk Co., NC
97-606-634	Martin, Dr. Joel	20–25	F?	N		Ellijay River (headwaters of), Gilmer Co., GA
97-606-635	Martin, Dr. Joel	11 ± 2.5	?	N		Ellijay River (headwaters of), Gilmer Co., GA
97-606-1285	Hardy, Dr. James Freeman Eppes	30–40	M	Y	"ball-player"	Mound, Cherokee Co., NC
97-606-1297	Hardy, Dr. James Freeman Eppes	45+	M	N		Mound, Cherokee Co., NC

Note: Cherokee skulls with information about the current catalogue number at Penn Museum, collector, age at time of death, sex (female, probable female, male, probable male, unknown), trauma (presence or absence), archival information about identity, and provenience.

tened in the antero posterior diameter | it must have been accidental, the result of early compression. I have directed the attention of other intelligent gentlemen traveling about the nation to similar enquiries & from their conversations with persons long resident here, capable giving information, all unite in the belief that no such form did exist here as Dr. A[badie]. has been led to suppose. (Martin 1838a)

In total, Martin sent Samuel the skulls of six Cherokees (Table 3.2). In the case of two skulls, the Medical Director's recruits set forth from Fort Butler, located along the Hiwassee River in Murphy, North Carolina. A cave[5] near Springtown, Tennessee, yielded two ideal specimens. No dirt or debris adhered to the skulls, suggesting they were deposited together but not buried in the cave. One individual, labeled specimen 632, was a possible female who had died at 15 years old ± 6 months. A second individual, specimen 633, was of unknown sex and 12 years old ± 6 months at the time of death.[6]

Martin's "citizen surgeons" acquired two other decedents near the headwaters of the Ellijay River in Georgia. These individuals were a possible female aged 20–25 years at the time of death and a child who died at 11 ±

2.5 years; Samuel designated these specimens 634 and 635, respectively. Martin (1838b) provided supplemental information about their identity: "They are crania of the mountain Indians & their forms strikingly characteristic of the full blood Cherokee of the present day. I think these as fine specimens as can be obtained of the Cherokee crania, tho' not as perfect as I could have wished them." The location placed them in the vicinity of Ellijay, a Cherokee town, and Fort Gilmer, a garrison used to temporarily inter the Cherokee families before the US Army marched them to Ross's Landing (White 1855, 152). Located along a stretch of the Tennessee River, Ross's Landing became a launching point for flatboats laden not with goods but subjugated Cherokees and the Blacks they had enslaved. White settlers and soldiers who remained in the area later rechristened the town Chattanooga. Described euphemistically as "emigration depots" (Rozema 2003, 22), today we may recognize Ross's Landing and Fort Cass, where Martin was stationed when he corresponded with Samuel, for what they were—internment camps from which Cherokee Indians set down the Trail of Tears.

Even before they departed, however, the Cherokee death toll was significant. The prevalence of cholera, dysentery, measles, and whooping cough were exacerbated by poor sanitation and inadequate food supplies (Johnston 2003, 69), and conditions in the camps resulted in the death of 2,000–2,500 individuals (McLoughlin 1989, 565). Children were a particularly vulnerable group, as attested to by the two Cherokee youths in Samuel's collection. Both have evidence of compromised health statuses. The decedent Samuel labeled 633 had slight cribra orbitalia (or skeletal lesions) in both eye sockets. Bone porosity developed on a number of surface areas: the alveolar sockets; maxilla's palate; inferior (lower) portion of the parietal bones; adjacent to the occipital condyles (which are located at the skull's base); temporal bones near the external auditory meatuses (the ear canals); and inside the temporomandibular joints (where the jaw connects to the lower skull). The child also appears to have slight hypervascularity on the endocranial (inner) surfaces near the superior sagittal suture. Taken together, this evidence suggests that in life this individual suffered from scurvy (Brown and Ortner 2011). The other young Cherokee, the decedent labeled 635, also displays the subtle marks of a precarious existence. While there is no evidence of cribra orbitalia, this youth did have significant dental disease. Alveolar resorption and porosity affect most of the maxillary (upper) arcade.

As for those Cherokee who opted to assimilate instead of relocating to Indian Territory, their Christian beliefs did not exempt them from objectification. In the case of two skulls labeled Cherokee, 1285 and 1297, Dr. James Freeman Eppes Hardy disinterred them from a mound in Cherokee County, North Carolina. According to a letter that Hardy sent Samuel on 13 July 1846, the individual labeled 1285 "was that of an Indian well known in the County, he has not been dead more than six years, he was one of the greatest ball players in the tribe. While playing ball he slipped + fell + dislocated his spine + died immediately, there is still a remnant of the tribe about seventy miles . . . they number about seven hundred, they have concluded to come under the laws of this state + remain on their land." Despite their assimilation, Hardy was not optimistic that the Cherokee who remained would thrive. His letter continued, "I have no doubt in time the Cherokee in this state will dwindle away as they have, unprepared while more are all the time endeavoring to take advantage of them + cheat them out of their property" (Hardy 1846). He said nothing about the desecration visited on the bodies of their decedents. Instead, these men fretted about how best to secure the safe passage of skulls to Samuel. From the hands of "citizen surgeons" or acting assistant surgeons, like Dr. W.I.I. Murrow, Martin received skulls, for instance. He then entrusted them up the chain of command. To Major Surgeon Dr. Richard Satterlee they first went. He left them in the charge of Dr. Thomas G. Mower, a senior surgeon and medical purveyor of the US Army, who was traveling to New York and would forward them to Samuel in Philadelphia (Martin 1838a, 1838b).

For the most part, however, Natives resisted removal, and warfare between them and the US Army ensued. These violent interactions subtly shifted medico-scientific practitioners' involvement in colonial necropolitics. Early on, physicians procured Indian skulls from the unfortunate decedents under their care. Or they pilfered skulls from ancient and historic burial settings and recently dug graves, removal having emptied the landscape of any Native occupants who might have protested. The opportunism afforded from "letting die" in time morphed into the making of the "future dead" (Hildebrandt 2016). After 1836—when deadlines to voluntarily migrate expired and Native peoples who refused to relocate retaliated out of desperation—medical officers took heads directly from their slain bodies, which US soldiers had killed and left to rot on battlefields. Nowhere is this better illustrated than in Florida. This frontier zone served as the setting for the Seminole Wars: three conflicts that occurred between US soldiers and the Indians of Florida and their Black allies that extended from roughly 1812 to 1858 (Missall and Missall 2004).[7] The events unfolding in this region were central to nineteenth-century nation-building. They also provided a backdrop for Samuel's acquisition of skulls labeled "Seminole."

The Indians of Florida

By the end of the eighteenth century, a distinct identity crystallized for those Creek bands that had moved into the northern Florida frontier (Weisman 2007). As Jack Martin (2011, 3) explains, "In the mid-eighteenth century, some Lower Creeks began moving into Florida. They and the escaped slaves who accompanied them were referred to by the Spanish name of *cimarrón* 'wild, untamed.' This term was borrowed into Creek as *simaló:ni* or *simanó:li*, and from there it was borrowed into English as Seminole."[8] Coexisting under the umbrella of Seminole were diverse groups with equally varied political agendas. Most groups, however, took issue with an increasing number of White settlers and the US military's violent interventions. Destructive and deadly conflicts followed from 1812 onward.[9] As a survival strategy, the Seminoles kept migrating south, reluctantly relinquishing their belongings, homes, and agricultural lands as they went.

The 1823 Treaty of Moultrie Creek, which created an inland-bound reservation roughly four million acres in size, offered a temporary solution for its begrudging signatories (figure 3.2). Although 32 individuals laid ink to paper on 18 September 1823, the treaty highlighted growing divisions among the Seminoles. Rather than viewed as a collective, members were identified in official verbiage as the "Florida tribes of Indians" (Missall and Missall 2004, 66). The United States' expansionist policies, however, produced only broken promises. Subsequent treaties negotiated with some Seminole leaders (not all given the divisions among the groups), specifically the 1832 Treaty of Payne's Landing, voided all Seminole land claims. In so doing, it worked to realize the aims of the Indian Removal Act. To avoid further violent confrontation with the US Army, which grew to a head in 1835, several Seminole groups emigrated to the west. Yet, like the Creek, circumstances had constrained the choices of this early wave of migrants. After 1836, the Indians that remained fiercely resisted removal.

White settlers living on the Florida frontier grew increasingly frustrated with the government's responses to "hostile" Indians. In an 1836 letter to Hardy Croom—a gentleman planter who counted among Samuel's collector—his half-brother William voiced concerns.

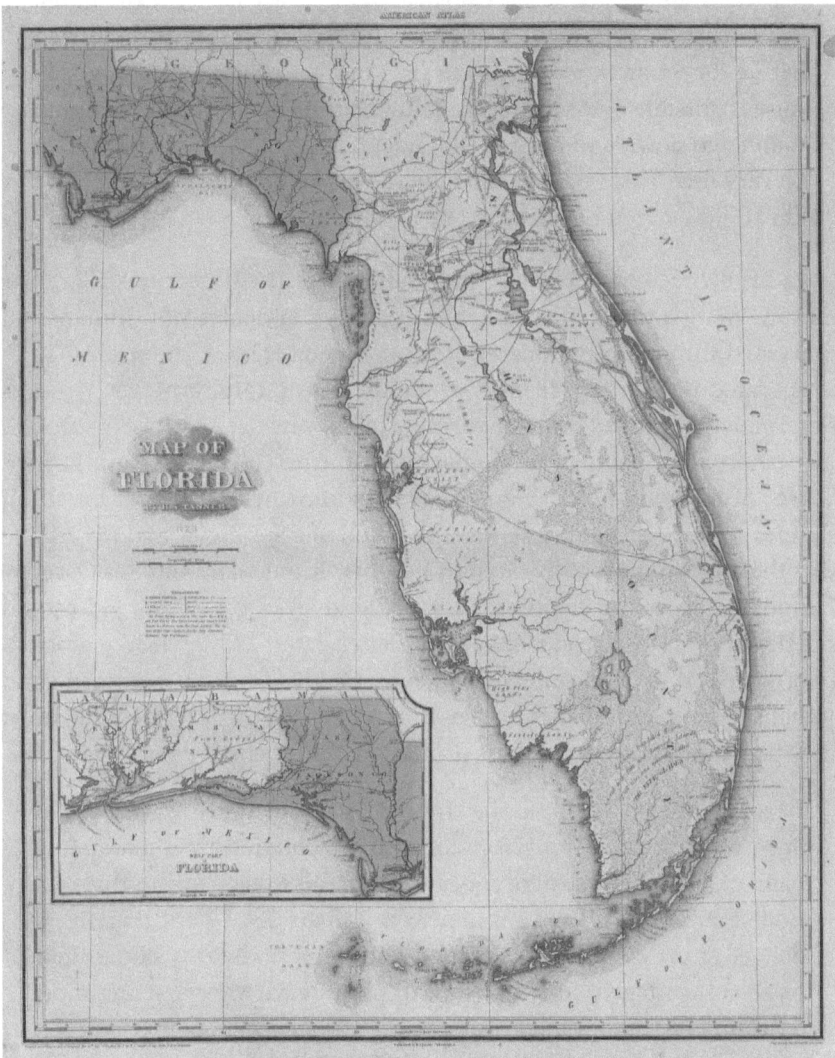

Figure 3.2. "Tanner's Florida, 1823," a map of Florida at the time of the 1823 Treaty of Moultrie Creek. State Archives of Florida, Florida Memory. Retrieved from https://www.floridamemory.com/items/show/323229.

We are a good deal excited here at present about the Indians. There is a rumour that the Creek Indians have committed several murders between the Flint and Chattahoochee and that they are making their way to join the Seminoles. The Governor had accordingly issued his orders to have them cut off by marching to Lowndes county in Georgia. The military are in a great stir making ready for the expedition, but I trust, as in a former instance the report will be contradicted before they march. The governor had another project in view, viz, to raise if possible by volunteering or by drafting an army of a thousand men to go down and destroy the Indian crop which is represented to be very fine. This I believe though is a very unpopular measure and I am afraid will not be effected. (W. Croom, 1836)

In his own letters, Croom's exasperation with the situation is a familiar refrain. Writing to his colleague John Torrey, he lamented how Indians had prevented him from botanizing in East Florida (H.B. Croom 1834–1837; letter dated 10 February 1836). Despite the disruptions, however, Croom's floral activities proved sufficient enough to impress the ANS; the institution made him a corresponding member that spring (1877, 21). He informed Torrey of the good news: "I am at a loss to know what I can do for them. Besides some fossils I have sent them a skull of a <u>Seminole</u>, and my regrets that the contribution is so small in <u>number</u>. If they had more of Osceola, Jumper, Alligator, Tiger-tail, the Little Cloud, <u>et id genus omne</u>, I should not be sorry" (H.B. Croom 1834–1837; letter dated 22 May 1836; emphasis in original). What had generated such ire that he now only regarded good Indians to be dead Indians? In that same letter, Croom described the threat they posed to the security of his plantation and its enslaved occupants.

I fear my summer will not be without its disquietude. A murder has been committed within 20 miles of my plantation by a marauding band of Indians, and there appears now to be some panic in that section of country. Still as I am so near to Tallahassee, I hope there is no danger to my people. How strangely, and how badly this whole affair has been managed! In truth, sir, I think we have the worst and most corrupt government in Christendom. . . . Paulo majora canamus, let us return to Botany! (H. B. Croom 1834–1837)

The federal government's inability to control a few Indians was an inconvenience but not a cause for alarm in his estimation, and he certainly did not regard it as a tragedy for Native peoples. Rather, Indian skulls were to be collected like so many plant specimens and then sent to the ANS for phrenological examination.

Once in Philadelphia, Samuel labeled the skull gifted by Croom specimen 456. In contrast to the latter's detailed descriptions of botanical samples, biographical information was not forthcoming. Skeletal analysis does indicate that this individual had been a possible male who was at least 35 years of age at the time of death. Extreme dental disease, healed cribra orbitalia in both eye sockets, and a small nasal fracture along the midline also hint at a life of adversity. Finally, specimen 456 had the perverse honor of being the first Seminole in Samuel's collection. As the war unfolded, however, that number grew.

Unpopular though the public may have found a scorched earth policy, the US Army did adopt one. The strategy had proven effective when Andrew Jackson, then a general, used it during the First Seminole War (Amos 1977). When troops implemented these tactics during the Second Seminole War, medical officers, sanctioned with fostering life, expressed little remorse. Abadie's postscript—so casual an afterthought—in a letter to Samuel is revealing: "P.S. I would have written before this, but since I left Miccanopy [sic] I have been with Col. Harney and 250 Dragoons on an expedition of 20 days to the Suwanee, Waccasassa, Weekiawa [sic], and Withlacoochie [sic] rivers; it is but a few days since we have returned having met no Indians, although we found two of their villages which we burned" (Abadie 1838b). The destruction, which certainly generated precarity for Seminoles, seems to have engendered no bioethical quandary for Abadie. Rather, the postscript demonstrates medical officers' complicity if not outright involvement in necropolitics—a transition from letting die to making living Indians the future dead. If anything, calculated destruction and indifference made collection of Seminole skulls all the easier. It certainly did for Abadie, who acquired nine of the 16 Seminole skulls in the Morton Collection (Table 3.3).

Abadie arrived in Florida in November 1837. Having performed admirably during Creek removal, the army promoted the physician to Medical Director and assigned him to the Fourth and Sixth Regiments of Infantry (Abadie 1838a). He traversed the Florida frontier until July 1839. His downtime afforded many opportunities to explore the local environs and carry out Samuel's request for skulls. Abadie recapped his findings in a letter to the physician in Philadelphia:

> You no doubt are aware of the manner in which the Seminoles bury their dead, they form 1st on the surface of the ground, a flooring of logs upon which is laid the body enveloped in cow hide with all its trinkets and weapons if a male, also some provisions to carry them, as they believe, to the end of their journey: they then built around the body a pen dove-tailed at the 4 angles 3 feet high with a roof of

Table 3.3. Seminole Skulls with Information

Current Catalogue #	Collector	Age	Sex	Trauma	Identity	Provenience
97-606-456	Croom, Hardy B.	35+	M?	Y		FL
97-606-604	Dimick, Captain Justin (primary) / Emerson, Dr. Gouverneur (secondary)	40+	M	Y	Warrior	St. Joseph's Plantation, St. Johns Co., 30 miles south of St. Augustine, FL
97-606-698	Abert, Colonel John J.	30–40	M	Y	Warrior	FL
97-606-707	Abadie, Dr. Eugene Hilarian	20–30	M?	N	Warrior; Eoklo Emathla	12 miles south of Sewannee River, vicinity of Tampa, FL
97-606-708	Abadie, Dr. Eugene Hilarian	30–40	F?	N	Warrior	FL
97-606-726	Abadie, Dr. Eugene Hilarian	30–40	F	N	"of rank"	Ft. Gardiner, Polk Co., FL
97-606-727	Abadie, Dr. Eugene Hilarian	7±24 mos.	?	N		Ft. Gardiner, Polk Co., FL
97-606-728	Abadie, Dr. Eugene Hilarian	4±12 mos.	M?	N		3 miles from Peas Creek (or Talak Hatchee), FL
97-606-729	Abadie, Dr. Eugene Hilarian	7±24 mos.	?	N	Fuke Luste Hadjo's (Black Dirt's) tribe	near Tampa, FL
97-606-730	Abadie, Dr. Eugene Hilarian	25–35	M	N	Warrior	Lake Okeechobee area, FL
97-606-732	Abadie, Dr. Eugene Hilarian	30–45	M	Y	Warrior	Lake Okeechobee area, FL
97-606-733	Abadie, Dr. Eugene Hilarian	30–40	F	Y	Micco-Sukie tribe	Ft. Basinger, Highlands Co., FL
97-606-754	Walker, Dr. Joseph	30–45	M	Y	Warrior	FL
97-606-1105	Robertson, Dr. Francis Marion	35–45	M?	N	Warrior	Dade's Battlefield, Bushnell, Sumter Co., FL
97-606-1286	Couper, Dr. James	35+	F?	N		FL
97-606-1840	Meigs, Dr. Charles Delucena	25–35	M	N		FL

Note: Seminole skulls with information about the current catalogue number at Penn Museum, collector, age at time of death, sex (female, probable female, male, probable male, unknown), trauma (presence or absence), archival information about identity, and provenience.

logs and raw hides; if the dead has rank they take much pains in the construction of this pen often digging a ditch around it throwing the dirt so as to incline from a level with the flooring. On our arriving on the Kissimee [sic] river 70 miles east of Tampa where Aligator [sic] camped all summer and Fort Gardner stands I obtained 3 specimens, in fine order of female heads. One of which evidently of distinction from the elaborate workmanship of her tomb and the many trinkets buried with her. (Abadie 1838a)[10]

Abadie's description is revealing, about Seminole communities' normative mortuary practices, but his disinterment also indicates the disruption wrought from warfare. Simply put, the Seminole did not bury their dead kin to later be disinterred. But the absence of living Seminoles in and around Tampa—mobile existences, high mortality rates, and forced relocations having depopulated the area—made scrutiny of graves' building materials and stratigraphic levels all the easier. We may understand the disinterment of Natives' bodies and heads from final resting places in terms of precarity. Political circumstances were at the root of these desecrations; they made military men act with impunity and produced transient, vulnerable peoples unable to confront them.

Abadie also took a page from Samuel's book at his various garrison posts.[11] Like inmates from the Philadelphia Almshouse bound for the cemetery but sidetracked by the dissecting table, Natives who perished at Florida's forts provided a source of skulls for Abadie. At Fort Brooke, near Tampa where Abadie was stationed, the cemetery held bodies of Seminole Indians and the Blacks who accompanied them (whether as enslaved people or tributary allies); most perished from myriad diseases to which they had little immunity (Piper et al. 1982). Near Fort Gardiner, in December 1837 (Buchanan 1950, 142), Abadie exhumed a child[12] 7 ± 24 months in age and woman who was aged 30–40 years old at the time of death (Abadie 1838a). Later written across the left side of her frontal bone were the words "Fort Gardner Seminole of rank," her elite status no safeguard against exhumation. Samuel designated her 726. The child, who he labeled 727, had extreme and active cribra orbitalia visible in both eye sockets, and porotic hyperostosis (or bone porosity) on the back of the skull (on the occipital and parietal bones near the lambdoidal suture). While posted at Ft. Brooke, Abadie secured the skulls of two more children; Samuel designated these specimens 728 and 729. The former had died between the age of 3–5 years and the latter had been 5–9 years old. Pathology also appears on both of their skulls. The younger child, 728, displays slight cribra orbitalia on the external surface of the left orbital roof. Slight cribra orbitalia is active in the orbital roofs of the child labeled 729, and there is porosity (or porous bone suggestive of generalized inflammation or infection) around the entrance of the external auditory meatus (or ear canal). Bioarchaeologists recognize that such pathological marks indicate malnourishment, chronic infections, and sub-standard living conditions (Walker et al. 2009). Situated within this historic moment, we may also read pathology as precarity; that is, nineteenth-century settler colonialism and the US government's expansionist policies gravely imperiled the developing bodies of Native children. Archival evidence offers additional support.

According to Abadie, one child (specimen 729) had been a member of the Alachua band lead by Black Dirt, or Foke Luste Hadjo (figure 3.3). "I obtained a boy's skull belonging to the tribe of Black Dirt . . . emigrated in 36 by Genl. Scott," he (1838a) wrote to Samuel.[13] Inked in capital letters across this child's forehead, just above the brow area, was "FUKE-LUSTE-HADJO" (a spelling variant of the Seminole leader's name). As early as 1832, Black Dirt had advocated for relocation west of the Mississippi (Covington 1993, 61). The death of children may indicate why some Seminole bands regarded voluntary migration as a viable option. In Black Dirt's particular case, his dealings with White settlers had endangered his and kin's lives, and he, ironically enough, sought protection from rebellious Florida Indians (Potter 1836, 69). Precarity constrained his band's choices, and Indian Territory may have held the promise of survival. Site unseen, they began their westward migration in 1836. Many perished on the journey, including Black Dirt's wife and daughter (Lancaster 1994, 21). The survivors arrived in Little Rock, Arkansas, on 5 May 1836, and settled near Little River where disease and death followed them (Lancaster 1994, 20, 25).

In the opinion of the US government, not all Seminoles were as accommodating as Black Dirt and his followers. The active resistance of these "hostile" Indians to removal was facilitated by alliances formed with Blacks, inclusive of Black Seminoles, freed Blacks, and Blacks enslaved by White plantation owners (Porter 1943; Wasserman 2010). One strong alliance was fostered between John Cavallo and Coacoochee (or Wild Cat). The Black Seminole and Seminole Indian, respectively, were associated with the child's skull that Samuel had labeled 728. Abadie (1838a) explained in a letter: "On reaching Pease Creek Nov. the 20th [1837] with the 4th and 6th Reg. Infy to which I was Med. Director, I obtained the skull of another boy belonging to the party of Seminoles headed by John Cavallo or Cow-

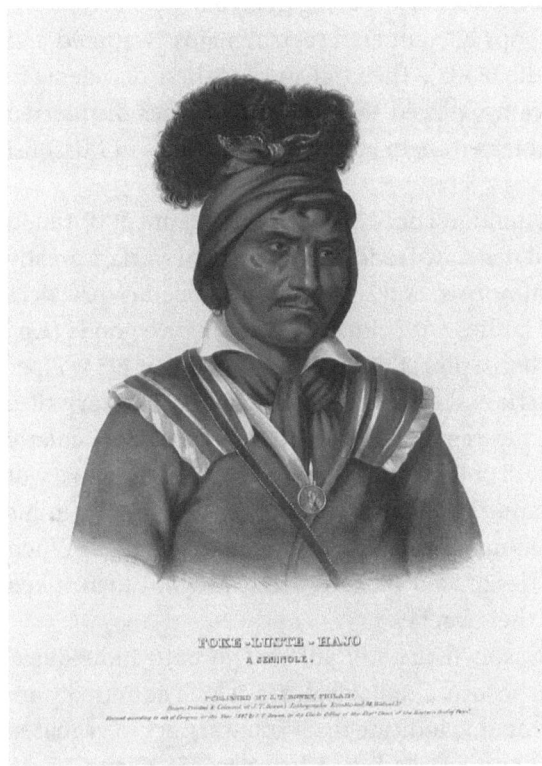

Figure 3.3. *Foke-Luste-Hajo a Seminole*, a lithographic portrait of Black Dirt by John T. Bowen, 1842. Library of Congress, Prints and Photographs Division, [LC-DIG-pga-07503]. Retrieved from https://www.loc.gov/item/2003656348/.

a-gee."[14] This information, abbreviated though it may be, hints at complex, intertwined life stories and hybrid existences that are often stricken from official historical accounts. These concerns are addressed more fully in the next chapter. Of pertinence here is John Cavallo's and Coacoochee's fierce defiance during the Second Seminole War (Mulroy 2007, 35–36). They were particularly effective against US troops at the Battle of Lake Okeechobee (Buchanan 1950; Lancaster 1994, 37, 84).

Seminole Warriors

"A Merry Christmas to all of my friends at home, and may they have many happy returns of the season!! Mine I am inclined to think will be more lively, but not so pleasant as theirs," so wrote Lieutenant Robert Buchanan in his journal the morning of the Battle of Lake Okeechobee. Fighting lasted two and a half hours and ranged along a mile of the lake's northeastern shore (Carr et al. 1989, 209; Missall and Missall 2004, 142). Twenty-five

US soldiers were slain and 111 wounded during guerrilla-style combat. A month later, Abadie and troops encountered their remains "scattered and bleaching in the sun" (Abadie 1838a). They transported these decedents to Colonel Zachary Taylor's camp, placed them in graves, later disinterred their remains, and then reinterred them at Jefferson Barracks in Missouri (Carr et al. 1989, 210).[15]

Such careful mortuary attention contrasts with the treatment of the 12 Seminole warriors who died that day. Trade, migration, and warfare greatly disrupted Seminole cultural norms, and so traditional funerary practices involving the interment of bodies with ritually "killed" grave goods (e.g., food containers, beads, earbobs, pipes) did not occur (Laxson 1954; Piper et al. 1982). Instead, for warriors slain at Lake Okeechobee, funerary rites went unperformed and bodies remained exposed, providing particularly ripe hunting grounds for skull collection. When he returned in January of 1838, Abadie selected for Samuel two of the least "offensive" skulls (in his words). He then boxed them up and sent them on to Philadelphia. When Samuel received them, he designated them 730 and 732 and then inked "SEMINOLE" across both of their forehead.

When I examined them, soft tissue still adhered to both individuals' palates, testifying to their exposure. Cranial features, which admittedly are less than ideal when assigning sex, indicate that both warriors were males; the individuals labeled 730 and 732 had died between 25–35 and 35–45 years of age, respectively. The former's skull had no ante- or perimortem trauma (markers of violence that occurred in life or were the cause of death), while the latter displayed an unhealed crescent shaped fracture located centrally on the frontal bone (or forehead). Additionally, in the case of the individual designated 732, the left zygomatic and maxillary bones appear to have been shaved as if a very sharp blade had sliced into the front of the face at a parallel and not perpendicular angle. If pathology discussed earlier in the chapter affirms how structural violence made certain lives precarious, the marks of trauma displayed by Seminole warriors signal the interpersonal and violent interactions that characterized the Second Seminole War's numerous conflicts. (In the next chapter, I return to the decedent labeled 730, as he has something to tell us about hybridity.)

The warriors slain at Lake Okeechobee were not the only individuals whose skulls physicians collected directly from battlefields. "I have, in my possession the skull of a Seminole Indian, which I will forward to you by the first opportunity," began a letter Dr. Francis Marion Robertson (1842) penned to Samuel. The two men's relationship had begun a year prior. Robertson, a stranger to Samuel at the time, had written to express his delight with *Crania Americana* (Robertson 1841). He had the good fortune to borrow a friend's tome, and now sought his own copy for the $30 subscription price. The subject was "deeply interesting," he explained. To vouch for his moral character, Robertson's postscript included the name of two friends who resided in Philadelphia. With phrenology and medicine as common intellectual ground, the physicians proceeded to strike up a collegial albeit spatially distant friendship. While Robertson's admiration is clear in correspondences, it is difficult to determine if the sentiment was reciprocated. In the *Catalogue* (1849a, 105), Samuel misidentified the physician as "Robinson." The surname confusion may testify to social indifference or just inadequate editing; all of Samuel's publications are rife with typographical mistakes.

Robertson typified a White, southern gentleman. He was born in South Carolina's Abbeville District on 12 December 1806. In 1822, he ventured north to enter the United States Military Academy at West Point (Robertson 2015, 19). His father William, who had served as a captain during the War of 1812 (Moore 1893, 18), encouraged this career path. But Robertson did not graduate from West Point, instead leaving in 1826 to pursue a career in medicine. He graduated from the Medical College of South Carolina in 1830 and soon after began to practice medicine in Augusta, Georgia. He married Henrietta (née Righton) in 1831, and the birth of two sons followed in due course. But political instability soon came to outweigh domestic responsibilities. In 1836, Robertson captained the Richmond Blues (Robertson 2002). The company volunteered its services to the US Army during the bloodiest year of all three Seminole Wars.

His service to country complete, he settled in Augusta, Georgia, to attend to his medical practice and growing family. Reflecting on his time in Florida, he elaborated on the skull's acquisition in a letter to Samuel:

> It was taken from the body of an Indian who was killed at the massacre of the lamented Dade and his brave companions in arms. . . . I regret that the shortness of our halt prevented me from obtaining several more specimens, as a number of other bodies were <u>covered</u> up (not buried) near this one.
>
> As a firm believer in the science of phrenology I considered it a great prize, and luged [*sic*] it with my baggage during many a hard day's march, and, for fear it might be stolen or lost, slept with it under my head every night. You, however, are welcome to it; and it will af-

ford me more pleasure to know that it occupies a place in your valuable collection than to have it remain neglected in my own office . . .

If I can possibly procure the skull of a native born African I will send it to you. (Robertson 1842; emphasis in original)

Robertson signed off by remaining Samuel's obedient servant. His deference may have been no more than professional courtesy, given the two men's recent introduction.

Skeletal analysis yields a possible male sex determination and an age at death of 35–45 years old. We may also infer that the US government regarded this individual as a "hostile" Indian given the circumstances of his death at Dade's Massacre—not Seminoles' Victory—on 28 December 1835. As reported, he would have been one of three Seminoles killed that day (Lucas 2011, 225). Though the skull bears no traces of trauma, the experiences precipitating his death indicate perimortem violence. But admittedly skeletal analysis produces incomplete and often inaudible narratives for most decedents in the Morton Collection, unsurprising since the methods used have historic origins in nineteenth-century medicine and natural history. I remain chagrined and frustrated. For physicians like Samuel, Abadie, and Robertson, however, inaudibility was intentional. To make the future dead required them to view skulls collected not as once living Indians but rather as depersonalized and fragmented objects, or specimens.

Becoming Object

As Robertson's casual tone indicates, collecting skulls was not undertaken in secret and it was not regarded as shameful (Fabian 2010). Nor did physicians frown upon retention of those skulls as souvenirs or pedagogical tools. In previous chapters, we learned how physicians' training generally involved courses of lectures in surgery and anatomy. As the nineteenth century got underway, these courses increasingly used pathological individuals or specimens to instruct on the abnormal. Medical institutions throughout the United States strove to accumulate anatomical (or pathological) collections large and varied enough to extend students' training. Hence, during this time, viewing bodies in parts and collecting those fragmented parts became normative medical practices.

The other nineteenth-century phenomenon that acted to transform skulls from subjects to specimens, as Robertson alluded to, was phrenology. Today regarded as a pseudoscience, adherents then examined skulls' morphology for information about their owner's mental faculties and character. But in phrenology's heyday, "respectable and intelligent gentleman" (Chapman 1822, 204) established societies of the likeminded throughout Europe and the United States, as discussed in chapter 2. Despite phrenology's increasing delegitimation as the nineteenth century wore on, the belief that measuring skulls communicated something about racial or national identity (i.e., a group's intelligence) persisted.

Finally, pragmatically speaking, skulls were transportable. They moved easily across landscapes with transient servicemen. Or skulls could be mailed to distant locations without incurring significant damage. Abadie, for instance, simply asked his quartermaster to ship them via post. As he explained to Samuel: "For our Quarter Masters are very punctual in forwarding any thing entrusted to their care: I saw it myself delivered to the shipping agent and directed to your address Arch St. as well as to the Acad. of Nat. Sciences: to be forwarded by Maj. Clark P[ost] . . . M[aster]. at N.O. I hope that my precautions have been successful and that the box has reached you safely" (Abadie 1838b). In Florida's case, the establishment of post offices in the mid-nineteenth century points to an increasing connectivity between this frontier zone and more northerly states, as well as a growing number of White settlers. From 1821 (the year it became a US territory) to 1859, Congress authorized the opening of 184 post offices throughout Florida (Winsberg 1993). Other men opted to pass skulls along to colleagues and friends bound for Philadelphia. These circuitous routes are one reason it is difficult to distinguish primary from secondary (or tertiary) collectors.

Once bodies and their parts were housed within scientific institutions, they were reidentified. The skull of the Seminole decedent that Robertson collected, for instance, was rechristened 1105 by Samuel. And in subsequent years this individual would be designated L-606-1105 and then 97-606-1105, a re-cataloguing that speaks to the dynamic nature of the Morton Collection (and all museum collections). After Samuel's death, his collection was purchased by colleagues on behalf of the ANS (see chapter 6). This institution loaned it to Penn Museum in 1966 and then granted formal ownership in 1997; hence the catalogue additions of "L" and "97." As it has moved—from institution to institution and storage space to storage space—parts have gone missing, albeit by accident: a central maxillary incisor here, a mandible there.

This brings up an additional aspect of colonial necropolitics—one tied to the processes that engendered transformation of identities. Mbembe (2019, 72) describes this process as "the becoming-object of the human being"—the somewhat counterintuitive notion that in being transformed from a human subject to an object one can acquire a modicum of social value.[16] Sovereign powers deemed certain bodies worthy of proper burial while Others—given class and/or race—were delegitimized as citizens. The worth they acquired only occurred after death and through a process of disinterment, fragmentation, and investigation by physicians with natural historic proclivities who were overwhelmingly White, male, and middle class.

Becoming object made skulls into analytically and pedagogically useful specimens—into "its." Placing a specimen into etic categories—male/female/unknown; infant/child/20–30/30–40/40+/etc.; idiot/criminal/slave/Indian; Negroid/Caucasoid/Mongoloid—facilitated this process. Individuals not easily categorized, those outliers, were often erased from samples or deemed deviant. In the specific case of race, Samuel's craniometric studies reified his categories as bounded and natural. He then calculated cranial capacity from the specimens sent his way and used data to rank the arbitrary racial categories he referenced. Big-brained Caucasians, he argued in the 1839 publication *Crania Americana*, were far superior to small-skulled Black Africans and American Indians, like 97–606–1105[17]—a scientific assessment that further legitimated state-sanctioned violence against races believed to be intellectually inferior. Researchers conducted these same kinds of assessments to distinguish between the sexes (Geller 2017, 33–6). Natural historians feminized the skulls of non-White males and racialized those of females (e.g., Ecker 1868; Vogt 1864; Welcker 1862). Gracility in both cases indicated arrested intellectual development, which was a sign of infantilization and inferiority. Or stated another way, women were on par with inferior races, and they were both subpar when compared to White males.

Perpetuation of these beliefs and practices occurred in pedagogical settings, as students learned the ways of racialization. Indeed, in the case of Samuel's skulls, handwritten script—now faded after so many years—attests to their use as teaching specimens. On 97–606–1105's cranium, for instance, he wrote "Oss Frontal" at the midpoint on the frontal bone, "Coronal Suture" at the coronal suture that connects the frontal to the parietal bones, and so forth. On the left temporal bone, Samuel inked metric information: "I.C. 82" to designate the cranium's internal capacity. In the case of other skulls, like 456 and 604, holes were drilled into the left and right parietals for analytical and display purposes. As Samuel explained: "The cranium is then taken from the instrument, and a hole, eighth of an inch in diameter, drilled through the pencil marks in each parietal bone, about two inches from the meatus auditorius: a stiff wire is then passed through these two holes, and the cranium nearly filled with white pepper seed" (Morton 1839, 255). Once his research was complete, Samuel exhibited the collection at the ANS's museum. The public could view it free of charge on Tuesdays and Saturdays (Morton 1840a, Note).

Samuel's work also established an important precedent for who could become object—decedents with low socioeconomic status as a consequence of racial stigma, indigent position, and/or mental instability. These facets of identity made it challenging for kin to claim bodies or hold researchers accountable for their studies. With this in mind, I put forward the idea—and thereby augment Mbembe's overview of necropolitics—that re-cataloguing, etic categorizations, and sustained analysis can signal a *maintaining object*, or the naturalization of structurally violent practices that affect disenfranchised and vulnerable groups comprising historic collections. Skulls then traveled between colleagues and institutions, like other nonhuman specimens in museum collections (Nichols 2014), to produce a "dynamic archive."

Official Sanction

The methods implemented by Samuel had long-term effects. On 4 April 1867, US Army surgeon general Joseph K. Barnes (1867–1868, 167) requested that medical officers amass:

1. Rare pathological specimens from animals, including monstrosities.
2. Typical crania of Indian tribes; specimens of their arms, dress, implements, rare articles of their diet, medicines, etc.
3. Specimens of poisonous insects and reptiles, and their effects on animals.

With this post in "Circular No. 2," the federal government officially sanctioned collection of American Indians' remains (in the same breath as monstrosities and poisonous insects). In Barnes's mind, the request was an uncontroversial one. Like Samuel, the surgeon general had graduated from the Medical Department at the University of Pennsylvania (class of 1838) where collections of anatomical and pathological specimens were familiar educational tools. After he graduated from medical school, he worked as a resident physician at Philadelphia's Old Blockley, the almshouse discussed in chapter 2. Samuel even acknowledged Barnes, among others, in *Crania Americana* for "the occasional attendance and aid" with information about measured skulls (Morton 1839, 261).

It is also more than likely that Barnes encountered the material and human remains of varied American Indian tribes while fulfilling the aims of Manifest Destiny. After a year at Blockley Almshouse, he was commissioned an assistant surgeon of the US Army. Barnes then proceeded to climb the ranks (United States Surgeon-General's Office 1883).[18] Over the course of a long military career, his active service took him to Florida, Louisiana, Texas, Mexico, Maryland, Kansas, Missouri, Mississippi, New York, California, Washington, and Oregon. "Circular No. 2," then, provided a pragmatic way for expanding and diversifying the Army Medical Museum's holdings, an institution established to teach physicians the basic principles of military medicine.[19] Whereas medical officers had initially culled medical and surgical specimens from White US soldiers, many of whom died on Civil War battlefields, they now turned to wild western frontiers. As detailed in an 1868 memorandum from Assistant Surgeon General Charles H. Crane, "The chief purpose had in view in forming this collection is to aid in the progress of anthropological science by obtaining measurements of a large number of skulls of the aboriginal races of North America" (as quoted in Lamb 1923, 117). To this end, the Surgeon General's Office, under the aegis of the War Department, took full advantage of its connections to medical officers stationed throughout "Indian country." This strategy was one that had proven effective in the recent past. The memorandum continued, "They have already enriched the *Mortonian* and other magnificent craniological cabinets by their contributions, and it is hoped they will evince even greater zeal in collecting for their own Museum" (Lamb 1923, 117; emphasis added).

Some two decades after Samuel's death, institutional forces still regarded his collection methods as foundational and worth emulating. His ideas about intelligence and race also remained influential. The Army Medical Museum's curator, Dr. George A. Otis, for instance, presented his findings before the National Academy of Science in 1870: "Judging from the capacity of the cranium, the American Indians must be assigned a lower position in the human scale than has been believed heretofore" (as cited by Lamb 1917, 56A). Evidence for Natives' inferiority did not circulate in a sociopolitical vacuum. As the nation continued to expand westward, the government, militia, and industry (e.g., railroad companies) utilized scientific data to justify violent subjugation of American Indians, negate their sovereign status, and consolidate national character.[20]

Rest in Peace

Rather than proper burial in mounds or cemeteries with kin, the bodies and fragmented pieces of "hostile" Indians and "rebellious" enslaved Africans were transported far from ancestral lands and final resting places. They were then housed in institutional settings—museums, scientific laboratories, classrooms. Samuel's collection of skulls instigates the normalization of these practices (see also Redman 2016). Such treatment offers a marked contrast to funerary rites for and interments of the White Americans who waged war against American Indians and Black Americans. For their heroism and service to the nation, military men received proper and uninterrupted burial when they died, an additional privilege of citizenship. (Though such deaths—violent, far from home, without family—did require the nation to grapple with the pragmatics of bodily preservation and the meaning of a "good death," reconfigurations that grew more urgent during the Civil War [Faust 2008]).

The nineteenth century brought a profound change not just in notions about bodies, and the ones deemed worthy of belonging to the larger body politic, but in the spaces associated with death. It was at the century's midpoint that the United States' "cemetery beautiful movement" commenced. In the eighteenth century, interment often occurred beneath the floors of urban churches and their attached yards, as well as in vacant lots (French 1974). Overcrowding and a growing concern about the threat dead bodies posed to public health put an end to these types of burials. Cities' boards of health became particularly proactive in prohibiting interment in these spaces.

In response, prominent members of urban communities throughout the United States advocated for the creation of rural cemeteries. The first of these garden cemeteries to open was Boston's Mount Auburn Cemetery in 1831. In turn, other prominent American cities advanced this cemetery beautiful movement. Situated on the outskirts of cities, these landscaped spaces were designed with functionality and aesthetics in mind. Mourning and socializing both occurred within their gates. Access was restricted, however, to upper- and middle-class White families. The potter's field or almshouse cemetery was still the most common resting place for cities' impoverished residents. Racial segregation also continued to remain the order of the day as evidenced by separate "Negro burying grounds" or separate areas within cemeteries for Black Americans.

When Abadie died, for instance, he was buried at Bellefontaine Cemetery, one scenic and carefully landscaped example in St. Louis. While the cemetery's founders did not explicitly address race, the price of lots and one's status as free or enslaved did contribute to an internal organization determined by socioeconomics (Smith 2020, 167). At the time of Bellefontaine's creation, the cemetery grounds were located on the city's rural outskirts. (Today a wrought iron fence demarcates its extensive grounds, 314 acres in total, from the urban neighborhood that has since grown up around the cemetery. The contrast between manicured green space and industrial decline is stark.) In 1849, when the cemetery opened, changing beliefs about bodies, their final disposition, and St. Louis's growth—the city was then the eighth-largest in the nation—provided impetus (Shepley 2008). With the passing years, Bellefontaine's burial population came to comprise mostly prominent White men and their kin.

After Abadie's inaugural interment in the family plot—the good doctor died in 1874 after a long and illustrious career in the military—other kin followed in turn. They rest in peace together atop a ridge that faces the Mississippi River. Adjacent to the Abadies are William Clark and his clan. Clark's activities, like Abadie's military service and skull collecting, are a testament to nation-building and mythmaking. When he set off from St. Louis in 1804 with Meriwether Lewis, the two men were charged with exploration of the western United States. The carved granite monument that marks Clark's grave site honors these efforts: "The expedition of Lewis and Clark across the continent in 1804-5-6 marked the beginning of the progress of exploration and colonization which thrust our national boundaries to the Pacific." Meant as eulogy, acknowledgment of colonization could easily be read today as victor's arrogance and the misfortune of the vanquished. The irony being that had it not been for the assistance Lewis and Clark received from various American Indian groups along the way, their survival and the expedition's success would have been unlikely. Indeed, Clark's negotiation of treaties with American Indians effectively disenfranchised them from their land and provided a model for future policy (Shepley 2008, 59).

As for Robertson's grave, it resides in a picturesque cemetery with a history similar to Bellefontaine. Magnolia Cemetery had once been a rice plantation on the outskirts of Charleston before its conversion into a final resting place for the city's esteemed White occupants. Robertson, who had relocated from Augusta in 1846, thrived in Charleston; he became a well-respected, slave-owning physician who specialized in obstetrics and gynecology (Moore 1893, 20). He even did another turn as a medical officer during the Civil War, acting as surgeon of the 16th Regiment of the South Carolina Militia (Moore 1893). After the war, he held numerous, prestigious medical positions: dean of the Medical College of South Carolina (later renamed the Medical University of South Carolina), president of the South Carolina Medical Association, and member of the American Medical Association (Knight 1917; Robertson 2015). When he died on 15 July 1892, he was regarded as a notable denizen of Charleston, a devout Christian, and a physician who had advanced the field of medicine. (For all his talk about phrenological prizes and skulls, Robertson's death certificate listed "softening of brain" as a secondary cause.) His obituary leaves the impression of a strict though tender patriarch, a wise and authoritative physician, and a moral, upstanding citizen (McGuire 1893). He would be laid to rest next to his wife, who had passed almost two decades prior. Five of his sons, who all proudly served the Confederacy and survived the Civil War, were also buried in the family plot at Magnolia Cemetery adjacent to their spouses.

And what of Samuel? Though I return to his death in this book's final chapter, there are some details germane to a discussion of final resting places. After his passing on 15 May 1851, family members and ANS colleagues gathered to bury Samuel's remains at Laurel Hill Cemetery. Samuel's brother-in-law John Jay Smith founded the cemetery in 1836. Impetus for its creation came from John Jay's inability to locate the grave of his beloved daughter Gulielma—she who Samuel had been at a loss to heal—in the overcrowded Quaker burying ground. Or so went mythmaking about the cemetery's establishment. "Philadelphia should have a rural cemetery on dry ground, where feelings should not be harrowed by viewing the bodies of beloved relatives plunged into mud and water," John Jay wrote (as quoted in Keels 2003, 21). His vision for Laurel Hill initially engendered pushback from the Quaker community, however. The *Rules of Discipline and Christian Advices of the Yearly Meeting of Friends for Pennsylvania and New Jersey* was clear on appropriate mourning and burial practices (Philadelphia Yearly Meeting of the Religious Society of Friends 1797, 16–17). Interment outside of the church's walls, in unconsecrated ground, was distressing, as was the burial of decedents not admitted to the Society of Friends. Additionally, grave markers were forbidden; the Society regarded them as "Marks of Superfluity and excess" and "inconsistent with the plain-

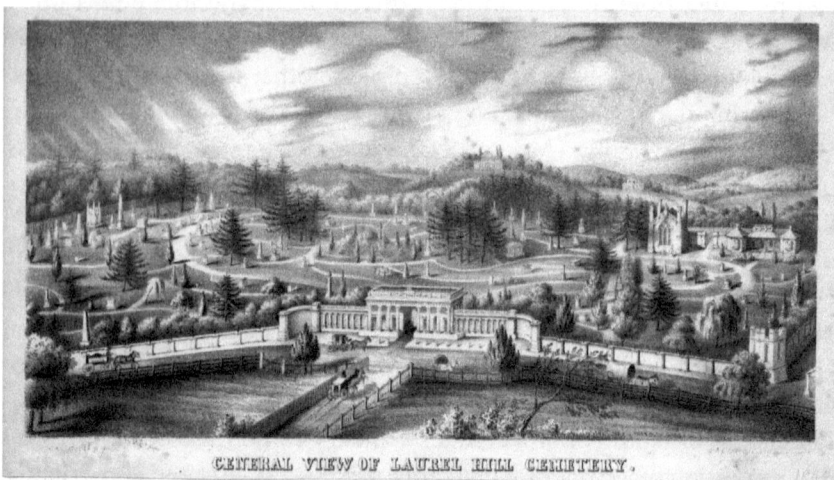

Figure 3.4. *General View of Laurel Hill Cemetery*, a lithograph by E. J. Pinkerton, 1847. The Library Company of Philadelphia. Retrieved from https://digital.librarycompany.org/islandora/object/digitool%3A65108.

ness of our Principles and Practice" (1797, 59). Refusal to remove tombstones from graves could result in removal from the Society of Friends.

Indifferent to the rules, John Jay transferred Gulielma's body to Laurel Hill in 1837 (Strachey 1980, 24). The cemetery's grounds, which had once been part of a large country estate on the outskirts of the city, represented the "supreme achievements of Philadelphia's 'cemetery beautiful movement'" (Cotter 1992, 201) (figure 3.4). Laurel Hill eventually catered to upper- and middle-class White families for whom sentimentality was as important as religion. Racial minorities, the poor, and other socially marginal people (i.e., unmarried lovers) were excluded (Keels 2003, 25; McDannell 1995, 111). And given the certainty of death, the venture became quite profitable for John Jay and his descendants.

After Samuel's passing, in keeping with the Greek Revival of the day, his kin erected a monument sculpted of marble. It continues to watch over his grave and the graves of family members, all of whom continue to rest in peace in the Morton plot, Section G, Lot 179. "Physician, Naturalist, and Ethnologist" reads Samuel's tombstone, his White, male, and nationalist privilege offering insurance that the physician-naturalist's skull would never become object or be subjected to the same regulatory techniques of necropower that he so deftly utilized on Others.

4

Border Making, Border Crossing

Note: [by Capt. Young] The material from which the following report has been prepared, were collected under all the disadvantages attending researches made during the operations of a very active campaign in an enemy's country. The author being engaged every day's march in surveying and measuring the route of the army, was unable to make many excursions, but every opportunity of examining the country was seized on.... It is hoped that the information derived from these sources will prove both interesting and useful—this memoir containing the only correct account which has been given of a section of country now rising rapidly into political importance.

So began Captain Hugh Young in *A Topographical Memoir on East and West Florida with Itineraries of General Jackson's Army, 1818* (Young et al. 1934). The topographical engineer's 1818 report was a record of observations made while mapping the Florida frontier, efforts undertaken as part of the campaign that (then) General Andrew Jackson was leading against the Seminoles. Young's description of the landscape across which he and his men trekked—classified into the hilly, the flat, the swampy, the marshy—is quite detailed, redolent even. His treatment of Florida's Indians, however, reads less like ethnography and more like military intel. It has breadth but lacks depth and is replete with disdain.

Of the "Okatiokinas," Young noted, "Their chief Hones-higa was a peaceable honest Indian who kept his warriors perfectly quiet during the late war.... In character they are warlike—but friendly to the whites" (Young et al. 1934, 85). Similarly, of the "Cheskitalowas," he commented, "They had sixty-five warriors and their chief Yaholamico is a good honest and sensible Indian, son of a half-breed. They are honest and friendly—cultivate good land, spin and weave and have a few cattle" (Young et al. 1934, 87). But Young did not mince words in his description of the "Tallehassas": "Character worthless, dishonest and inveterately hostile" (Young et al. 1934, 88). And he drew a comparable conclusion about the Tallewheanas; they were "keeping up a show of friendship but inveterately hostile to the whites" (Young et al. 1934, 88). Friendly or hostile—the rhetorical distinction that Young evoked—glossed over complex ancestries, identities, and experiences of Native peoples dispersed throughout the southeastern United States in the nineteenth century. It became strategic discourse adopted by the US War Department to justify an expansionist national agenda, which topographical engineers helped realize (or materialize) through border making. As one influential example with connections to Samuel, this chapter discusses John James Abert.

Without American Indians' hostility—whether real or imagined though always deemed gratuitous—how could US soldiers perform acts of heroism? The rationalization for such violence is best illustrated by stories describing their clashes with Natives peoples and escaped slaves living in Florida's frontier. In defense of White settlers, men like Captain Justin Dimick scouted, soldiered, and slayed enemies during the Second Seminole War.

Like chapter 3's medical officers, military men tasked with producing information about Florida's landscape also acquired skulls for Samuel. The friendly/hostile distinction that facilitated their collection was rendered moot once skulls had become objects. "Specimens" put up no resistance to their use in scientific research or anatomy classrooms. Instead, Samuel created bounded categories with racialized significance; differences between groups were presented as natural and hierarchical. His investigation of hybridity also muted conversation about miscegenation and the messiness of social and sexual interactions.

Yet, as Michel-Rolph Trouillot (1995) reminded us, recounting alternative narratives—those used to subvert or extend the official, the mythological, the epic—is feasible. The strategies for doing so are multiple and more easily executed when scholars attend to history's materiality. Trouillot recognized that repositioning evidence is also quite effective (1995, 27). For skulls comprising the Morton Collection, they may have become objects, as outlined in chapter 3, but they also make visible traces of the past. They invite possibilities for "retrieving minor lives from oblivion," in Saidiya Hartman's words, that can redress "the violence of history" (2019, 31). To this end, the named individuals in the Morton Collection are instructive, as well as those decedents who hint at alliances between Blacks and American Indians. The latter, I argue, are suggestive of a hybridity that reveals the fallacy of purity, the transgression of borders, and the fragility of an exclusionary nation-building project.

Friendly and Hostile

Captain Young's rhetorical distinction between friendly and hostile was not without earlier precedent. Europeans in the sixteenth century vacillated between the two terms in their descriptions of Natives throughout the Americas, though they did always agree on their primitiveness (Nash 1972). In their chronicles, friendly was a catchall for gentle, kind, and pastoral, while hostile encompassed savage, cannibalistic, barbarous, and bestial, among other negative qualifiers. These designations were contingent on the imperial ends sought by Europeans—whether mercantile prospects, Christian conversion, sexual relations, or possession of land. Into the early nineteenth century, White Americans continued to evoke the distinction in their descriptions of American Indians (e.g., Potter 1836; Simmons 1822; Sprague 1848; White 1950). But the impetus for Young's assessments was neither religious fervor nor satiation of wants and needs (though Christianization and an expansion of market opportunities certainly provided some incentive for his superior officers and the congressional leaders who authorized their activities). Rather, as a member of the US Army Corps of Topographical Engineers (hereafter corps), he operated at the intersection of the military (as an operative for the War Department) and science (as a gatherer of geographic and natural historic information). The techniques of topographical engineering—reconnaissance, surveying, mapping—functioned to demarcate boundaries between people and places in the service of Manifest Destiny.[1]

With the passage of the Indian Removal Act, Indians characterized as friendly were amenable to moving beyond state borders or willing to stay within them and assimilate. Several examples were discussed in the previous chapter. To circle back to one, John Lee Williams, a White settler instrumental in establishing Tallahassee as Florida's territorial capital, made the following observation about Black Dirt: "FuctaLuste Hajo—Black Ragged Clay—is an old chief of Chicuchatty; was at one time principal war chief. He is usually called Black Dirt. He has at all times been friendly to emigration, and finally headed the Indians that removed during the last year" (1837, 35–36; see also Potter 1836, 82). Migration to Arkansas in 1836 ultimately did little to benefit Black Dirt and his band, as the reader may also remember. "FUKE-LUSTE-HADJO" was the name inked across the forehead of "specimen" 729 in the Morton Collection, a child who died between the ages of five and nine years. When US Army surgeon Eugene Abadie (1838a) exhumed the child from a grave near Tampa two years after Black Dirt's departure, there was no kin left to object.

In contrast, allegedly hostile Indians balked at White settler encroachment, demarcated boundaries, and negotiated relocations. Written accounts—in national newspapers, private correspondences, and governmental reports—took up this rhetoric. The *Jacksonville Courier*, for instance, included a weekly column titled "Indian Hostilities." It kept local readership abreast of the "latest intelligence" about the growing threat posed to their property (terrestrial and enslaved) and their personal wellbeing. In their private correspondences, White settlers repeated these claims, though their experiences do nuance a more complex set of circumstances. "It is feared the Creek will join the Seminoles," Corinna Brown wrote to her brother Mannevillette in Ithaca, New York. Her 1836 letter continued, "If they should, they will make havoc, I reckon. The Creeks are blood thirsty and the Seminoles brave—at least they have proved themselves of late. . . . They say it will take 5,000 to subdue the Creeks—and there are 5 or 6,000 of them—Scott could not quell 1,000 Seminoles with 2,000 men. Great General! His talent for tactics is quite bewildering!" (Denham and Huneycutt 2004, 32; emphasis in original).

She wrote from Mandarin, a community situated on the eastern banks of the St. Johns River. Like many before, Corinna, her sister Ellen, and brother Charles came to eastern Florida in the fall of 1835 for two reasons: economic opportunity and a reprieve from northern winters (Denham and Huneycutt 2004, xxiii). (Some things about migration to Florida have not changed after almost two centuries.) Their aunt had married a wealthy plantation owner who gifted them some acreage on which to live and grow crops. Despite this windfall, the Brown family was not financially well-off. They were, however, well-educated. And their affinity for writing engendered thoughtful correspondences about White settlers' lives on a frontier, which was often isolated, largely unregulated, and rapidly changing. An amalgam of personal musings, journalistic reports, and official word, their letters contain pervasive tropes about American Indians' hostility and savagery. They arrived in Florida at the outset of the Second Seminole War. In the intervening years, houses were built, Black slaves purchased, trees planted, gardens cultivated, marital matches made, and babies born. There was even time for collecting skulls, though more out of idle curiosity and less for scientific purposes as was the case for Samuel.

"They killed two Indians—E. brought home a scalp & three heads from some graves he opened near Lake Eipopka of a man, one woman very large & one little papoose with all the hair on," Corinna wrote to Mannevillette in 1840 (Denham and Huneycutt 2004, 113). "E." referred to her husband, Dr. Edward S. Aldrich. Originally, he arrived in Jacksonville from the Medical College of South Carolina intent on doctoring. But on 4 July 1837, in a moment of patriotic spirit, he joined up as surgeon with the First Regiment of Florida Mounted Volunteers (Adjutant General's Office 1838, 39–43) (figure 4.1). Two months later, Aldrich and Corinna were wed. Like the medical officers discussed in chapter 3, his downtime was spent exploring. Her letter recounted the fruits of his labors—details about graves opened, goods and bodies positions within, and states of preservation. As to what became of her husband's war trophies, however, Corinna's letters are silent.

Although the Brown family's accounts hint at the constant and violent threat posed by Florida Indians, they experienced nothing directly. Corinna wrote to Mannevillette in 1841: "I wish we may be in the U.S. to meet you—*for this place called Florida does not seem a part or portion of the Union.* The Indians are still at large & cutting capers & throats at pleasure. I see no hope of a termination to their game this year. Of course there is a bar to all improvement. We trust in Gen. Harrison & the new administration for an end of these things" (Denham and Huneycutt 2004, 143; emphasis added). Despite her exasperation, Corinna remained in Florida throughout the duration of the Second Seminole War. Like many White settlers, she was not deterred by American Indians' actions though she did regard them as disruptive and deadly. Such a portrayal—whether it was accurate, fabricated, or exaggerated—stoked fear among the wider American citizenry.[2] Corinna's observations about the imminent threat of hostile Indians and Florida's tenuous ties to the Union are also suggestive of the significance, contingency, and creation of boundaries during this moment in time.

Mapping National Borders

Although Captain Young's untimely death in 1822 precluded further involvement in boundary making efforts, subsequent topographical engineers soldiered on. In the figure of Colonel John James Abert (b. 1788, d. 1863), we can see how mapmaking continued to reinforce a distinction

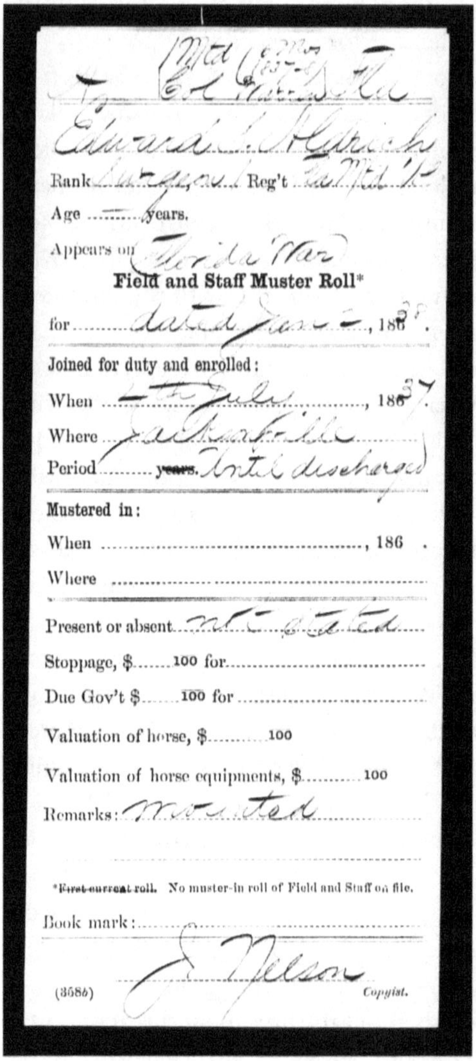
Edward S. Aldrich

Rank Surgeon Reg't Fla Mtd Vo

Age ...... years.

Appears on Florida War

Field and Staff Muster Roll*

for dated Jan 2, 1838.

Joined for duty and enrolled:

When 4th July, 1837.

Where Jacksonville

Period ...... years. Until discharged

Mustered in:

When ......, 186 .

Where ......

Present or absent not stated

Stoppage, $ 100 for ......

Due Gov't $ 100 for ......

Valuation of horse, $ 100

Valuation of horse equipments, $ 100

Remarks: mounted

*~~First current~~ roll. No muster-in roll of Field and Staff on file.

Book mark: ......

(3586) J. Nelson Copyist.

Figure 4.1. Service record for Dr. Edward S. Aldrich, a surgeon with the First Regiment of Florida Mounted Volunteers. Source: Compiled Service Records of Volunteer Soldiers Who Served in Organizations from the State of Florida during the Florida Indian Wars. Records of the Adjutant General's Office, 1780s–1917, pp. 39–43. National Archives (Record Group 94, Microfilm M1086).

between friendly and hostile Indians, as well as expedited the process of becoming object. The latter entailed a rhetorical shift from subject to specimen. For some 32 years, Abert oversaw the corps' activities. Not coincidentally, he also donated two skulls to Samuel's cause. It is not clear how the two men first met. Born in Frederick, Maryland, Abert attended West Point, graduating in 1811. He then moved to Washington, DC, with a plan to study law, but the venture proved short-lived. As an alternative, Abert found employment with the War Department. Under the department's aegis, in November 1814, he was made a topographical engineer at the rank of major. Come 1829, his superiors selected him to head up the Topographical Bureau. Thereafter, Abert actively worked to have the corps recognized as a distinct branch of the War Department; he succeeded in 1831. The appointment set him down a long and productive career path (Beers 1942; Cullum 1891, 101–102; Wilson and Fiske 1887, 8).

From 1828 to 1833, Abert and his family lived in Philadelphia; *Desilver's Philadelphia Directory and Stranger's Guide* placed them in the vicinity of 11th and Market Streets (1828, 1829, 1831, 1833).[3] Given his professional obligations in DC, however, his time in the city must have been sporadic over that span. Two major family events likely drew him back to Philadelphia. Abert's wife, Ellen Matlack Abert, gave birth to their fourth child Silvanus "Thayer" Abert on 22 July 1828. Nine months later, on 16 April 1829, Ellen's grandfather, Timothy Matlack, died at the age of 95 (Abert 1890). (Matlack is best known for his penmanship, excellent enough that the Continental Congress selected him to transcribe the original US Declaration of Independence.) Abert and Samuel's paths would have crossed periodically at the city's various scientific institutions. The topographical engineer became a member of the ANS in 1828 (Academy of Natural Sciences 1877, 3) and was elected to the APS in 1832 (Abert 1832). In his capacity as corresponding secretary for the ANS, Samuel also reached out to Abert about the various corps expeditions. Expeditions, he realized, allowed for collection of geological and geographical information about the expanding nation, as well as fossils, faunal specimens, and American Indians' skulls. In an 1833 letter, for instance, Samuel inquired about the possibility of attaching a naturalist to an expedition being "fitting out by government for ascertaining the southwestern boundary of the U.S." In his replies, the topographical engineer dispensed with the formality of titles and full names; letters were brief, mostly illegible, and always signed with "J. J. Abert" (figure 4.2).

In contrast to the abbreviated letters he wrote Samuel, Abert corresponded frequently, at great length, and over the course of many years with his military colleagues. By all official accounts, he was adept at his vocation. Come the fall of 1832, as cholera raged across the North American continent, he was also appointed special commissioner of emigration. Orchestrating Indian removal necessitated much letter writing to various secretaries of war and their underlings. Detailed correspondences flowed back and forth between his many field stations and Washington, DC—about surveying landscapes, logistics of mapping national borders, establishment of new reservations' parameters, certification of contracts and

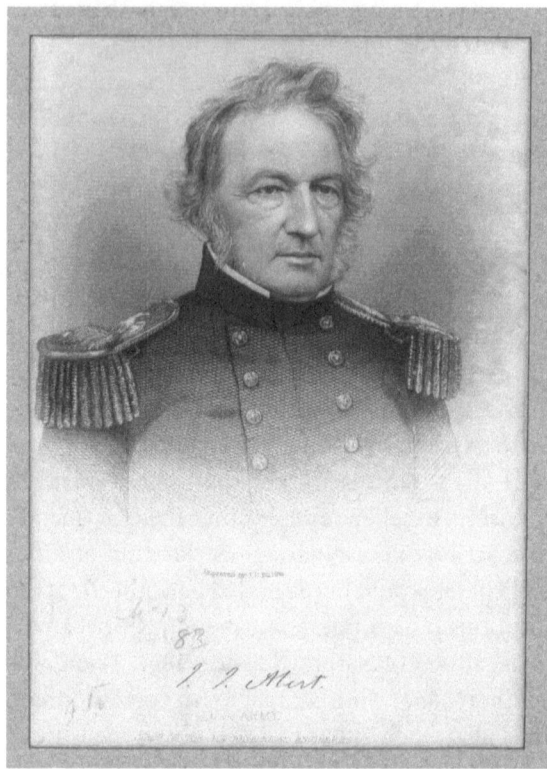

Figure 4.2. Portrait of Colonel John James Abert titled "J. J. Abert, U.S. Army, chielf [sic] of topographical engineers" (1886). The Miriam and Ira D. Wallach Division of Art, Prints and Photographs: Print Collection. New York Public Library. Retrieved from https://digitalcollections.nypl.org/items/510d47da-fee6-a3d9-e040-e00a18064a99.

treaties with American Indians (e.g., Commissary General of Subsistence 1834, 1835). That Abert held seemingly incongruent positions is no accident. National borders could not be conceived until Native peoples ceded their lands and were resettled elsewhere, the government maintained.

Abert had a hand in the emigration of the Pottawatomie, Ottawa, Chippewa, Shawnee, Winnebago, Creek, Cherokee, and Seminole. While formal and deferential, his letters initially convey an ambivalence about implementing colonial settler policies. Given "the state of want and misery" that he observed among the Creek, for instance, Abert proposed changes to the treaty he was negotiating between them and the US government (Commissary General of Subsistence 1835, 704–705). His statements about the Cherokee also conveyed remorse about the precarity he witnessed. "You cannot have an adequate idea of the deterioration which these Indians have undergone during the last two or three years, from a general state of comparative plenty to that of unqualified wretchedness and want," he wrote in 1834 (as quoted in Foreman 1972, 119). Advocacy on these groups' behalf was strongly rebuffed by President Jackson, however (Commissary General of Subsistence 1835, 704, 718, 720–22).

For acquiescing to the chain of command, the Department of War promoted Abert from lieutenant colonel to colonel on 7 July 1838 (Jones 1839, 111–12). He was to head up the Corps of Topographical Engineers, an organization where scientific inquiry, political strategy, and military intervention converged. The corps, historian William Goetzmann (1959, 17) argued (or, rather, lauded with little critical reflection in his exhaustive treatment of the subject), "was an instrument of self-conscious nationalism." As such, it directly advanced Manifest Destiny. While chief of the corps, Abert went on to organize and oversee the mapping of the American West (Goetzmann 1959; O'Brien and Diefendorf 1864, 181). His ability to do so effectively can be traced to events in Florida.

Despite earlier forays like those documented by Young, the Florida frontier was relatively unknown to the US Army. So, by order of General Zachary Taylor and under Abert's direction,[4] topographic engineers began to map the seat of the Second Seminole War in 1839 (figure 4.3). Reconnaissance and surveying yielded essential information about the lands where Seminoles sought refuge and carried out guerrilla warfare (Beers 1942). Thus, by the time Abert's men arrived in Florida, any prior qualms he had about the removal of southeastern American Indians seem to have dissipated. Instead, the activities he and his topographical engineers carried out exacerbated necropolitical conditions, and the skulls he gifted Samuel—one from Florida and later one from Michigan[5]—suggest that resignation had replaced empathy.

Samuel labeled the skull Abert sent him from Florida 698. He then inked "Seminole" across the left parietal. Archival documentation described the decedent as a "warrior," and skeletal study supports this designation. Analysis indicated that he had been a male aged 30–40 years old who died when a musket ball, presumably fired by a White soldier given the circumstances surrounding its collection, lodged in his brain.[6] On the left portion of the occipital bone (the back of the skull) a circular entry hole appears that measures 18.2 mm in diameter. Its outer edge is sharp and inner margin slightly beveled. There is no exit hole, though—and keeping in mind the projectile's direction—the musket ball's internal impact produced an external crack that runs the length of the left frontal, sphenoid, and temporal bones (the side of the skull).

This perimortem trauma, evidence of the Seminole warrior's cause of death, materializes the necropolitics of nation-building laid out in the

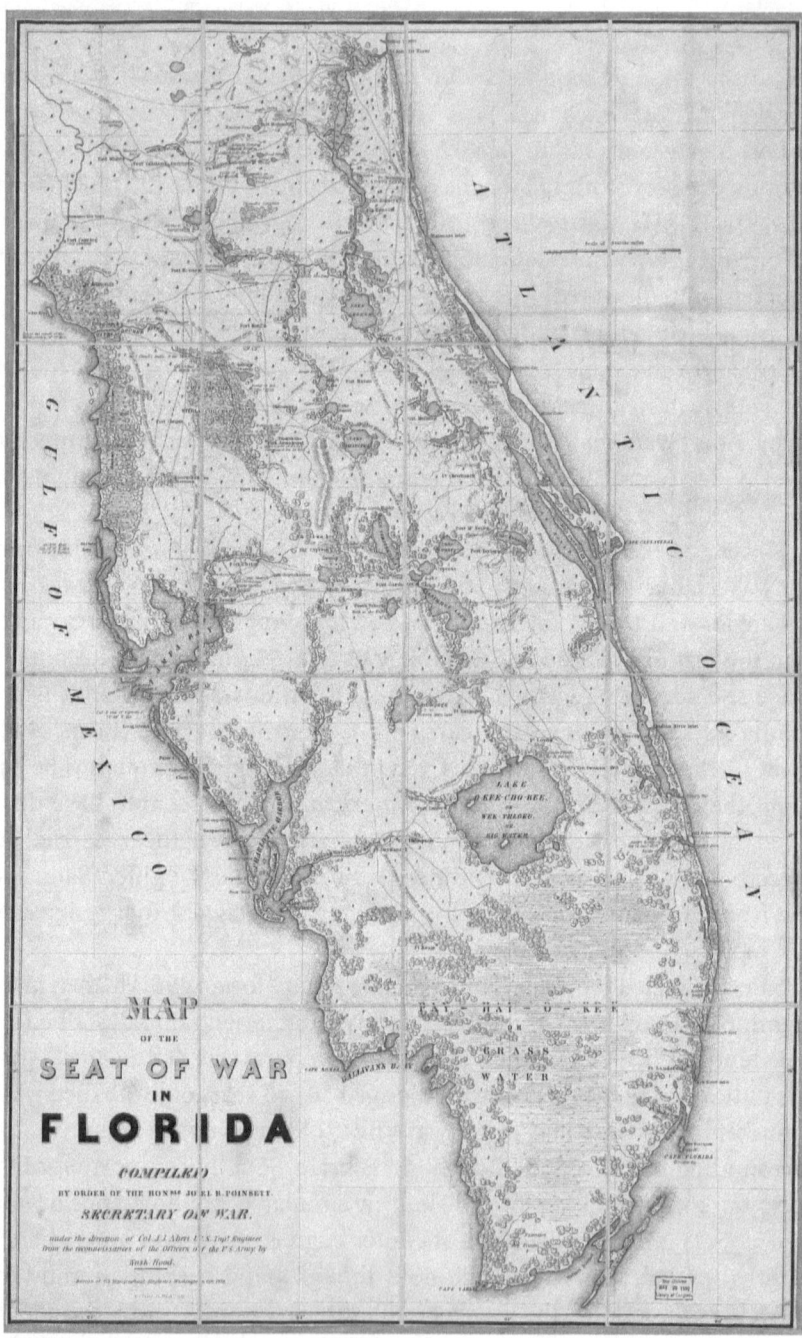

Figure 4.3. "Map of the seat of war in Florida." Created by the Bureau of US Topographical Engineers under the direction of Colonel J. J. Abert, 1838. Library of Congress, Geography and Map Division. Retrieved from https://www.loc.gov/item/2018588050/.

previous chapter, as well as the rhetorical boundaries drawn between "friendly" and "hostile" Indians discussed here. Such politicized and public discourse was strategic. American Indians' rebelliousness and violence—rarely, if ever, were their actions qualified as perseverance—provided justification for US soldiers to slay them, detach their heads from their bodies, and send said heads along to Samuel in Philadelphia. Qualifying Indians as hostile also presented opportunities for these White men to perform heroic acts. Safeguarding the nation necessitated enemies against whom they could test their valor and strength.

Heroism

The wide circulation of stories about Indians' hostility served to lionize the bravery and violent deeds of US soldiers. Accounts of Justin Dimick's exploits during the Second Seminole War are demonstrative, as well as pertinent to Samuel's research and cranial collection. Dimick received his appointment as captain in the spring of 1835. Less than one year later, on 4 February 1836, he was bound for the Florida frontier. There he was placed in charge of scouting activities.[7] More than organized warfare, the US Army's objectives primarily involved the protection of settlers' property—land, livestock, crops, homesteads, and enslaved Blacks—from raids by Seminole bands. In May, Dimick and company were sent to contend with the disruptive activities of "enemy" Indians, who, among other things, had helped enslaved Blacks escape from two plantations near St. Augustine. In the aftermath, General Winfield Scott reported to the War Department that the Seminoles were successfully subdued. As published in the *Army and Navy Chronicle* (Homans 1836, 346):

> On the morning of the eighth, we received a report that a party of Indians were at the Matansas; had captured the slaves of [Joseph Marion (Jose Mariano)] Hernandez and [Abraham] Dupont; and would no doubt destroy the fixtures at both plantations. Capt. Dimick was again hastily mounted and despatched. At a little distance from Dupont's place, a small party of the enemy were overtaken; at least three killed and seven wounded. Dimick lost a private killed, and had a sergeant and three privates wounded. Two of his horses were also killed. The Indians, as usual, availed themselves of a near hammock, and fought better than they have commonly done.

Among the literate American citizenry this official chronicle, vocal in its praise of Dimick and company's actions, was widely shared.

For example, in the journal he kept of his own experiences during the Second Seminole War, Dr. Jacob Rhett Motte, an assistant surgeon with the US Army, described Dimick's modesty, gallantry, and levelheadedness during the skirmish. He added that the Indians were superior in number, huge in stature, fear inducing, and desirous of White scalps (Motte 1953, 115). Similarly, periodicals across the nation—the *Gloucester (MA) Democrat* (1836), *Boston (MA) Courier* (1836), *New-London (CT) Gazette* (1836), *Richmond (VA) Enquirer* (1836), and more—offered an embellished narrative or one peppered with errors. Writers often misspelled Dimick's name (sometimes as Dimmick or Dimmock). Or they represented the actions of those who served under him, if mentioned at all, as superfluous. Reports also contained inconsistencies in dates, locations, and the number of attacking Indians (anywhere from a couple to 7–10). Of course, authenticity and accuracy were less important than the dissemination of notions about singular heroism and inevitable victory. These retellings, imperfect though they may be, indicate just how individual memories solidify into a collective's history—one tied to White men's individualistic effort, patriotism, and violent bravery. This variety of masculinity was rewarded and deemed necessary for realizing nationalist agendas. In the aftermath, Dimick was promoted to major "for gallant and meritorious conduct in the war against the Fla. Ind." (Sprague 1848, 552).

Unsurprisingly, the story of Dimick's heroism was also rehashed in the scientific circles of the day. Samuel included a version in *Crania Americana*:

> Seminole warrior, slain at the battle of St. Joseph's, thirty miles below St. Augustine in June 1836 by Captain Justin Dimmick of the First Regiment United States Artillery. At the commencement of the action Captain Dimmick rode forward, and received the fire of the Indians at a distance of about thirty yards. The Captain's horse being struck on the neck and flank, he dismounted: and the Indians, supposing him to be badly wounded, rushed towards him to scalp him. At that moment Captain D. raised his gun, (a double-barrel fowling piece.) and shot both of the Indians in succession: he then seized the musket of a soldier who stood near him, and sprang upon his enemies, one of whom . . . he found already dead, by a ball through the head, while the other was merely wounded. The latter was at once despatched by

a thrust of the bayonet: and thus by the singular bravery of Captain Dimmick these two savages lay dead, and side by side, in a few moments after the action began. (Morton 1839, 166–67)

This account came from Dr. Gouverneur Emerson. He had ripped the handwritten description (replete with doodled faces) straight from his medical notebook to share with Samuel.[8] Emerson was also kind enough to pass along the cranium from one of the two Indians described in the passage (Emerson 1837). Samuel labeled the "specimen" 604. This reidentification—a facet of the process involved in becoming object—further diminished the threat of hostile Indians and effaced the decedent's identity. What we do not learn, however, is how the slain Seminole's head was detached from his body. Nor do letters, notebook entries, or news reports include a discussion of how Emerson acquired the skull. The Philadelphia physician seems to have had no direct connection to Captain Dimick, and he never visited the Florida frontier.

These multiple retellings of Dimick's defensive actions and the slaying of hostile Seminoles tell us something about the production of American History. "Power is constitutive of the story," wrote Michel-Rolph Trouillot (1995, 28). What we see is how power works to produce events and actors. This process has a two-fold outcome; it conjures cause for official celebration, as well as actively silences. Some peoples and things, Trouillot observed, become "absent in history" (1995, 48–49). What then goes unaccounted for in the historic narratives that originated with military personnel and later circulated among men of science?

Samuel and his colleagues carefully curated their descriptions of violences perpetrated against Others; they deemed some acts appropriate and even laudatory, while they sanitized or disappeared others altogether. There is, for example, no suggestion that the "captured slaves of Hernandez and Dupont" were freedom seekers, joining with Seminole Indians to rebel against their enslavers. Nor do we hear of Seminole Indians' desperation, defensive strategizing, or resilience in the wake of White settler encroachment. Instead, they are categorized, reductively so, as friendly or hostile. And while we may learn of Native warriors' last breaths, sources suppress information about their lives and the postmortem violation of their bodies. (In the almshouse's hospital, as discussed in prior chapters, a comparable muting occurs. The clinical language of medicine served to efface the identities and suffering of inmates while concealing the acts physicians performed at the dissecting table's edge.)

To reposition evidence, however, can make for an alternative historical narrative, as Trouillot (1995, 27) recognized. From the fact of collection, detailed in chapter 3 and reiterated by Emerson's gifting of a story and skull to Samuel, something more nefarious can emerge. Rather than professional collegiality and scientific curiosity, the silences surrounding the appropriation of Native decedents' skulls call into question the morality of physicians sworn to foster life. Their active role in advancing necropolitics—letting die and the making of the future dead—is instead brought to the fore. Additionally, from the fact of perimortem trauma, we may counter discourse about Seminole hostility. In the case of the warrior labeled 604, for instance, forensic analysis confirms the interpersonal violence described in official accounts. An entry wound for the killing shot fired by Dimick appears on the decedent's left parietal; its outer edge is characteristically sharp, and the inner margin is beveled. A larger exit wound appears on the right parietal with the inverse, a sharp inner edge and beveled outer one. If we read against the grain, such evidence chronicles valiant resistance—heroism—by Seminoles despite years of precarious living and insurmountable odds.

"Nothing Is Known"

The Seminole slain by Dimick is just one of many examples of individuals in the Morton Collection for whom stories are difficult to craft. Of the skull he labeled 707, Samuel (1839, 168) states: "Seminole warrior, of whose history nothing is known." Yet despite the disclaimer, Samuel does provide some additional information. The skull's point of collection—to Abadie he was again indebted—took place "twelve miles south of the Suwannee River" (Morton 1839, 168). His *Catalogue*'s 1849 edition also notes that the warrior died at around 30 years of age. A paucity of details, for sure, but not "nothing." Forensic analysis supplements historic or archival sources. Cranial features indicate that the decedent was a male who died between 20–30 years of age.[9] While this individual possessed no perimortem trauma, we may assume he died violently given his warrior designation and inclusion in the Morton Collection. Curious and unexpected were the bold letters **"EOKLO-EMATHLA"** I found inked across his frontal bone; archival or published sources make no mention of this name. What then to make of an alias handwritten as such but intentionally stricken from official texts?

"Inequalities experienced by the actors," Trouillot (1995, 48) observed, "lead to uneven historical power in the inscription of traces." Certainly, copious source materials exist about the White men who collected skulls for Samuel. Biographical documentation on Abadie's family, for example, is traceable from the present back to a noble heritage in sixteenth-century France (Lippincott 1919; Pittman 1903; Virkus 1925). But the same cannot be said of decedents comprising the Morton Collection. One hindrance is the fact that Samuel referred to only a few individuals by name.[10]

As one eulogist later noted, "Nothing short of positive certainty, however, would induce him to place a name upon a cranium" (Patterson 1854, xxxviii). As listed in the *Catalogue* (1849a), named decedents are:

59 ANGLO-SAXON head: skull of Pierce,* a convict and cannibal who was executed in New South Wales, A. D. 18–. F. A. 85°. I. C. 99 . . .

80 Skull of an ENGLISHMAN named Samuel Gwillym, a convict in Australia . . .

579 ATHLA-FICKSA; a Muskogee or Creek chief, ætat. 50 . . .

639 Skull of James Moran, an ENGLISHMAN, who was executed at Philadelphia for piracy and murder, May 19, 1837. Ætat. 20 . . .

1227 COTONAY (Blackfoot) chief, named the "Bloody Hand," ætat. 50 . . .

1319 Skull of John Voorhees, a Mulatto porter, born in Chester county, Pennsylvania, and died of consumption in the Blockley Hospital, November 5, 1846, aged 35 years. About an hour before his death, he called the nurse to him, and confessed as follows: That eighteen or twenty years before, having a hatred against another boy of his own color, two years younger than himself, he strangled and killed him . . .

1323 The skull of Vicente Rivaz, an Otomie Cazique of the pure MEXICAN race, born and died in the village of San Piedro Flaxcoapan, in the department of Tula, 20 leagues from the city of Mexico . . .

1327 AUSTRALIAN of Port St. Philip, New South Wales. This man, whose name was Durabub, was killed in a fray after having himself killed two savages of a hostile tribe, A.D. 1841. His skull is the nearest approach to the Orang type that I have seen. Ætat. 40 . . .

1330 Sumboo-sing, a HINDU of the Brahmin caste, hanged at Calcutta for murder, December, 1840. Ætat. 40 . . .

1332 Gunga-Govind: HINDU, ætat. 40. I.C. 86.

Most of these individuals were identified as executed criminals. The inscription of their names in publications does not serve to celebrate but to further stigmatize and sensationalize; naming in these instances may be read as an act of violence. Yet, for the Americans Indians identified, two to be exact, naming functions differently; it reinforced the day's rhetoric (though, no doubt, a more subtle type of violence is at work here). For the Cotonay (or Blackfoot) chief, the "Bloody Hand" who Samuel catalogued as 1227, he was "fierce, crafty and courageous" and displayed an "uncompromising hostility" (1839, 201). Samuel is a bit more gracious in his characterization of Athlaha Ficksa. From *Crania Americana:* "This plate is taken from the skull of Athlaha Ficksa, a full-blood chief of the Creek nation. He fought with great bravery in the United States service, and against the majority of his own countrymen in the present Florida war. He died in Mobile, in 1837, whence I received his cranium through the kindness of Dr. Henry S. Rennolds, of the United States Navy" (Morton 1839, 170). In his *Catalogue* (1849a), Samuel supplements this information: "579 ATHLA-FICKSA; a Muskogee or Creek chief, ætat. 50." But he did not go as far to ink this name on the cranium's surface. Perhaps, for Samuel, Athlaha Ficksa's status as a "friendly" Indian inclined him to couple collection of his skull with additional explanation, whereas abridgment was deemed appropriate in the case of hostile Indians like Bloody Hand. But how to explain the erasure of Eoklo-Emathla by Samuel?

Some silences are indeed stubborn. As Saidiya Hartman notes, the archive has its limits—"on what can be known, whose perspective matters, and who is endowed with the gravity and authority of historical actor" (2019, xiii; see also 2008). Given these limits is it possible to make visible individuals intentionally excluded from or muted in the archives? To conceive of their lives in terms other than death, violation, and victimization? And, when bringing skeletal data into the evidentiary fold, how does one avoid compounding negative outcomes? Contemporary scientific studies may seem neutral, prescriptive, necessary. But processes and people considered in previous chapters have revealed the history of such work (i.e., bodily fragmentation, labeling, categorizing, analyzing) as the exercise of necropower—the power to disappear, the power to constitute a scientific specimen, the power to exert ownership. Hartman wonders, "If it is no longer sufficient to expose the scandal, then how might it be possible to generate a different set of descriptions from this archive? To imagine what could have been?" (2008, 7). In answer, she suggests that critical fabulation, a more speculative narration, makes possible a deeper engagement with the inscriptive traces left on paper and bone. From an appellation inked on a cranium, Eoklo-Emathla, an alternative historical narrative is imaginable. One that contextualizes while working to subvert anonymity and objectification.

To make legible the name Eoklo-Emathla is to represent a cultural system with complex naming patterns (Moore 1995; Swanton 1928; Toomey 1917; Wickman 2006). Emathla, according to John Moore (1995), has several versions—Homarty, *emathlî*, Emarthla, Emarthi, and Emarthlee—and translates into "war leader." It was not a title that Maskókî speakers designated at birth, nor did they use Emathla in a casual, familiar setting. As a "man's civic title," an individual had to earn this honorific (Wickman 2006, 46). Thus, given its association with age, gender, and social status, Emathla signals becoming—not a becoming object but becoming an esteemed, authoritative member of one's community. Connecting this term to historical circumstances, we can also see how its meaning changed. English speakers came to mistranslate Emathla as a surname (Wickman 2006, 46), and so its traditional significance became a casualty of colonialism.

There are many Emathlas discussed in historic texts. In the run-up to the Second Seminole War, the Miccosukee leader Tuckose Emathla (or John Hicks) voiced discontent about removal and White settlers' capture of Blacks who allied with the Seminoles (Klos 1989, 60). Accounts of the Seminole chief Charley Emathla describe how Osceola executed him in November 1835 for supporting emigration to Indian Territory (Missall and Missall 2004, 92). Echo Emathla, originally from the Tallahassee area, is documented as having relocated to Indian Territory by the 1840s (Lancaster 1994, 58). Histories also contain mention of Oclo Archo-Emathla, a Creek warrior (Drake 1854, 436). But, in the case of Eoklo-Emathla,[11] I have yet to come across his appellation in any phonetic form. To evoke his name then is not to recount a personal biography. Nor is it to rechristen, as Samuel did when he designated the skull 707. Rather, the naming of Eoklo-Emathla humanizes a life ended and then expunged by necropolitical conditions and scientific opportunism. Such resurrection is an acknowledgment of ancestral agency. It also reminds us to attend to other aspects of identity and experience erased in the name of science.

On Hybridity

Upside down and on the left parietal of a cranium labeled 408 by Samuel appears the word "Tack." No historic or archival sources mention what, where, or who Tack might have been. Perhaps, like Eoklo-Emathla, this notation represents another name erased from the historic annals. In front of Tack, though right side up and written in a different hand, is "*Negro A.M.*" The racial categorization would be typical were it not for the fact that Samuel's first edition of the *Catalogue* identified the cranium as "Choctaw" (Morton 1840a, 11), which also appears inked across the skull's forehead (or glabellar region). Clarification comes only later, in the form of Samuel's handwritten annotation of the *Catalogue:* "Dr. Wilson, who dissected this man, assures me that he was a full-blooded Choctaw. The skull, however, strongly indicates a mixture of the Negro" (Morton 1840b). The physician in question was Thomas Bellerby Wilson (b. 1807, d. 1865), a Philadelphia local, alumnus of Penn's Medical Department (class of 1830), and naturalist (Ennis et al. 1865). Wilson was an esteemed peer—the two men were emmeshed in the business of the ANS[12]—and so Samuel did not dismiss him outright. Rather, in the revised *Catalogue*, as a concession to categorical ambiguity, he re-identified 408 as "Choctaw and Negro?" (Morton 1849a). The inclusion of a question mark presents an assessment of race that is simultaneously (and confusingly) authoritative, tentative, and more than skin deep.

While the idiosyncratic aspects of "specimen" 408 are intriguing, he is by no means singular. Skulls categorizable by Samuel as "mixed races" presented an especial conundrum for him. In the *Catalogue*, they include "Hispano-Peruvian," "Mulatto," "Negro and Indian," and "Negroid Egyptian," as well as terms like "Cholo" and "Sambo" (Morton 1849a, vi).[13] These individuals were excluded from his calculations of cranial capacity (Morton 1849a, viii–ix), presumably because they complicated Samuel's understanding of race.

In his estimation, race was natural, hierarchical, and discrete. Boundaries based in biology separated different groups. His understanding built on Johann Blumenbach's five-part system of racial division—Caucasian, Mongolian, Malay, American, and Ethiopian. Samuel took the liberty to further subdivide "races" into "families," however, as he explained in the 1839 publication *Crania Americana* (Morton 1839, 4). This finer-grained classification accounted for physical attributes as well as national origin, moral character, and language. In a subsequent publication, he offered a clear, expanded definition of race: "By this term is only meant an indigenous relation to the country they inhabit, and that collective identity of physical traits, mental and moral endowments, language, &c." (Morton 1849a, ix).

Dissimilar from Blumenbach, whose observations fixated on aesthetics, Samuel ranked races' intellectual endowments from superior to inferior (Gould 1981). About the "Caucasian Race," he (1839, 4–7) wrote of their "naturally fair skin" and "highest intellectual endowments." (With his white complexion and British ancestors, he would have fit squarely within this category). Next were "ingenious" Mongolians (Asians) and Malays (Melanesians, Polynesians, and Aboriginal Australians). Members of the "American Race," New World inhabitants like American Indians, possessed a "brown complexion" and were "slow in acquiring knowledge," while black-skinned Ethiopians did "present a singular diversity of intellectual character, of which the far extreme was the lower grade of humanity." Into this latter racial category Samuel slotted the United States' enslaved or freed Africans, situating them in the "Negro Family."

It is more than coincidence that the racial categories recognized as inferior to Caucasians were formally excluded from US citizenship. The nation's body politic was exclusively "White," a designation that went well beyond skin color. In the nineteenth century, Whiteness was an emergent fiction referring to those who were fair of skin, northern European in origin, Anglo-Saxon in heritage, and Protestant in belief (Jacobson 1999; Takaki 1993). During this time, immigrants of southern or eastern European or Celtic background, and Catholic or Jewish religion, qualified as members of the "Caucasian Race," but a racial hierarchy slotted them as lesser variants (or "families" in Samuel's classificatory schema). To reinforce this idea, for the 1850 census, Congress authorized additional questions about place of birth, a first step in distinguishing "native Whites" from "foreign born" ones (figure 4.4). It was also the first census to introduce gradations of Blackness, distinguishing "black" from "mulatto" (evidence of the one-drop rule's official though implicit inception). The prior census only saw "Black" and "White" and divided the former into "Slaves" and "Free Colored Persons."[14] Congress's addition of mulatto to the 1850 census occurred after much debate in the Senate (United States Congress 1850, 671–77). Senator William Dayton from New Jersey, for instance, was an outspoken proponent:

> That, in a word, the mulatto in a certain degree is a *hybrid*! I am informed, too, that the pure black has, in the South, an admitted greater value than the mulatto; that he consumes more, and can do more; that the power of endurance of plantation labor diminishes in proportion to the admixture of white blood. . . . These become important physiological facts, if they be facts. Professor Agassiz, I believe, and others, have even held them and the whites as of an originally different race. . . . I know of nothing that can be incorporated in these census

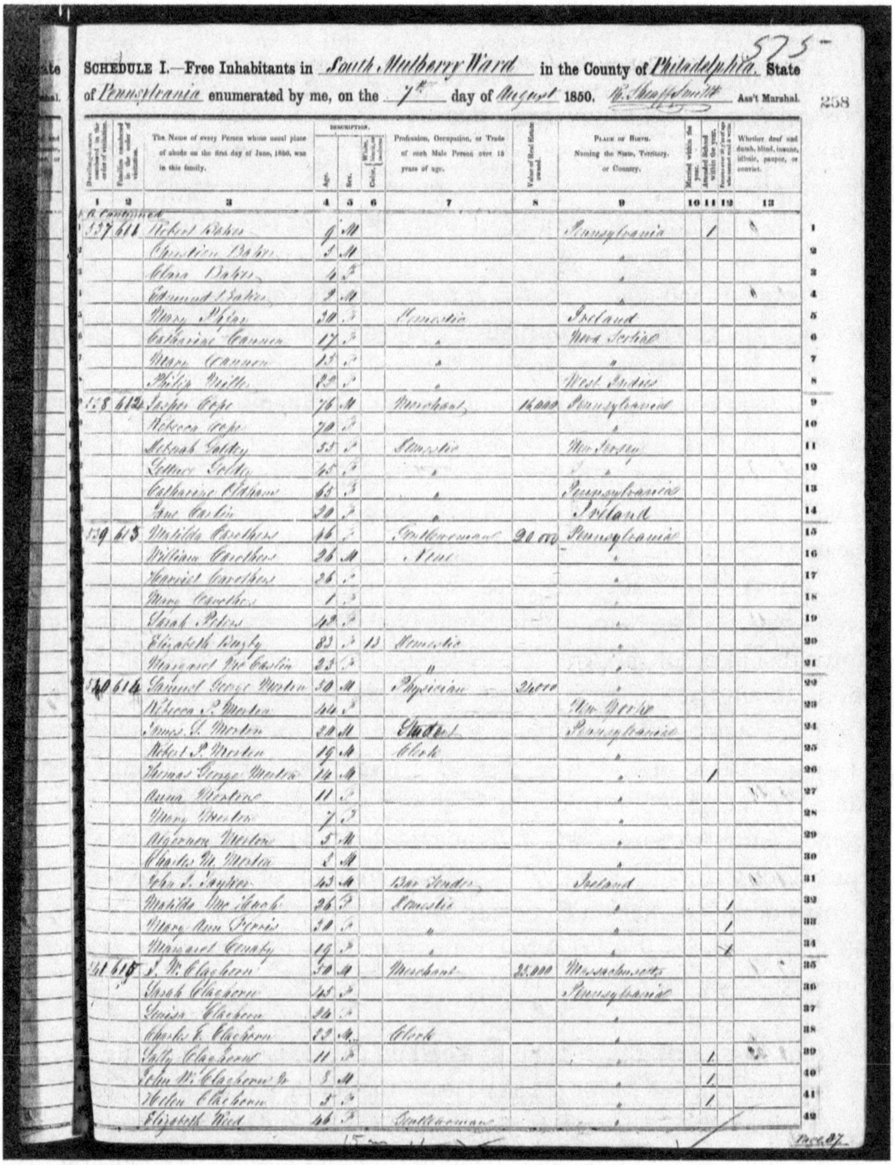

575

SCHEDULE I.—Free Inhabitants in South Mulberry Ward in the County of Philadelphia State of Pennsylvania enumerated by me, on the 7th day of August 1850. [illegible] Ass't Marshal.

258

Dwelling-houses numbered in the order of visitation.	Families numbered in the order of visitation.	The Name of every Person whose usual place of abode on the first day of June, 1850, was in this family.	Age.	Sex.	Color, white, black, or mulatto.	Profession, Occupation, or Trade of each Male Person over 15 years of age.	Value of Real Estate owned.	Place of Birth. Naming the State, Territory, or Country.	Married within the year.	Attended School within the year.	Persons over 20 y'rs of age who cannot read & write.	Whether deaf and dumb, blind, insane, idiotic, pauper, or convict.	
1	2	3	4	5	6	7	8	9	10	11	12	13	
537	611	Robert Baker	9	M				Pennsylvania		1			1
		Christian Baker	3	M				"					2
		Clara Baker	4	F				"					3
		Edmund I. Baker	2	M				"					4
		Mary Phelan	30	F		Domestic		Ireland					5
		Catharine Cannon	17	F		"		Nova Scotia					6
		Mary Cannon	13	F		"		"					7
		Philip Miller	22	F		"		West Indies					8
538	612	Jasper Cope	76	M		Merchant	16,000	Pennsylvania					9
		Rebecca Cope	70	F				"					10
		Deborah Goldey	55	F		Domestic		New Jersey					11
		[illegible] Goldey	45	F		"		"					12
		Catharine Oldham	63	F		"		Pennsylvania					13
		Jane Carlin	20	F		"		Ireland					14
539	613	Matilda Carothers	46	F		Gentlewoman	20,000	Pennsylvania					15
		William Carothers	26	M		None		"					16
		Harriet Carothers	26	F				"					17
		Mary Carothers	1	F				"					18
		Sarah Peters	42	F				"					19
		Elizabeth Wigby	83	F	B	Domestic		"					20
		Margaret McCaslin	23	F		"		"					21
540	614	Samuel George Morton	50	M		Physician	24,000	"					22
		Rebecca P. Morton	44	F				New York					23
		James S. Morton	20	M		Student		Pennsylvania					24
		Robert P. Morton	19	M		Clerk		"					25
		Thomas George Morton	14	M				"		1			26
		Anna Morton	11	F				"					27
		Mary Morton	7	F				"					28
		Algernon Morton	5	M				"					29
		Charles M. Morton	3	M				"					30
		John J. Taylor	43	M		Bar Tender		Ireland					31
		Matilda McHugh	26	F		Domestic		"			1		32
		Mary Ann Ferris	30	F		"		"			1		33
		Margaret Cenaty	19	F		"		"			1		34
541	615	J. M. Clachorn	50	M		Merchant	25,000	Massachusetts					35
		Sarah Clachorn	45	F				Pennsylvania					36
		Louisa Clachorn	24	F				"					37
		Charles E. Clachorn	22	M		Clerk		"					38
		Sally Clachorn	11	F				"		1			39
		John M. Clachorn Jr	8	M				"		1			40
		Helen Clachorn	5	F				"		1			41
		Elizabeth Weed	46	F		Gentlewoman		"					42

Figure 4.4. Page from the 1850 Census with columns' categories and information about Samuel Morton's household. Records of the Bureau of the Census, pp. 49b. National Archives (Microfilm Publication M432, Record Group 29).

statistics that will be more interesting than this very fact to which attention has been called . . . if it does not increase the trouble and expense, the facts ought to be ascertained; for there certainly can be no bad use made of them. (United States Congress 1850, 676)

Hence, legislators had census takers collect information about hybridity to extend research undertaken by scientists like Samuel and Louis Agassiz, to whom I will return shortly. Opponents, on the other hand, argued that such data collection would incur additional and unnecessary expenses for the government; would lack any usefulness; and could be marshaled to "make war on southern institutions" (i.e., enslavement).

Hybridity complicated the matter of race in the day's political and scientific circles. For his part, Samuel grappled with the idea in lectures and publications (Morton 1847, 1850a, 1850b, 1850–1851). Animals were his starting point, though he extrapolated to humans. Mating between distinct species, or races, Samuel argued, resulted in sterile offspring. How then to explain fertile hybrid progeny, those unnatural exceptions to the general law? Much of the answer to this question hinged on one's definition of "species" and acceptance (or dismissal) of fertility as a key trait. With polygenist faith as a foundation, Samuel maintained that fertility was inconsequential. Rather, he argued "that the faculty possessed by different species of animals of producing fertile hybrid offspring, is in proportion to their aptitude for domesticity" (Morton 1847, 22). The extent of domestication and proximity between races could surmount their "natural repugnance" for each other. In his conclusions, Samuel remained adamant about separate origins for distinct human racial groups: "The mere fact that the several races of mankind [sic] produce with each other, a more or less fertile progeny, constitutes, in itself, no proof of the unity of the human species" (1847, 23).

Samuel's ideas on hybridity reached a wide audience. There were fans. Dr. John Perkins Barratt (1846), a medical colleague residing in South Carolina, wrote to Samuel with enthusiasm:

> Mr. Phillips informs me you are preparing a work on hybrids. I congratulate the scientific world on the prospect of such a book by Samuel G. Morton. I have rested satisfied for 25 years that amalgamated races, sooner or later are destined to disappear. The female Mulatto in this country are comparatively barren, while the full blooded Negress breeds like a rabbit. The Genus Homo appears to me to exist under the same laws of geographical distribution—that is presented in the

whole Animal Kingdom. Negroes were created negroes. Education has only beautified them but has not lengthened their nose, or chin, or changed their frizzled wool . . . hair, or done or wrought any other physical miracle. The mixed race exhibits more of the Mother, physically and mentally than of the Father.

Samuel's belief in a plurality of origins for humans resonated with Barratt, who was an avid polygenist and enslaver (Stephens 2014). Indeed, he offered his services should Samuel require additional firsthand observations about hybridity and Black inferiority. Southern towns were a rich source of knowledge, as were the 54 enslaved persons who resided at his plantation. Barratt was more than willing to help in any capacity, he assured Samuel, having long tried to procure skulls for him but with little success. (His enthusiasm for polygenism [and flattery] may be the reason that the ANS made him a correspondent a year later [Academy of Natural Sciences 1877, 18; Stephens 2014, 264].)

Louis Agassiz also shared Samuel's sentiments on hybridity. The Philadelphia physician had left a marked impression on the Swiss scientist when he visited the city in fall of 1846 (Agassiz 1893, 417, 437–38). Over the course of Agassiz's two month stay, the men conversed often and at length in Samuel's library where Samuel's poor health kept him confined (Marcou 1896, 29). But not everyone regarded their relationship in so favorable a light. After Samuel's death, the author of one obituary decried the ungodly, intellectual influence wielded by Agassiz (rather than vice versa): "It is a subject of regret that he adopted Professor Agassiz's theory of the human race, which we regard as of infidel tendency, although we have every reason to believe that it affected not Dr. Morton's views of Bible truth, or diminished his reverence for the Christian religion" (Anonymous n.d. b). Regardless of whose ideology swayed whom, when the United States became his adopted nation, which occurred well after Samuel's death and during the Civil War, Agassiz railed against the threat posed by "half-breeds."

> Conceive for a moment the difference it would make in future ages for the prospect of republican institutions, and our civilization generally, if instead of the *manly* population descended from cognate nations the United States should be inhabited by the *effeminate* progeny of mixed races, half Indian, half negro, sprinkled with white blood. Can you devise a scheme to rescue the Spaniards of Mexico from their degradation? Beware, then, of any policy which may bring our own race to their level. (Agassiz 1893, 603; emphasis added)

The subtle misogyny in his statement is also worth contemplating; hybridity threatened to redefine the body politic in terms of the hybrid *and* the feminine. Somewhat counterintuitively, he regarded "half-breeds" as reason enough for abolishing slavery. To do so would preserve pure races. Half-breeds' sterility would naturally reduce their numbers, while establishment of a national policy, in Agassiz's estimation, would redress miscegenation.

Samuel also had his critics. Charles Darwin, for instance, expressed disapproval after reading his thoughts on hybridity. He was glad to have encountered these ideas, wrote Darwin to Charles Lyell, but they were quite deficient. Particularly troubling to Darwin was Samuel's misunderstanding of hybridity in certain species, a consequence of cherry-picking facts and superficial engagement with original sources. "In conclusion, therefore, I do not think Dr. Morton a safe man to quote from, without going to his authority; nor has he discovered any recondite authorities" (Darwin 1847). Perhaps it is more than coincidence that Darwin, unlike the fawning Barratt, did not become a correspondent in the ANS until 1860, several years after Samuel's death (Academy of Natural Sciences 1877, 21). His writings—first with *On the Origin of Species* (1859) and then *The Descent of Man* (1871)—effectively debunked notions about the plurality of humans' origins, which Samuel had so zealously advanced. Instead, the theory of natural selection elegantly explained the common origin and continued unity of *Homo sapiens*.

Darwin was not the only one to find fault with Samuel's ideas. The Lutheran minister and naturalist John Bachman took him to task in print (1850). Prior to this, Bachman had a long and amicable acquaintance with Samuel (his correspondent membership with the ANS began in 1832). But eventually he came to question much about the Philadelphia physician's take on species, hybridity, and racial differences. One issue Bachman raised pertained to the relationship between facts and theory. "We are fully aware that Dr. Morton intended no more than to present fairly such facts as he supposed could be relied on, in favour of his theory," critiqued Bachman (1850, 42). That is, Samuel labored to consecrate polygeny citing selective examples rather than using theoretical ideas to explain hybrid phenomena. Bachman read those facts—compiled by Samuel in a manner similar to the skulls he collected, secondhand and without on-the-ground observation—in quite a different way. For him, they were evidence of the unity of *Homo sapiens*.

Initially, Samuel was reticent to engage in further discussions with Bachman. But the editors of the *Charleston Medical Journal and Review*, Daniel Cain and Francis Porcher (1850), appealed to his ego. And so, he countered criticisms and clarified his statements about fertile hybrids. He did, however, remain wedded to a plurality of origins for humans (Morton 1850a, 1850b, 1850c). In what was to be one of his last public statements on the matter—remarks made to the ANS less than a month before his death—Samuel suggested that half-breeds were evidence of how miscegenation limited the fertility of pure races (Morton 1850–1851). At the time, he was president of that venerable institution. Samuel's words carried weight. And they continued to after his death, which I turn to in chapter 6, contributing in some capacity to the effacement (or denial) of miscegenation in an expanding United States.

Comparable to the work of topographic engineering, medico-scientific investigations of hybridity solidified boundaries between bodies. The focus was on White superiority and racial purity, or at least advancing these ideas as intrinsic to a founding national myth. To cordon off Whites from Others, social and legal thought promoted anti-miscegenation as early as the seventeenth century (Moran 2001)—the execution of "elaborate boundary work" per Stephan Palmié (2013, 469). But these policies did change over time, reflecting dynamic sociopolitical circumstances and cultural perceptions of different racial groups. Interracial desire between Whites and Blacks was long subject to harsh punishment, but many Whites regarded intermarriage with American Indians as a way for the former to effectively assimilate and civilize the latter (Moran 2001, 18–28, 48–50). There was, however, no legislative regulation of intimate interactions between Blacks and Natives, though their relationships did generate much cause for concern among members of the US government and the public.

Black–American Indian Alliances

The sheltering swamps of Florida offered a refuge to Blacks freed from or enslaved in more northerly states (Missall and Missall 2004, 10). It also presented a prime opportunity for fostering "borderline conditions" (Bhabha 1994, 9)—a hybridity that translated and negotiated geographical permeability, cultural entanglements, and biological confluence. The frontier was a colonial hybrid space though relations between Whites and Others followed a hierarchical racial trope. Interactions between Blacks and American Indians, on the other hand, took myriad forms; hierarchical organization was not the default. Individuals were brought into the fold of Seminole Indian bands through marriage or adoption and then birthed hybrid progeny (see also Forbes 1993, 89; Mulroy 2007, 30, 233). Or groups, known as maroons, formed independent communities and acted as tributary allies (Weik 1997, 2009) and advisers (Porter 1943). Some Seminoles also re-enslaved Blacks (Mulroy 2007; Porter 1943; Simmons 1822).

The US government and White settlers alike had long feared what might come of relations between Blacks and Seminole Indians. The anxiety was warranted. Historian Kenneth Porter (1996, 28) deduced that 15 percent of warriors who fought during the Seminole Wars were Black. The military alliances they fostered with Seminoles were not without good cause. The constant threat of enslavement corroded ontological security and stoked precarity. The Treaty of Moultrie Creek, for instance, required Seminole Indians to apprehend and return enslaved Blacks seeking refuge in Florida (Missall and Missall 2004, 65). But they were reticent to do so. When Indian removal began in earnest, the issue came to a head. Seminole Indians refused to forsake Black allies who risked re-enslavement by Whites and Creeks (Missall and Missall 2004, 83). At the Second Seminole War's outset, Black Seminoles, freed Blacks, and Blacks enslaved by White plantation owners joined with Seminole Indians in rebellion. Together they destroyed 21 plantations in the St. Johns River region, effectively laying to waste the sugar industry in eastern Florida (Potter 1836, 116–20; Wasserman 2010, 242–50). This region was home to Corinna Brown and served as the backdrop for Captain Justin Dimick's celebrated exploits.

Mass-produced pamphlets and broadsides did not represent the actions of American Indians and subjugated Blacks as resistance, rebellion, or emancipation. Instead, captivity narratives, a genre of thinly veiled propaganda that circulated among the American citizenry, described them as "horrid massacres." For example, the graphic foldout *Massacre of the Whites by the Indians and Blacks in Florida* appeared in the pamphlet *An Authentic Narrative of the Seminole War; and of the Miraculous Escape of Mrs. Mary Godfrey, and Her Four Female Children* (figure 4.5). It depicts a composite of prints from other sources, some of which had nothing to do with the Seminole Wars or Florida.[15] Similarly, the pamphlet's written narrative combined news reports about the Second Seminole War with an overview of the tribulations suffered by a White woman and her daughters (though many question Mrs. Godfrey's existence and the story's authenticity). Forced to hide in a Florida swamp, they are rescued by a "humane

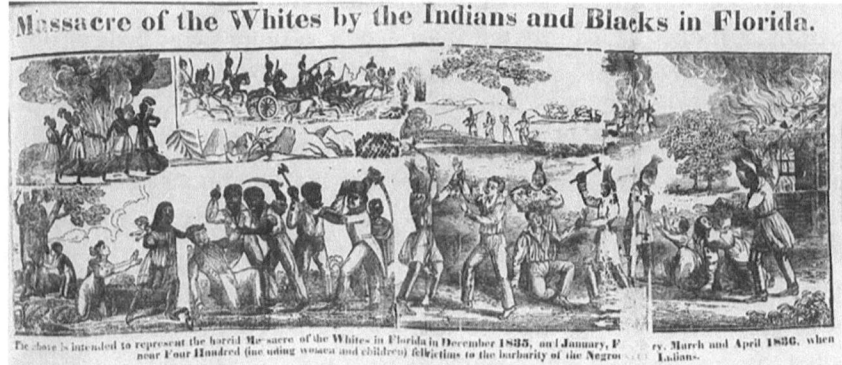

Figure 4.5. *Massacre of the Whites by the Indians and Blacks in Florida* in *An Authentic Narrative of the Seminole War; and of the Miraculous Escape of Mrs. Mary Godfrey*, 1836. Rare Book Division, The New York Public Library. Retrieved from https://digitalcollections.nypl.org/items/510d47db-bbc1-a3d9-e040-e00a18064a99.

African (our deliverer)" (Godfrey 1836, 12); thoughts of his own children, who remained the property of White enslavers, provoked his empathetic response.

For its wide readership, Mrs. Godfrey and her children's suffering was intended to simultaneously evoke horror and support for the war. So went one passage, "The frightful whoopings of the Indians had not ceased; nor were our prospects of escaping with our lives any better, should we attempt leaving our hiding place. Before the close of the day my youngest children began to complain of hunger and thirst; a few wild berries and a little stagnant water was all that could be procured with which to appease either . . . their dreadful forebodings of being seized and murdered by cruel Indians" (Godfrey 1836, 11). The takeaway for readers: even innocents were not safe from the hostility of Indians. As the passage also suggests, most captivity narratives were unapologetically racist, sensationalized, and reiterative in their portrayal of gender (Shire 2016). But in Mrs. Godfrey's tale there is an interesting complication that speaks to the complexity of those times. While Indians were decried as "cruel" and "savage," her savior is depicted as a "friendly negro" (Godfrey 1836, 11). Yet advocacy for abolitionism is not the narrative's aim. Rather, we may read the Black man's actions as a play on the hostile/friendly trope and a portrayal of his deficient parenting. So the story went, he had left his own two children in bondage: "to enjoy his own liberty he had left them to their fate" (Godfrey 1836, 10). Hence, guilt and shame, not an altruistic spirit, compelled his actions.

Mrs. Godfrey's salvation aside, White settlers felt imperiled by both American Indians and Blacks. Major General Thomas S. Jesup, then commander of the US Army, assessed the situation in Florida. "This, you may be assured, is a negro, not an Indian war; and if it be not speedily put down, the South will feel the effects of it on their slave population before the end of the next season," he proclaimed in an 1836 letter to Acting Secretary of War B. F. Butler (as quoted by Montgomery 1839, 269). His words came as no surprise to settlers and soldiers already entrenched in Florida, though they may have alerted government officials in Washington, DC, who resided far from the frontier. So as to circumvent a large-scale slave revolution birthed from the Seminole Wars, Jesup went on to broker various treaties, starting in March 1837 with the Camp Dade accord. These supported westward emigration of Blacks with Seminole Indians (Mulroy 2007, 46–50). But in the accords, Jesup flip-flopped; should Blacks be emancipated once removed to Indian Territory or remain the "bona fide property" of Indians (Mulroy 2007, 48)?

Given the US government's inconsistent positions and persistent violence, Black and Seminole warriors became even closer allies. US Army surgeon Jacob Rhett Motte witnessed the scale of their involvement during the Battle of Lake Okeechobee. "The number of Indians engaged," he wrote (1953, 195), "were estimated from two to three hundred warriors and there were with them probably as many negroes." Casualties for the US Army included seven dead and thirty wounded, but Motte was uncertain about the enemy. "We found one warrior shot through the head; but it might be presumed that they carried off and concealed their dead, according to their custom," he reported (Motte 1953, 195).

Neither of the skulls Abadie collected from the battlefield for Samuel bore gunshot wounds (see chapter 3). But there is evidence to suggest that the decedent numbered 730, a man who died between the ages of 25 and 35 years, was a Black Seminole warrior. Using comparative craniometric analysis to reassess Seminole skulls in the Morton Collection, Christopher Stojanowski and I (2017) identified this individual as "African American" whereas the six other Seminole warriors allocated as "Native American" (per our original wording).[16] If not a Black Seminole, perhaps the decedent had been a freed Black or one "captured" by Natives from a plantation who did not want to be re-enslaved. Such might explain why his body was left on the battlefield and not recovered or concealed in keeping with Seminole practices.

Abadie's collecting proffered additional evidence of hybridity between Blacks and Natives. As mentioned in the prior chapter, he sent Samuel the skull of a boy who had belonged to a Seminole group led by either John Cavallo or Coacoochee (Abadie 1838a). Information about these two men's exploits was extensively chronicled in official documents, news reports, personal correspondences, and more. Yet the volume of writings about John Cavallo and Coacoochee (or Wild Cat) do not guarantee clarity. (Silence, as was the case with Eoklo-Emathla, is not the only factor that can obfuscate a life.) Contingent on the author, they were variably characterized as hostile, brave, audacious, violent, cunning, or tenacious. And variant spellings of their names proliferated.

Historic documents identify John Cavallo as John Horse, Juan Caballo, Cohia, John Cowaya, John Ca-wai-yie, Pease Creek John, and Gopher John, among others (Dixon 2007, 151–54; Mulroy 2007; Wickman 2006, 25, 103). While his identity as a "half-breed" was not in question (Porter 1944, 114), details about his parentage are hazier. Historic sources indicate hybridity all the way down. John Cavallo's mother was Black and his father—who may or may not have been her owner Charles Cavallo (or Imotley)—was Seminole. Mulroy (2007, 35) suggests that John Cavallo's parents also had hybrid identities. His mother may have been Black and American Indian, and his father American Indian and Spanish. After Charles Cavallo's death, John Cavallo's ownership was transferred to a collective of Seminole leaders. Despite enslavement, John Cavallo managed to acquire wealth and authority as the head of a maroon band living on the Ocklawaha (or Oklawaha) River. During the Second Seminole War, he fiercely defied US troops with Coacoochee, a Seminole leader described in several sources as an effective warrior (though prone to performance) (e.g., Denham and Huneycutt 2004, 274; Forry 1928 [1837], 90; Porter 1944, 130; Sprague 1847, 98).

Both men escaped from Fort Marion in St. Augustine following their imprisonment in October 1837. While the event was an important moment in the war, Porter (1944, 114) found that the widely circulated story only highlighted Coacoochee's actions, eliding John Cavallo's part altogether. After their escape, the men formed a tight alliance. They led groups into battle at Lake Okeechobee. And when defeated later in the war, they begrudgingly emigrated (Lancaster 1994, 37, 84). After relocating to Indian Territory, John Cavallo was emancipated in 1842, a reward for financing the move. Coacoochee vouched for his freed status when the proper papers could not be located (Mulroy 2007, 70). They also clashed with Creek Indians who were raiding Black Seminoles' homesteads with the intention of selling them as slaves in Louisiana (Porter 1944, 133). This continued threat of re-enslavement is perhaps one reason John Cavallo led a group of Black Seminoles to Mexico. In 1849, he migrated south joined by Coacoochee and his band, and there they established the village of Wewoka (Porter 1944, 133).

Women and Children

Stories about John Cavallo and Coacoochee's deep friendship bring hybridity, mobility, resistance, and resilience to the fore—a crossing of borders (real and imagined) that counters the making of them by settlers, soldiers, and scientists. But the narrative that links them to Samuel, as communicated by the skull Abadie collected for him, is quieter and far more heartbreaking (see also chapter 3). Analysis indicates that the child had died between the ages of three and five years. Slight cribra orbitalia appears in the left orbital roof, pathology suggestive of malnourishment, chronic infections, and substandard living conditions (Walker et al. 2009). A biohistorical marker of precarity. Though the *Catalogue* contains scant information—it only notes "728. SEMINOLE BOY. Florida. *Dr. Abadie*" (Morton 1840a, 22)—the skull is layered with handwriting. On the child's left frontal and parietal bones, Abadie inked information about provenience:

Boy—3 miles
From Talokc ... Hatchee[17]
or Peas Creek
Lake
...
Seminole
Boy

While we may never know the exact nature of his relationship to John Cavallo or Coacoochee, this child did share with them the experience of a landscape and way of life in dramatic transition.

In the early nineteenth century, American Indians and Blacks settled in the vicinity of Tampa; the former resided closer to Peace River's headwaters while the latter lived near the bay (Rivers and Brown 1997). Prior to the Second Seminole War, around 1826, Charles Cavallo established a village on Lake Thonotosassa where John Cavallo spent his formative years (Mulroy 2007). But, come 1836, US troops—like the Fourth and Sixth regiments that Abadie trekked with as an army surgeon—had destroyed most of the region's villages and crops (Rivers and Brown 1997, 8). For a militia bent on subduing hostiles, these necropolitical strategies proved effective. For Seminole Indians and Blacks, they proved tragic. From destruction came perverse opportunities for Abadie—the skull of a child whose death he regarded as ungrievable. There is a matter-of-factness in his letter to Samuel and a cruelty suggested by the morphing of this subject into a textual object. Abadie's indifference to innocence lost and ontological insecurity spawned contrasts markedly with emotions evoked by captivity narratives like Mary Godfrey's. Whether real or crafted for purposes of propaganda, in her story the White children were ultimately rescued from dislocation, starvation, suffering, and imminent death by a Black man unable to save his own enslaved children.

In circling back to captivity narratives, I wish to stress how they communicate ideas about nationalist enterprise as it pertained to race, gender, and age. Much of this chapter (and the previous one) has recognized how White, heroic, and violent masculinity is at the core of American nation-building. But essentializing narratives about the US body politic also relied on a notion of femininity defined by maternal instincts and domesticity, as well as an understanding of children as future possibility. In the next chapter, I consider how Samuel's colleagues used his craniometric methods to study sex differences, and in so doing buttressed ideas that promoted women's second-class status. Like the racial hybridity these men grappled with in their medico-scientific work, the nineteenth-century United States also included diverse and not easily categorizable socio-sexual lives, those in-between identities that subverted a gender ideology defined by the cult of true womanhood.

5

The Beloved Woman

Dr. Morton was married to Miss Elizabeth Piersoll [*sic*], of Philadelphia, in 1827. From that time, his home was the secure abode of peace, unity, and concord; and the happiness of that charmed intellectual circle was broken only when Disease or Death could burst through the sacred spell of love and hope that bound, as in a protecting zone, its sweet repose![1]
—*New York Daily Times*, 17 January 1852

If Samuel G. Morton has long been a caricature, Mrs. Samuel G. Morton (née Rebecca Grellet Pearsall) is a stubborn silence. As is so often the case for women married to men of science (or politics or law or "great" men in general), their identities are reduced to that of supportive wife. Diminution was certainly applicable to Rebecca. In a portrait, the only one that I uncovered of her during my research, she stares intently and straight on. Rebecca's eyes are expressive and clearly rendered, but her image gradually disappears into the background (Figure 5.1). We see her becoming a trace through the whims of preservation . . . and historic machinations. In written accounts, Rebecca has received minimal and often misspelled mention, the above excerpt from Samuel's obituary being one example. Her furtive effacement presents a contrast to Captain Justin Dimick, whose misidentification occurred after repeated narrations of his heroic, violent deeds undertaken in the service of the nation (see previous chapter). In the few sources that acknowledge Rebecca, her identity—distilled down to daughter, sister, aunt, wife, mother—always and only is represented in terms of the domestic and religious. As I discuss in this chapter, from her life we may learn about Euro-American ideologies of sex, gender, and sexuality in the nineteenth century that reinforced women's second-class citizenship in the body politic.

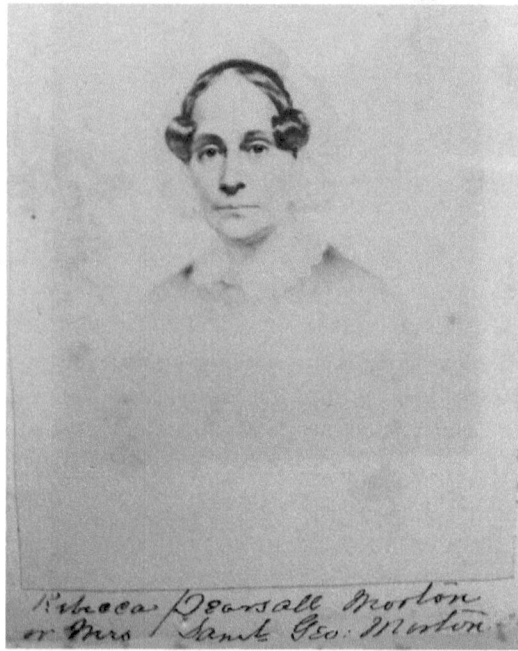

Figure 5.1. A portrait of Rebecca Pearsall Morton, or Mrs. Samuel George Morton, included among the personal correspondences and family photographs compiled by Elizabeth Pearsall Smith; these were interspersed throughout *Recollections of John Jay Smith*. Image courtesy of the Library Company of Philadelphia.

The traces of Rebecca's biography, gleaned from archival materials, indicate that she adhered religiously to the cult of true womanhood. We may also consider how beliefs about appropriate gender identities and actions shaped Samuel's and colleagues' treatment and study of bodily differences. These medical men were instrumental in reifying ideologies that framed nineteenth-century socio-sexual lives; they contributed to a nascent biomedical bodyscape that represented the ideal female body in terms of reproduction, pathology, and disability (Geller 2017). During this juncture, the biopolitical regulation of women's bodies is evident by the growing legitimacy and intervention of medical specializations like obstetrics and gynecology. Limits placed on the bodily autonomy of women deeply constrained their political and economic involvement in American society. But not entirely.

As a counterpoint to Rebecca, this chapter also makes visible sociosexual lives that subverted heteronorms in the nineteenth century. One Philadelphia acquaintance of the Mortons who actively worked to do so was Lucretia Mott. Her commitment to suffrage and abolitionism aimed to expand the definition of American citizenship by bringing women and Blacks into the body politic. Additionally, and beyond the binary of femininity and masculinity, the likelihood of Native warrior or "Beloved" women in the Morton Collection brings us back to hybrid identities not easily categorizable, an issue raised in the previous chapter's consideration of Black Indians. Here "Beloved" represents a title bestowed on certain female-bodied individuals who were active in warfare and political life. Samuel's narrow and analytically expedient classifications of sex could not make sense of these Natives who performed identities or activities he believed masculine. And so, the physician was complicit in their erasure from the nation's historic annals. Yet, in American Indian cultures, this type of socio-sexual variance has historic veracity. Importantly, though, it was not homogeneous across tribal groups. In the nineteenth century, such persons have much to relate about the necropolitical conditions that transformed Native communities' sex/gender systems during European colonialism, Christianization, and US nation-building.

Mrs. Samuel G. Morton

Much of what we know about Rebecca comes from personal recollections penned by other people. She was born in Flushing, Long Island (New York) on 18 June 1805. The youngest of four siblings—three sisters (Rachel, Mary, and Elizabeth) and one brother (Robert Jr.)—Rebecca grew up in a well-respected and tight-knit Quaker family. Her parents Robert W. Pearsall and Elizabeth (née Collins) Pearsall were of English descent and could trace their occupation of the American continent back to the mid-seventeenth century (Jordan 1911, 1405). Her great-great-grandfather, Henry Pearsall was among the first Europeans to settle in Hempstead, Long Island. The land on which he settled, under Dutch jurisdiction at the time, had been purchased from American Indians in 1643 (Jordan 1911, 1404). Soon after arriving in New York, Henry Pearsall and family entered into the Society of Friends. In short order, they manumitted their enslaved Blacks, which, according to Rebecca's eldest sister Rachel, "greatly impaired their fortunes" (Smith 1892, 379). (Rachel and her family were prolific writers, and from their recollections we can extrapolate much about Rebecca's life.)

By all accounts, the Pearsall siblings had an idyllic childhood. "Long Island was the day-dream of my early happiness," wrote Rachel (Smith 1892, 381). While their brother attended the Westtown School in his youth (see chapter 1), the Pearsall sisters were educated closer to home. Robert Jr. did not overlap with Samuel at the boarding school, but he did meet John Jay Smith, who would become his close friend, business partner, and brother-

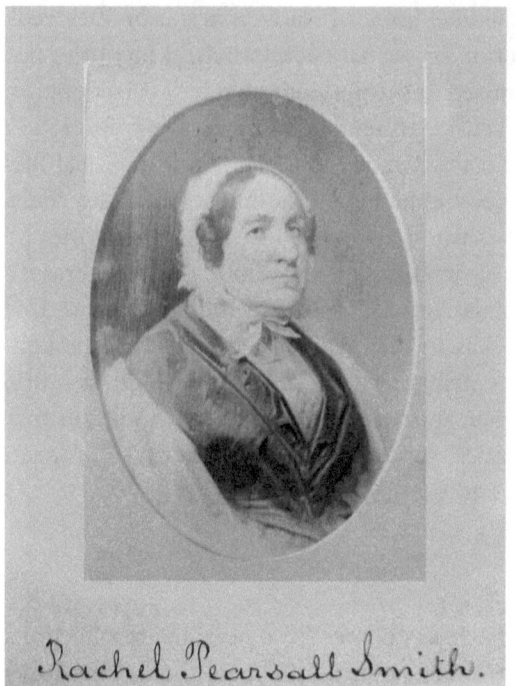

Figure 5.2. A portrait of Rachel Pearsall Smith included among the personal correspondences and family photographs compiled by Elizabeth Pearsall Smith; these were interspersed throughout *Recollections of John Jay Smith*. Image courtesy of the Library Company of Philadelphia.

in-law (in that order). Rachel and John Jay married on 12 April 1821 and took up residence in Philadelphia (figure 5.2). Despite the distance, Rachel stayed in close contact with her family in New York. She returned home often and sent her children for extended stays under the watchful and loving eye of Rebecca. "Aunt Becky" was also a frequent guest in the Smiths' Philadelphia home.

When Robert Sr.'s health began to fail in 1826, the family relocated to Philadelphia.[2] There Rebecca met Samuel, a close friend of both her brother and brother-in-law. At six feet tall with flaxen hair, blue eyes, aquiline nose, and fair complexion (as documented for his passport [Biddle 1833]), Samuel's appearance likely attracted Rebecca as much as his professional potential. Unlike the amorous correspondences that preceded the marriage of Samuel's parents (see chapter 1), the family archives preserved no love letters penned by Rebecca to her husband-to-be, or vice versa. Whether a marriage of convenience or affair of the heart, the two were nevertheless wed in late October of 1827. It was a small gathering. The mayor of Philadelphia, Joseph Watson, officiated at his City Hall office. Friends and family members convened: Rebecca's brother Robert Jr.; sisters Mary,

Elizabeth, and Rachel; her brother-in-law John Jay Smith, Samuel's sister Anna, cousin William R. Clapp, colleague Caspar Wistar Pennock, and Susan Shoemaker (most likely Robert Jr.'s wife who went by Ann).

Despite the happy occasion, their marriage displeased the Philadelphia Quaker community. Rebecca, like Samuel's mother Jane, was chastised for her decision to wed a non-Quaker. "Rebecca P. Morton, late Pearsall," the meeting minutes from 19 December 1827 state, "has deviated from the order of our discipline in the accomplishment of her marriage with a man who is not a member of our religious Society and with the assistance of a Magistrate" (Anonymous 1827b, 232). That neither Samuel's name is mentioned nor his family ties to the Society of Friends suggests a substantial falling out. Despite her husband's removal, Rebecca continued to have a right of membership with Philadelphia's Society of Friends. Her position in the religious order, however, remained uncertain and she vacillated. In the summer of 1843, she was disowned by the Society of Friends. But she did not forsake Christianity, having been brought further into the fold of the city's Episcopalian community (Anonymous 1843).

A little less than a year after marrying, Rebecca was pregnant with the first of her and Samuel's nine children. They named their newborn son James St. Clair (b. 24 September 1828). In due time, Robert Pearsall, George, Thomas George, Anna, William Henry Harrison (who did not survive infancy), Mary Elizabeth, Algernon, and Charles Mortimer followed. Rebecca's fertility and maternal tendencies were likely cause for celebration and emulation. In the first half of the nineteenth century, White women, on average, had six children over their life course (Hacker 2003). Rebecca was above average. Like other women of her generational cohort, race, and class, she spent the majority of her adult life birthing and rearing children, as well as suffering silently in the face of their untimely deaths (Theriot 1996, 22–23). To maintain their growing brood and family home,[3] Rebecca had hired help; the 1850 census, for instance, listed three Irish domestics in residence at the Morton home. Her husband's professional pursuits in medicine and the sciences ensured that the family could afford this bourgeois convenience. The irony being that while Irish immigrants and their labor helped realize a middle-class lifestyle, which became a crucial facet of national identity, they were often denied the full benefits of American citizenship (Warner-Smith 2024).

We may not know the degree to which Rebecca shared Samuel's affinity for skulls. Nor is it clear if she knew about the acts of violation and desecration that preceded their arrival at her door. For many years, Samuel stored the skulls he acquired in his home office (Wood 1853, 13). But this arrangement became less and less tenable as the collection grew, and so Samuel rehoused it at the ANS. As of 1847, it occupied two-thirds of a gallery space. For those skulls that remained in the Morton residence, Rebecca must have tolerated their presence at the very least. As a good Christian wife and mother her deference was expected.

True Womanhood

The rise of true womanhood, an ideology that dominated American gender relations in the first half of the nineteenth century (1820–1860), demanded "piety, purity, submissiveness and domesticity" (Welter 1966, 152). Since Barbara Welter's initial arguments about this cult, subsequent feminist scholars have further attested to and honed ideas about the complex, institutional transformations wrought with the advent of labor's industrialization (e.g., Conway 1982; Cott 1977; Kerber 1988; Kraus 2008; Roberts 2002; Rotman 2009; Ryan 1975; Smith-Rosenberg 1985; Spencer-Wood 1999; Wall 1991). Most indicative were the separate and differentially valued spheres that arose, constraining White, middle-class women to private spaces and granting men the freedom to navigate public ones. For the bourgeoisie, the family as an institution was nuclear in constitution and heteronormative in organization. With time this arrangement became naturalized. Additionally, as connected to a larger project of US nation-building, moralizing—a feminine value informed by religiosity and middle-class values—acted to ameliorate or legitimate the rapacity of masculine activities, like competitive capitalism and violent, colonial expansion (Winter 2004).

More recently, writers have found the trope of true womanhood lacking. Because it glosses over intersectional differences, they stress, this analytical frame cannot address how race, class, religious affiliation, and sexual inclinations informed women's lived experiences (e.g., Cutter 2003; Faulkner 2019). For Rebecca—a White, middle-class, Christian woman, wife, and mother—the traditional framing of womanhood is applicable. While radical activists, prostitutes, actresses (who were on par socially with prostitutes save for Charlotte Cushman), and Indigenous war-women, all of whom I discuss later in this chapter, reveal how ideological aspects of this cult (e.g., separate spheres, passivity, domesticity, compulsory heterosexuality) were immaterial and not absolute. If Samuel is emblematic of the White, Christian, heterosexual, and middle-class men of science who exercised biopower in the nineteenth century, then these women's lives demonstrate the varying effects that anatomo- and biopolitics had on American womanhood in the nineteenth century.

Men traversed boundaries between the public and private sectors with greater ease regardless of their location or class (though not race). Some of this boundary crossing was pragmatic; men may have labored elsewhere, but they returned to the family home at day's end for respite. Such was certainly true for Samuel. As one eulogist wrote: "Quiet and unobtrusive in manner, and fond of the retirement of study, it was only in the privacy of the domestic circle that he could be rightly known; and those that were privileged to approach nearest the *Sanctum Sanctorum* of his happy home, could best see the full beauty of his character" (Patterson 1854, xx). (And for this eulogist, Samuel's affability more strongly defined his character than his intelligence.) In contrast, middle-, and to a certain extent upper-, class women were dissuaded if not outright forbidden from intruding into most public, institutional settings. The church, which provided a pretext for social reform activism, granted a freedom of sorts to women living in the North (Smith-Rosenberg 1985, 109–28). In the South, enslavement and an emphasis on gentility and chivalry reaffirmed White men's paternalism, as well as the dependence, inferiority, and weakness of women (and the enslaved) (Fraser 2013). These regional differences aside, physicians increasingly became an authoritative source about women's socio-sexual experiences and abilities.

The ideology of separate spheres had a profound impact on the field of medicine, most evident in its treatment of reproductive bodies. Prior to the eighteenth century, childbirth fell under the purview of women, midwives, and female kin who fostered a sense of solidarity, a "social childbirth" in the words of Richard Wertz and Dorothy Wertz (1977). Midwives' training was informal, gleaned from personal encounters and maintained by knowledge transmission from generation to generation (McIntosh 2012; Wertz and Wertz 1977). Rather than financial compensation, interactions were of a reciprocal nature; emotional and practical support occurred during labor and into the post-partum period. Midwives' authority, however, did not go uncontested. Indeed, the first person executed in the colony of Massachusetts was the midwife Margaret Jones. Accused of practicing witchcraft, she was hanged in 1648 (Haggard 1929, 69).

A century plus later, when medical schools were established in the American colonies, women were expressly forbidden from enrolling. Were they to acquire medical degrees, they might compete economically with their male counterparts and circumvent biopolitical control of their reproductive capabilities. (The latter fear festered over the years. Come the 1860s, the American Medical Association in collusion with the Catholic church and Protestant clergy first politicized the issue of abortion, advocating for legislation that made it illegal [Smith-Rosenberg 1985, 217–44; Theriot 1996, 45]. Pushback against women's bodily autonomy may have also been a reaction to their entrance into medical schools in the 1850s, sex-segregated though they may have been; see chapter 1's discussion of Sarah Mapps Douglass.) Midwifery counted among the first courses offered to aspiring male physicians at Penn's Medical Department (Medical Faculty of the University of Pennsylvania 1839, 90). Dr. William Shippen Jr. provided instruction. An advertisement he placed in the *Pennsylvania Gazette* (1 January 1765) made clear his opinion of the risk engendered by childbirth and the ineptness of female attendants:

> Having lately been called to the assistance of a number of women in the country in difficult labors, most of which was made so by the unskilled old women about them; the poor women having suffered extremely, and their innocent little ones being entirely destroyed, whose lives might have been easily saved by proper management; and being informed of several desperate cases in the different neighborhoods which have proved fatal to the mothers as to their infants, and were attended with the most painful circumstances, too dismal to be related. (as quoted in Haggard 1929, 71)

In 1810, faculty designated midwifery a stand-alone specialty with Dr. Thomas C. James appointed professor (Shippen had died two years prior). Courses in midwifery became a curricular requirement by 1813 (Medical Faculty of the University of Pennsylvania 1839, 97). Come the late-1830s, the field was linked with children[4] and women's diseases and the term used interchangeably with obstetrics. There was no comparable specialty in men's diseases. Physicians presumed the female body was destined for motherhood, inherently pathological, and required curing in ways that the male body did not.

That medical school did not involve firsthand experience in obstetrics— knowledge was theoretical not practical—did little to deter physicians from practicing it. With a disease model framing their perspective, they portrayed pregnancy as risky and their intervention as necessary. The irony was that risk was in large part generated by medical "advances" (Theriot

1996, 54–56). Forceps endangered newborns. The presence of strange men in an age of sexual modesty induced anxiety for laboring women. Postpartum bacterial infections like puerperal fever, introduced by physicians, increased the likelihood of maternal mortality. Standardized treatments, which came to qualify natural differences as either normal or pathological, were inflexible in the face of variable physiology and life experiences. Reducing women to their pathology and parts—uteri from which hysteria originated, prolapsed pelvic organs, leaky breasts—also made it easier to dismiss them as authoritative sources of knowledge.

Despite the drawbacks, male physicians eventually replaced midwives as childbirth attendants and repositories of knowledge about the female body. What needs explaining is the normalization of a medicalized birth. Stated another way, we may deliberate about symbolic violence—how did women come to relinquish their bodily autonomy? Beyond the sway of gender ideology, there are other plausible explanations. Silvia Federici (2004, 200–206) has historicized this transition, showing how state violence preceded symbolic violence; torture, trials, and execution for witchcraft deterred women from practicing midwifery. For her part, feminist historian Nancy Theriot (1996, 50–51) has pointed to bourgeois women's concern with affirming social status, the seduction of formal training from respectable institutions, and the false hope of new technology (e.g., obstetrical forceps, anesthesia). Physicians also vilified midwives; the former claimed that the latter were ignorant, drunk, and dirty. Rather than a robust corpus of knowledge accumulated over generations, midwifery as practiced by women was represented as a primitive throwback that exacerbated suffering and fatalities.

As an important addendum, much of this discussion is only applicable to White women. Within Black communities, for instance, "granny midwives" continued to serve laboring women well into the early twentieth century (Wilkie 2003). Black women were also far more reticent to embrace the lure of obstetrics and gynecology, having historically fallen victim to necropolitical practices couched as medical experimentation during their enslavement (Owens 2017; Washington 2006). Racial segregation also meant that granny midwives were of limited economic threat to physicians. By the early twentieth century, however, the medical profession's tolerance for Black midwives waned. Physicians effectively campaigned—in the court of public opinion and through political lobbying efforts—to delegitimate their activities while expanding medical authority (Bonaparte 2015; Wilkie 2003).

After usurping control of childbirth from midwives, male physicians did bring female attendants back into the "lying-in chamber" but only as nurses in subordinate positions. With an unapologetic arrogance (or nascent medical paternalism), Dr. Joseph Warrington, a prominent Philadelphia obstetrician, explained in his *The Nurse's Guide* (1839, 14) this de facto hierarchy:

> Since the general concession, that the duty of superintending and aiding a female at the interesting and critical period of parturition, devolves rather upon well-instructed physicians than uneducated midwives, the opinions of a nurse are not unfrequently demanded by the nervous and timid lady, and ingenuity or superstition may often be exercised in the absence of true knowledge; the nurse should, therefore, in all cases, decline any opinion as to the condition of the inquirer, and refer her to the accoucheur [i.e., male physician], who should be regarded as the only person suitable to explain the condition, and direct the conduct of the pregnant or parturient female.

These points were ones that Warrington reiterated throughout the treatise. Nurses were important, he conceded, though not equals. It was the male attendant's education not women's subjective or professional experiences—whether midwife, nurse, or birthing mother—that was valued.

Perhaps the most influential American professor of obstetrics during this time was Dr. Charles Meigs (b. 1792, d. 1869). His thesis on "Prolapsus Uteri"[5] earned him a medical degree from Penn in 1817 (Medical Faculty of the University of Pennsylvania 1839, 52). He went on to translate and publish several books on midwifery, obstetrics, females, and their diseases (e.g., Meigs 1838, 1848, 1849; Velpeau 1831). Though he failed to land a faculty position at Penn's medical school, he was appointed professor of midwifery and the diseases of women and children at Jefferson Medical College. There he taught many cohorts of physicians-in-training from 1841 to 1862 (Bell 1873, 174). He also had a prosperous private medical practice. It is possible, though difficult to confirm, that Meigs, a close friend of Samuel's (he was one of his eulogists), served as Rebecca's obstetrician for at least a few of her nine births.

Meigs was a valued medical colleague to many. The aforementioned Dr. Warrington, for instance, cited him copiously throughout *The Nurse's Guide* (e.g., 1839, 59–62). And after his death in 1869, eulogies followed.

One writer noted that the obstetrician was so committed to his specialty that he willingly compromised his own health in its service (Bell 1873, 172). But Meigs also had vocal critics. They rebuked him for his arrogance and tendency to speculate. Particularly controversial and eventually upended was his position that puerperal fever, which had reached epidemic proportions in Philadelphia during the 1840s, was not a contagious disease (Aptowicz 2014, 164, 254–61; Loudon 2000, 54–55). Also contentious was his take on anesthesia during childbirth. "*What* do you call the pain of parturition? There is no name for it but *Agony*," he lectured (1847, 18–19; emphasis in original). And yet he saw no reason to administer pain relief to women in distress (Meigs 1849, 316–19).

Underpinning Meigs's lessons in female anatomy and best clinical practices were ideas about the cult of true womanhood. In a lecture to the all-male graduating class of Jefferson Medical College, the one in which he remarked on the agony of childbirth, Meigs waxed lyrical on Woman's "gentleness, her docility, her submissiveness, and patience" (1847, 11).[6] She was predisposed to domesticity, he continued. "The household altar is her place of worship and service" (Meigs 1847, 10). In contrast, his statements about men, the "hardier" sex, call to mind the ambition, individualism, and violent heroism discussed in prior chapters. "He pursues the devious track of politics with a resolute will; reaching ever onwards to the possession of fame and patron age, and rank and wealth," Meigs (1847, 15) stated. Men need not worry themselves with religiosity since women were far more inclined: "Hers is a pious mind . . . her confiding nature leads her more readily than men to accept the proffered grace of the Gospel" (Meigs 1847, 13).

Much of what Meigs articulated about womanhood was received wisdom, a biological determinism presumed rather than proved. Though he did marshal scientific studies of certain body parts as further support. Samuel had been kind enough to present Meigs with "one of the most perfect specimens of the female pelvis that" he had ever seen (Meigs 1849, 455). The pelvis had come from a tomb in Thebes containing the burial of a noble Egyptian woman. (Meigs would reciprocate, though a year after Samuel's death, by sending along a skull—taken from a Seminole male from Florida who was 25–35 years old at the time of his death—for inclusion in the cranial collection.[7]) In his textbook *Obstetrics*, Meigs used the pelvis for comparative purposes; this ideal, ancient specimen brought into stark relief modern pelvic deformities that necessitated medical interventions.

On skulls, Meigs and Samuel seem to have been of one mind. "Woman has a head almost too small for intellect but just big enough for love," claimed Meigs (1847, 17). The craniometric assessments that Samuel conducted contributed to this hierarchization of sex (and gender, for during this period they were regarded as one and the same). Yet Samuel did not discuss his methods for determining the sex of the skulls he received. This was not terribly surprising since the development of formal techniques was forthcoming (e.g., Ecker 1868; Welcker 1862). During the first half of the nineteenth century, in absence of biographical information, many scientists seemed to have simply assessed a skull's size. And craniometric methods developed by Samuel likely reified the assumption that a male skull was larger than a female one. Though one eulogist did remark on Samuel's examination of morphological traits. "A small piece of the occiput served as a basis, upon which he put together all the posterior portion of the cranium, showing it by characteristic marks to be that of an adult Indian female," Patterson (1854, xxxix) wrote of a fragmentary, reconstructed skull from the Yucatan.

While readers generally lauded these craniometric studies, some did critique Samuel for failing to deliberate about the link between sex and race (e.g., Hamilton 1850; Hyrtl 1857, 9). In response to an 1850 publication authored by Samuel, a follow-up to *Crania Americana*, William Hamilton (1850, 330–31) stressed: "It is impossible to compare national skulls with national skulls, in respect of their capacity, unless we compare male with male, female with female heads, or, at least, know how many of either sex go to makeup the national complement." To a certain extent the criticism was valid; on average, females' crania are smaller than those of males. But, as aforementioned, this observation (though not universal truth since a bimodal distribution is not the same thing as an absolute binary) was a value-laden one. These scientists presumed that like racial groups, men and women possessed *inherent* differences in intelligence, behaviors, and morality. And they believed that smaller skulls, whether a consequence of sex or race (or both), indicated an arrested stage of intellectual development (e.g., Ecker 1868, 355; Welcker 1862). "We may, therefore, say that the type of the female skull approaches, in many respects, that of the infant, and in a still greater degree that of the lower races," wrote the German scientists Carl Vogt (1864, 81).

Scientific authorities' infantilization justified restricting women's access to education and maintaining their sociopolitical status as second-class citizens. Like children, they were financially dependent, unable to vote, and prohibited from owning property, among other things. Resistance to this narrative grew, however. By the mid-nineteenth century, American feminists proposed a more radical attack on ideologies that maintained separate, unequal spheres between men and women.

Women's Rights

Social angst about sex, gender, and sexuality was part and parcel of a larger national debate about "the social, civil, and religious condition and rights of woman" (Stanton 1848), which formally got underway at the 1848 Seneca Falls Convention in New York. Samuel and Rebecca were certainly not ignorant of these events and the growing women's rights movement. Located a few short blocks from the Mortons' home was the family residence of James Mott and his wife Lucretia Coffin Mott, the famous feminist, abolitionist, and Quaker minister; the couple had chaired and co-convened the convention.[8]

The outcome, the powerful Declaration of Sentiments and Resolutions, advocated broadly for women's equality. Given many attendees' abolitionist activism, the declaration also supported racial equality: "That the equality of human rights results necessarily from the fact of the identity of the race in capabilities and responsibilities" (Stanton 1848). Some signers did balk at the resolution pertaining to women's elective franchise, however. Fredrick Douglass, one of the 32 male signatories, orated in favor of suffrage, helping to swing enough votes for the resolution's passage (McMillen 2008, 93–94). Not at issue was the final, twelfth resolution, which Lucretia had proposed. Convention goers unanimously agreed to secure "woman an equal participation with men in the various trades, professions, and commerce." The success of the women's movement, she stated, was dependent on economic autonomy and access to public spheres.

After the convention, newspapers throughout the United States were quick to report on the events and resolutions that had transpired in Seneca. Some accounts were quite laudatory. The *Seneca County Courier*, for instance, wrote of Lucretia and her political activism in especially glowing terms: "The lady is so well known as a pleasing and eloquent orator, that a description of her manner would be a work of superserogation" (McMillen 2008, 98). Other news outlets condemned the growing women's rights movement. According to the *Philadelphia Public Ledger and Daily Transcript*, a local newspaper that may have passed through the Mortons' household, Lucretia's activism was unnatural. "A wife is everything.... The ladies of Philadelphia . . . are resolved to maintain their rights as Wives, Belles, Virgins, and Mothers, and not as Women," one journalist proclaimed (McMillen 2008, 99).

Archival documents suggest that Samuel and Lucretia were acquainted. Surprisingly, the two had several things in common. Both were raised within the Society of Friends and had spouses from well-connected Quaker families. Lucretia, like Samuel's mother, was a well-respected minister. And both had a complicated relationship with the religion. As Lucretia's abolitionism and involvement in the women's rights movement unfolded, she came to repudiate orthodox Quakerism for a more humanist version preached by Elias Hicks (Faulkner 2011, 42–58; Smith-Rosenberg 1985, 134). (Presumably, Rebecca's religiosity aligned her with the former, more evangelical sect of Quakerism.) Hicksite Quakerism allowed Lucretia to reconcile her religious beliefs and activism. "Among Quakers there had never been any talk of woman's rights—it was simply human rights," she reflected at the twentieth anniversary of the inauguration of the women's rights movement (Mott 1871, 31). She did, however, come to find aspects of Hicksite Quakerism "retrograde," and so Lucretia sought other avenues for contending with intolerance and inequality (Faulkner 2011, 58–59).

Aside from religion, Lucretia and Samuel had also forged a relationship with the phrenologist George Combe. In a January 1845 letter from Combe to Samuel, he implored the latter: "If you chance to meet Mrs. [Anne D.] Morrison or Mrs. Lucretia Mott will you be so kind as present kind remembrances from Mrs. Combe + me to them, and with the same to you and Mrs. Morton." Lucretia reciprocated by making mention of Samuel in her letters to Combe.[9] All three individuals shared an interest in phrenology (see chapter 2). Lucretia initially became intrigued after hearing Combe lecture on the subject during his 1838 visit to Philadelphia (Faulkner 2011, 102; Palmer 2002, 139). Dissimilar from Samuel, however, she embraced those aspects of phrenology that supported her anti-slavery arguments.

Combe and Lucretia's correspondences indicate a mutual respect and general fondness. When he and his wife, Cecilia, were in Philadelphia, they had visited with the Motts. The former returned the hospitality when Lucretia and James traveled England to attend the World's Anti-Slavery Convention in 1840. In an 1841 letter, Combe sought Lucretia's "honest" opinion on his publications, while commending her abolitionism—"the great cause in which your soul is engaged," he wrote. Years later, in 1852, he wrote about her commitment to the women's rights movement. (This letter also lamented the death of Samuel, described by Combe as "a valuable man to science, + one whom we much esteemed.")

> I am glad that you + I agree more nearly than I supposed on the sphere + rights of woman. I think the chief difference between us lies in your taking your own brain and the brains of women equal to your own in size, form, + temperament, as specimens of the average brain of your sex. Such women as you, have brains like men, with the addition of more Philopro. Adhesiveness, + Veneration, + generally less Com[b]ativeness + Destructiveness, although not always so. In consequence, you and your like, are fitted to fill any situation in which insight of character, intellect, + morality are the elements of success, and to such women such places should be open. But the great majority of women have much smaller brains, and are positively unfitted for offices of responsibility, in which energy, deep sagacity, powers of endurance in exertion, + other vigorous efforts are required.

Lucretia Mott by any standards was an exceptional person. But from his statements, it is clear Combe regarded her as exceptional for her sex. Lucretia's abilities and intelligence in his estimation indicated a masculinity, which he did not regard as the general rule. While Combe may have been willing to concede that Lucretia was of superior intelligence, the additional faculties that she possessed (and lacked) reiterated aspects of femininity central to the cult of true womanhood. Philoprogenitiveness, for instance, referred to paternal attachment for one's offspring with an emphasis on maternal love; boys' adhesiveness focused on pets or animals and girls' on dolls (Combe 1825). Such an assessment, one that regarded the female sex as deficient overall, was hardly the fervent support needed to make a case for women's equality.

Regardless, Lucretia's intellectual inquiries and political activism did give rise to a first wave of feminism that eventually resulted in women's suffrage, rights of contract, and property rights. But, similar to Rebecca, there were aspects of her life—her marriage, six children, and domestic responsibilities, for instance—that did little to challenge the day's heteronorms, which most presumed to be biologically determined. Much about sexuality, beyond the monogamous and procreative, also remained a taboo topic for respectable middle-class, White women. Rebecca's sheltered bourgeois existence likely kept her in ignorance of sexual affairs that were transactional or non-conjugal, whereas social reformers like Lucretia championed the salvation of prostitutes as a worthy cause (Klepp 2021, 253–54; Smith-Rosenberg 1985, 109–28).

Fallen Women

Prostitutes appeared "as the most dissolute and lawless of the undeserving poor, as women whose surrender to unlicensed and immoral sexuality threatened the very fabric of society in the new republic" (Newman 2003, 32). Their antisocial behaviors troubled the day's ideas about sex, gender, and sexuality. Their bodies were presumed to be syphilitic, their socioeconomic activities immoral, and their sexual inclinations deviant. Their fall from grace often involved time spent in the almshouse as a punishment. As unbeloved women who advertised love for sale, they generated little compassion in comparison to other varieties of inmates (Newman 2003, 33; Rosenberg 1982, 120–21).

Given his time as a staff physician at the Philadelphia Almshouse's hospital, Samuel interacted often with prostitutes (see chapter 2). The inclusion of one's skull in his collection suggests an indifference to their situation. In his *Catalogue*, Samuel identifies this specimen as "24. ANGLO-AMERICAN Female; a fille-de-joie, aged 26. Died of mania á potu." His use of the euphemism *fille-de-joie* belies her desperate poverty, the precarity of her life. Her cause of death, *mania à potu*, suggests that this fallen woman's final days were spent in the institution's Insanity Department, social and medical norms having long linked alcohol abuse and insanity.

Mania à potu, or delirium tremens, refers to a type of alcoholic insanity, a madness derived from habitual alcohol consumption. As Ric Caric (2007, 453) describes, its symptoms "included tremors over the whole body, intense fearfulness, and hallucinations of walls falling, devils on one's skin, and attacks by murderers as well as intense efforts to ward off hallucinatory threats." He argues that in the first half of the nineteenth century, the condition predominantly affected men. They overconsumed alcohol to ameliorate anxiety induced by the rapid socioeconomic changes of early industrialization. Such gendered associations then worked to further stigmatize women who suffered from its ill effects.

These variations on womanhood—true, radical, and fallen—in the nineteenth-century United States, while suggestive of the messiness of lived experiences, still relied on a heteronormative understanding of sex, gender, and sexuality. Bodies were rigidly dimorphic and divinely designed for different types of labor. Biology was social destiny that transpired in separate spheres. Intimate relationships occurred between opposite sexes and were ideal when contractual, monogamous, and for reproductive purposes but stigmatized when commercialized. For women who deviated from true womanhood, whether intentionally or inadvertently, social repercussions or economic hardships often resulted. White women from the bourgeoisie could better weather the backlash, their class providing a measure of protection. But working and impoverished women, who were already quite vulnerable, could not. As for those individuals of female body and masculine gender identity, a socio-sexual variance that transgressed heteronormativity altogether, they were largely erased from the official versions of American history.

Socio-Sexual Variance

The Walnut Street Theater was just a 15-minute stroll from the Mortons' home. There, in 1842, the renowned American actress Charlotte Cushman took over as stage manager and leading actress. By all accounts, Charlotte was tall (for the day) at five feet and six inches, angular, square-jawed, gray-eyed, and deep-voiced (Merrill 1999, 116). As her career progressed, biographers recount, audiences at home and abroad celebrated her for performing masculine roles, notably tragic Shakespearean ones (Merrill 1999; Wojczuk 2020). For instance, to much acclaim, she played Romeo to her sister Susan's Juliet (figure 5.3). Susan's status as a divorcee was far more controversial than her sister's gender bending performances.[10] Perhaps because her "true" identity as a woman was never in question and her transgressions largely confined to the stage, Charlotte's donning of masculine breeches and bearing was not regarded as a socially subversive act. (Though sentiments would change come the late nineteenth century [Wojczuk 2020].) And her intimate relationships with women, which might have compromised her vision of the theater as a space defined by "respectable" middle-class values, was not public knowledge (Merrill 1999, 52–53). Charlotte's was a strategic approximation of true womanhood. As a working woman—a woman celebrated widely for her work, in fact—she promoted publicly bourgeois sensibilities. If she appeared sexually chaste, a pointed contrast to other actresses of the day, it was only because men held no erotic attraction for her.

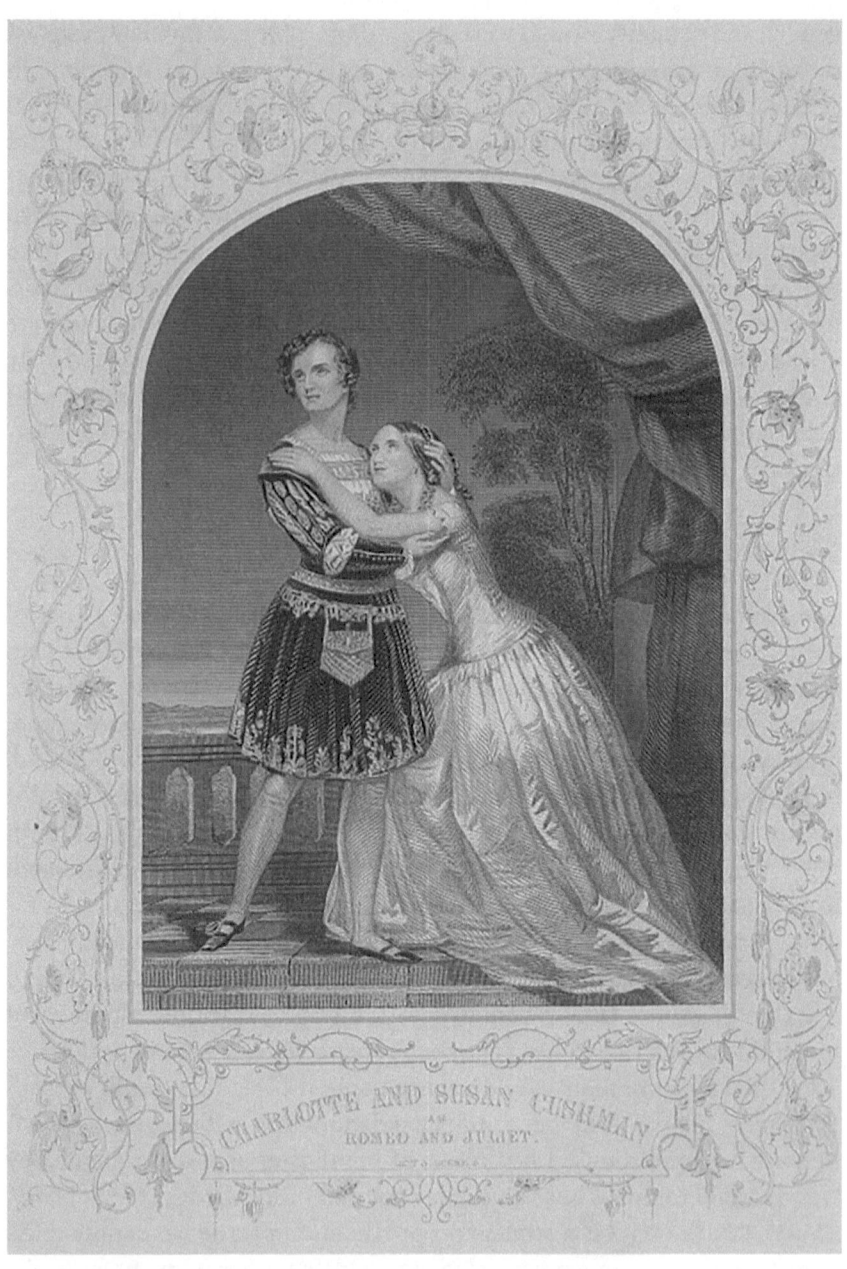

Figure 5.3. The sisters Charlotte and Susan Cushman as Romeo and Juliet. Sketch by Margaret Gillies from an 1846 performance, published by *John Tallis & Company, London & New York*. Library of Congress, Prints & Photographs Division, [LC-DIG-ppmsca-54262]. Retrieved from https://www.loc.gov/item/2017652172/.

For other women, female masculinity was a calculation that reaffirmed heteronormative romance. Narratives about nation-building recount the stories of women who disguised their sex and soldiered on. Patriotism played a part as did financial incentive, but by and large many women fought in the name of love (Blanton and Cook 2002; Hall 1993). During the Civil War, for instance, Frances Clayton passed as a soldier named Jack Williams. She had enlisted in 1861 with her husband and the two fought for the Union until 1862 when he was killed and she was wounded (Tsui 2006, 66–68).

More relevant to the players that populated Samuel's world is a part legend, part ghost story in which Justin Dimick has a crucial part (chapter 4). Like the tales that circulated about his Florida exploits, these accounts also contain various spellings of his surname and emphasize his savvy in the face of ferment (e.g., Baltrusis 2016, 61–65; Snow 1935, 29–33). So it goes, during the Civil War, Dimick commanded Fort Warren on Boston Harbor's Georges Island. Imprisoned within was a young Confederate lieutenant from North Carolina. In an attempt to free him, his newlywed wife, Mrs. Melanie Lanier, traveled to Boston, dressed as a man, and gained access to his cell. With help from other prisoners, they were to tunnel to freedom. The prison break, however, ended in tragedy. Melanie accidentally shot her husband before being captured by Dimick, the intended target of her bullet. With reticence, he sentenced her to hang as a spy. Melanie's last request was that she do so dressed in women's clothing. To avoid her complete disgrace, she was provided with a black robe as a makeshift dress (for acquiescing to this request, Dimick's "humanity" is also described in accounts). Well into the twentieth century, soldiers and visitors to the fort claimed to see her ghost, dubbed the Lady in Black, haunting its corridors. Whether fact or fiction, female masculinity tied to military prowess was not easily squared with ideological beliefs about sex, gender, and sexuality in the nineteenth-century United States. If Melanie Lanier's demise tells us anything, it is that emboldened women wearing breeches suffered the consequences of their actions. Even if those actions were motivated by romantic, heteronormative love.

As for those cultural contexts where such socio-sexual variance was socially acceptable, Euro-Americans took issue. In their historic accounts of Indigenous communities throughout North America, for instance, Christian proselytizers and European colonizers conflated *two-spiritedness* with homosexuality, transvestism, and hermaphroditism. In so doing, they oversimplified the complexities of these socio-sexual lives. These writers failed to see how Two-Spirits conveyed important cultural information about occupational specializations, spiritual sanction, gendered norms, and personal predilections (Jacobs et al. 1997b; Roscoe 1988a, 1988b, 1991, 1998).

Among North America's Indigenous peoples, socio-sexual variance involving female-bodied individuals included queens, warrior women, women chiefs, manly hearted women, and beloved women (Roscoe 1998). In the particular case of warrior women, this category of personhood was not uniform across communities. Some groups recognized Two-Spirits that were anatomically female; they may have been involved in cross- or mixed-gender socioeconomic behavior, partial and/or occasional cross-dressing, and intimate same-sex relations (Roscoe 1998, 73). Other groups had no linguistic designation for warrior women, an absence that suggests gender was situational and fluid—contingent on social circumstances, historical context, and political events.

For Samuel, it would have been difficult if not impossible to comprehend such socio-sexual lives in an age of separate spheres. His dichotomous and deterministic understanding of sex provided no frame of reference. The theater aside, a female-bodied individual wearing breeches, symbols of masculine power and autonomy, was seen as a socially subversive act (Mullenix 2000). And while physicians had much to say about hysteria—his colleague Charles Meigs devoted an entire chapter to the topic in his book *Females and their Diseases* (1848)—they never identified rebellion or anger as acceptable feminine qualities. As a pointed contrast to docile and virtuous White ladies, women of color, like Pocahontas (Green 1975) or Sarah Baartman, the "Hottentot Venus" (Fausto-Sterling 1995), could be (hetero) sexually lustful and conquerable. But female masculinity was another matter altogether. It is not surprising, then, that Samuel failed to identify such gender variant individuals among the skulls he amassed.

A biohistorical analysis has proven useful for revealing the traces of socio-sexual variance in the Morton Collection. Two individuals—one identified as Sioux, the other as Seminole—are intriguing. Samuel labeled them 605 and 708, respectively. I deal with them in turn. Seeing that these individuals come from distinct tribes, they are evidence of the heterogeneous nature of socio-sexual variance in North America. Additionally, their presence invites consideration of the dramatic changes wrought to Native sex/gender systems by settler colonialism and necropolitical conditions.

"Sioux Warrior of Bad Character"

> The *wasicun* do not speak the truth. Their tongues are always forked. They stole our land, our ponies, our way of life and killed the buffalo and our self-respect. They have murdered our women, children, and old people. They burned our tipis, carved our sacred stones, and spat upon the *wicasa wakan* and the *winkte*. They did all of this while talking sweetly to us and promising many things.
> —Little Hawk (1988, 193)

As Samuel explained in *Crania Americana*, the skull he labeled 605 belonged to a "Dacota" or "Sioux warrior of bad character . . . who was killed by some act of violence on the northwestern frontier" (1839, 198) (figure 5.4). Though Samuel's statement about the events precipitating this individual's death seem perfunctory, we can recognize US expansionism at work, as well as the destabilizing effects it had on Sioux communities in the nineteenth century (Westerman and White 2012).

Said Siouxan warrior had come from Dr. William Cox Poole, a fellow graduate of Penn's Medical Department (class of 1824) and respected druggist (DeSilver 1833; Medical Faculty of the University of Pennsylvania 1839, 61). He provided little background information to Samuel, and his untimely death at the age of 39 precluded expansion. Regardless, Samuel later identified the individual as a man from Wisconsin who had died at the age of 20 years (Morton 1849a). He offered no supplemental information about his methods for estimating sex.

Though Samuel seemed certain, additional archival information calls this decedent's sex into question. In the ANS Ledger, the original document cataloguing the institution's holdings, the skull was sexed as a young female. Skeletal analysis also indicates that all dimorphic cranial features were slight, supporting a female sex estimation.[11] The decedent's young age—based on dental calcification and eruption, this person was 17 ± 3 years old—may be one reason characteristic male features were not pronounced, as would be the case with an older individual. But confusion about this decedent's sex may be the point. Given his ideological beliefs about sex (and gender), Samuel would have rejected the notion that this "warrior of bad character" was female.

Traditionally, a division of labor characterized Sioux gender relations; men were hunters and warriors, while women's labor involved caring for

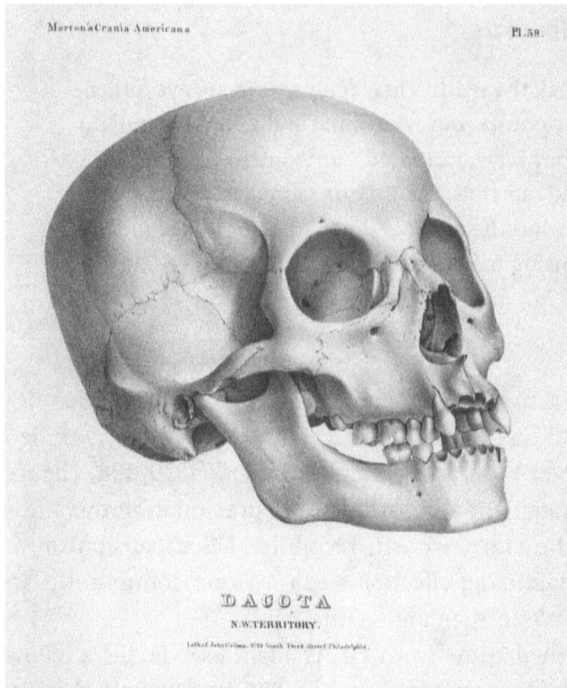

Figure 5.4. "Sioux warrior of bad character... who was killed by some act of violence on the northwestern frontier"; this lithograph of *Dacota, N.W. Territory*, plate 39, by John Collins was described as such and included in *Crania Americana* (1839). General Research Division, The New York Public Library. Retrieved from http://digitalcollections.nypl.org/items/7cf9f2eb-2560-fae1-e040-e00a1806480b.

kin and community through craftwork, homework, food preparation, healing, and so forth (Gagnon 2011, 109–13). But socio-sexual variance was also a facet of Sioux culture with social and ceremonial functions (Brokenleg 2006; Kenny 1988, 29–30; Medicine 2002; Williams 1985). Individuals identified as such represented an ambiguity that was accepted and *wakan*, a concept that conveys mysteriousness, power, and holiness (Walker 1980, 68–74). For male-bodied Two-Spirits, the Lakota used *wi'i'nkte*,[12] a "man who speaks with women's language" (Brokenleg 2006, 5–6), while those of female body included the *lila witkowin*, or "crazy woman" (Kenny 1988, 17; Roscoe 1998, 13–14, 216). The Eastern and Western Dakota labeled the latter *winox:tca' akitcita*, or "women police" (Roscoe 1998, 216). These female-bodied Two-Spirits also had an aversion to opposite-sex marriage and an affinity for same-sex desire (Roscoe 1998, 72). The *lila witkowin* possessed attributes similar to the Double Woman, as Thomas Tyon related:

> But then the woman is very much like a crazy woman (*lila witkowin*). She laughs uncontrollably and so time and time again she acts deceptively (*knayan xkinyelo*). So the people are very afraid of her. She causes

all men who stand near her to become possessed (*wicayuknaxkin*). For that reason these women are called Double Women. They are very promiscuous (*lila hinknatunpi s'a*, repeatedly have many husbands). But then in the things they make nobody excels them. They do much quillwork. From then on, they are very skillful. They also do work like a man. (quoted in Walker 1980, 165–66)

It is possible that this Sioux warrior of supposedly bad character was such a "crazy woman." More certainly, this individual's short life had been a stressful one, as evidenced by active cribra orbitalia. Malnourishment, chronic infections, and substandard living conditions—all possible causes for cribra orbitalia (Walker et al. 2009)—present a type of embodied violence that signaled the precarity of the Sioux Nations' colonial experiences. And with Christian proselytizing and government oversight, the sacred transmuted into the stigmatized and eventually forgotten. Writing with disgust about the "Dance to the Berdashe," which he observed among the Sioux and Sac and Fox, the artist George Catlin declared, "I should wish that it might be extinguished before it be more fully recorded" (as quoted in Donaldson 1886, 313). His statement proved prescient.

Two-Spiritedness in the Southeast

Since the treaty at Fort Jackson there has been several murders Committed above the line by Soldiers & by Citizens. One in particular at the Council house (Tookabatchee) I did not think the murderer would be carried out of the country, but would be executed; but instead of that he was taken over the line. . . . I think hard about the female killed at Tookabatchee, she was a beloved woman.

—Big BW Warrior, Speaker for Upper Creeks, 16 April 1816
(as quoted in Moser et al. 1994, 20)

As in the Sioux Nations, Two-Spirits played an active part in Indigenous communities throughout the Southeast. And, similarly, European writers represented them through a lens distorted by Judeo-Christian beliefs, binaries, and sexual hang-ups. In Florida, sixteenth-century chroniclers described "effeminate youths" and "hermaphrodites" of the Timucua Indians who dressed in feminine garb, carried provisions during war, buried the dead, and cared for the ailing (e.g., Laudonnière 1869, 172, 237, 306; Bry et al. 1591; Roscoe 1988b, 48–50). Of those who participated in warfare, the

French explorer René Goulaine de Laudonnière (1869, 172) wrote, "There are, in all this country, many hermaphrodites, which take all the greatest pain, and bear the victuals when they go to war. They paint their faces much, and stick their hair full of feathers, or down, that they may seem more terrible." The Caddo, Chickasaw, Cherokee, Choctaw, Creek, Natchez, and Yamasee also recognized variants of male Two-Spirits (Roscoe 1988a, 218, 220, 222; Smithers 2014; Williams 1986, 70, 289n22). For Bernard Romans, an eighteenth-century explorer and naturalist, the concern was not uncategorizable bodies (though these individuals' "hermaphroditism" does remain in question) (cf. Adair 1775, 23). Rather, his comments about Indigenous groups in the Southeast reduced their two-spiritedness to sexuality: "Both sexes are wanton to the highest degree, and a certain fashionable disorder is very common among them. Sodomy is also practiced but not to the same excess as among the Creeks and Chicasaws [sic], and the *Cinædi* among the Chactaws [sic] are obliged to dress themselves in woman's attire, and are highly despised especially by the women" (Romans 1776, 82–83; emphasis in original). More than confusion about the socio-sexual variance he witnessed, Romans's characterization betrays a deep aversion to Indigenous sex/gender systems—one that underpinned European and Euro-Americans' efforts to eradicate two-spiritedness and institute heteronormativity.

As for female-bodied Two-Spirits, these socio-sexual lives were not uncommon among Southeastern groups. Among the Choctaw, as Romans observed, some women went to war. "I have several times seen armed women in motion with the [war] parties going in pursuit of the invading enemy, who having completed their intended murder, were flying off," he wrote (1776, 75). In Cherokee communities, "War Women" also earned social prestige from their bravery in combat (Driskill 2016, 160; Miles 2009; Palencia 1987; Perdue 1998; Smithers 2014). Writing in the mid-eighteenth century, the British colonial officer lieutenant Henry Timberlake (1765, 70) took note: "These chiefs, or headmen, likewise compose the assemblies of the nation, into which the war-women are admitted. The reader will not be a little surprised to find the story of Amazons not so great a fable as we imagined, many of the Indian women being as famous in war, as powerful in the council." He continued, "Old warriors likewise, or war-women, who can no longer go to war, but have distinguished themselves in their younger days, have the title of Beloved" (1765, 71). While some writers have conflated War Women and Beloved Women, or *Ghighau* (e.g., Palencia 1987), others have distinguished between the two (e.g., Miles 2009; Perdue

1998). Less is known about the Creek, however. Historic documents held forth on single women's promiscuity but made only abbreviated mention of "Beloved Women" and their involvement in political life (Braund 1990, 22–23, 242; Corkran 1967, 30–31). Given the cultural connections between Southeastern groups, certain beliefs and practices may have been retained in the wake of Seminole ethnogenesis, like women who warred and became Beloved. The decedent that Samuel labeled 708, for instance, may have had such a lived experience.

This decedent's skull was among the "specimens" that US Army surgeon Eugene Abadie shipped to Samuel from Florida. During his time in the frontier zone, from 1837 to 1839, landscapes became depopulated of Native inhabitants while violent military encounters facilitated skull collection from graves and battlefields (see chapter 3). In his *Catalogue*, Samuel identifies 708 as a "SEMINOLE warrior of Florida: woman, ætat. 30. F.A. 730. I.C. 91. Dr. E. H. Abadie" (Morton 1849a). (Though inexplicably, the 1840 edition only notes: "708. SEMINOLE. Florida. *Dr. E. H. Abadie.*") My skeletal and analyses support an age at death between 30 to 40 years old and a female sex estimation. All dimorphic cranial features were intermediary; that is, morphological traits are neither decisively male nor female.[13] This individual also exhibited no marks of trauma but did have evidence of pathology; there was slight, healed cribra orbitalia in both eye sockets and porotic hyperostosis on the posterior portion of the parietal bones.

Seminole women played a crucial role in tribal life. "Like other southeastern Native peoples in the nineteenth century," Laurel Clark Shire (2016, 111–12) relates, "the Seminoles defined all social relationships through matrilineal clan membership." And, as occurred throughout the region, gender complementarity structured relations between women and men (figure 5.5). Seminole women managed and nourished *huti*, or neighboring, clan-related households and their associated lands (Shire 2016, 111–13; Weisman 1989, 47). They did so through farming, trading, childcare, tanning hides, pottery and basketing making, weaving, and more. As described in chapter 3, Seminole women likely sustained the villages and fields that Abadie so casually mentions burning in his postscript to Samuel. Men, on the other hand, traditionally hunted, herded, and engaged in warfare.

As the US government's violent expansionist policies intensified, land disenfranchisement and war came to overshadow all aspects of the Seminoles' way of life. The Seminole Wars "had particularly severe effects on Seminole economy and social and political organization" (Sturtevant and Cattelino 2004, 434). Not least of which, Shire (2016, 113) states, was the

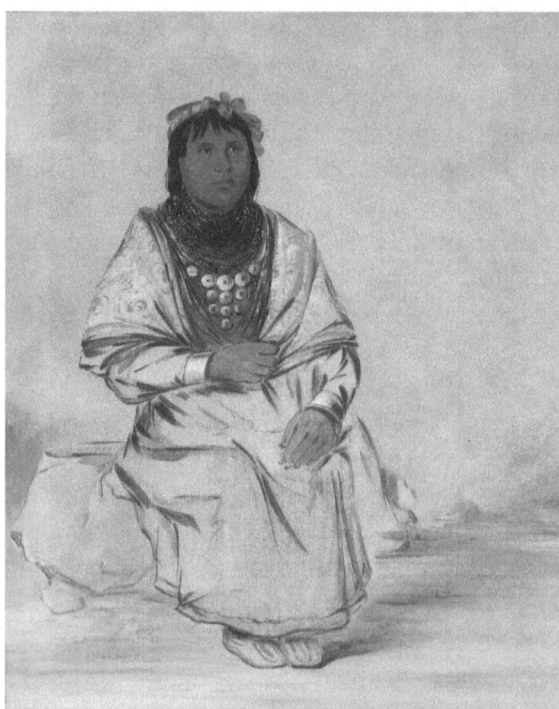

Figure 5.5. *A Seminole Woman*, portrait by George Catlin, 1838, oil on canvas. Smithsonian American Art Museum, gift of Mrs. Joseph Harrison Jr.

creation of a gender imbalance. Based on her in-depth research, she also suggests that US soldiers engaged in martial rape of Seminole women, a desecration of their individual bodies and clans (2016, 119–22). As Private Bartholomew Lynch (1837–1839, 30) lamented in his journal, "If the officers in Tampa would be half as mad to fight Buck Indians as they are to buck Indian Squaws, they would unquestionably be the bravest and gallantest officers in the world. The way they pitch into the squaws is a sin." (Lynch was an Irish immigrant stationed on the Florida frontier from 1837 to 1839 whose criticisms of the US Army touch upon topics that many deemed conversationally impolite or socially inappropriate—soldiers' engagement in prostitution, drunkenness, and thievery, for example.) Accordingly, these moments of cultural crisis and historical trauma generated sociosexual outcomes that either evolved from traditional roles (in the case of the Sioux) or had no earlier precedent (like the Seminole). Regardless, both "crazy" and Beloved women in the nineteenth century—as suggested by the skulls that Samuel labeled 605 and 708, respectively—may have been a strategic response to sociopolitical circumstances characterized by racism, sexism, homophobia, and necropolitical aspects of nation-building.

"Blessed Are the Dead Which Die in the Lord"

After his death, one-third of Samuel's estate transferred to his "beloved wife." As penned in his last will and testament, the meaning of "beloved" departed from its usage among Indigenous tribes. Rebecca was beloved for her devotion to husband, household, and God. Instead of ambiguity and agency, her socio-sexual life was defined by humility and docility. Nevertheless, Samuel made Rebecca keeper of his prized skulls. She seems to have attached no sentimental value to the collection, however, and her curatorial role was short-lived.

It is possible that she saw the whole skull business as a financial liability. Publication of *Crania Americana* had cost the family. Remarks penned in Samuel's will indicate a business deal gone sour. "I take occasion to add that I have lost up to this time upwards of One thousand dollars by said publication owing to the faithless conduct of that person to whom I originally confided the sale of it" (Morton 1849b). An act of God also seems to have intervened, as a handwritten note included in the Morton family's genealogical documents recapped: "Many copies of his 'Crania Americana' lost at sea in a voyage from Phil to Boston—no insurance—a loss he could ill afford to bear" (Anonymous n.d. a, 4). Moreover, Samuel spared little expense when it came to his skulls. He had relied on the kindness of colleagues and friends to cover the freight charges of skulls shipped from distant locales (Patterson 1854, xxx). But when the collection grew too large to house in his office, he paid out of pocket for glass cabinets at the ANS (McFarland and Bennett 1997, 26).

He seems to have regarded his financial woes as a greater impingement on the ANS than his family. Per his will: "I much regret that my large family and the serious losses I had sustained, during the past few years, will not permit me to leave a monied legacy to the Academy of Natural Sciences, an Institution which I have endeavored to serve with my time, and other resources during a period of twenty nine years" (Morton 1849b). The sale of skulls to Samuel's colleagues in 1853, as discussed in the next chapter, only seems to have eased some of the family's financial straits. Thomas, for instance, was forced to leave the University of Pennsylvania at the end of his freshman year. To earn a living, he took a job at J. B. Lippincott & Co.'s publishing house (Anonymous n.d. a, 147). Only after borrowing money from his brother James was Thomas able to afford Penn's enrollment fees and return to medical school (Anonymous n.d. a, 280). He eventually graduated in 1856 and became a prominent Philadelphia surgeon.

Rebecca was more reticent to part with Samuel's many correspondences, a rich trove of information about the decedents included in his collection. While she did consent to his colleagues accessing unpublished manuscripts and letters at the "home-circle" (Gliddon 1854, x), family members did not formally donate his papers to the APS until the mid-twentieth century, well after her death. (The bulk of the correspondences Samuel received are housed at this institution.) Perhaps she thought the letters too revealing about the flexible ethics Samuel exercised in his dogged pursuit of skulls. Or maybe Rebecca was sentimental, the letters invoking her husband in a way that the skulls did not. As a sign of respect, Samuel's ANS colleagues permitted her to visit the library and museum whenever she so desired. We do not know if Rebecca ever took advantage of this offer. It seems unlikely, though. After her husband's death, the family moved from their Philadelphia home on Arch Street to Shoemaker Lane[14] in Germantown (Anonymous n.d. a, 316), a neighborhood situated about eight miles northwest of the city's center. John Jay Smith had built a house for his sister-in-law across the street from the Smith family residence, Ivy Lodge.

Rebecca died on 20 January 1864 at the age of 58. Her funeral was held at St. Luke's Episcopal Church in Germantown. After recording her day of death (mistakenly listed as the 28th of January) and name ("Rebecca P. Morton"), the church's log added the following notation: "(widow of Dr. S. G. Morton)" (Anonymous 1864). Kin then buried Rebecca next to Samuel at Laurel Hill Cemetery, which her brother-in-law had established several decades prior (see chapter 3). Like other family plots at the cemetery, the Mortons' became a shrine to the sacredness of that institution (McDannell 1987, 296). Many offspring birthed by Rebecca were interred within this "dynasty" plot as it expanded with the passing years.

Within a few months' time, James, Rebecca's first-born son, joined her. His burial marks a shift in mortuary practices compelled by the Civil War. James had graduated from West Point the same year Samuel died, 1851. He then went on to serve in the US Corps of Engineers. Come the Civil War, his primary responsibilities involved supervising the construction of defensive fortifications and surveying for the Union Army (Hagerman 1967). While scouting around Petersburg, Virginia, on 17 June 1864, he was shot in the chest and killed. The irony being that James died fighting a war to end the peculiar institution, enslavement of Black Americans, that his father's scientific work had justified. (His brother Thomas also served the nation as an acting assistant surgeon to Philadelphia's general hospitals, caring for sick and wounded Union soldiers [Lewis 1914]). James's body was then preserved and transported back to Philadelphia for burial in the family plot (figure 5.6).

All of these graves lie in the shadow of a stone monument, the details of which contain some latent and significant symbolism. Atop the monument are four neoclassical columns, Doric in design. They "symbolized the durable character of republican virtues" and middle-class values (McDannell 1987, 292). One of the four panels encircling the monument was dedicated to Rebecca (figure 5.7). The epitaph reads:

>REBECCA PEARSALL
>
>WIFE OF
>
>SAMUEL G. MORTON, M.D.
>
>BORN JUNE 18, 1805
>
>DIED JAN. 20, 1864
>
>"BLESSED ARE THE DEAD WHICH DIE IN THE LORD"

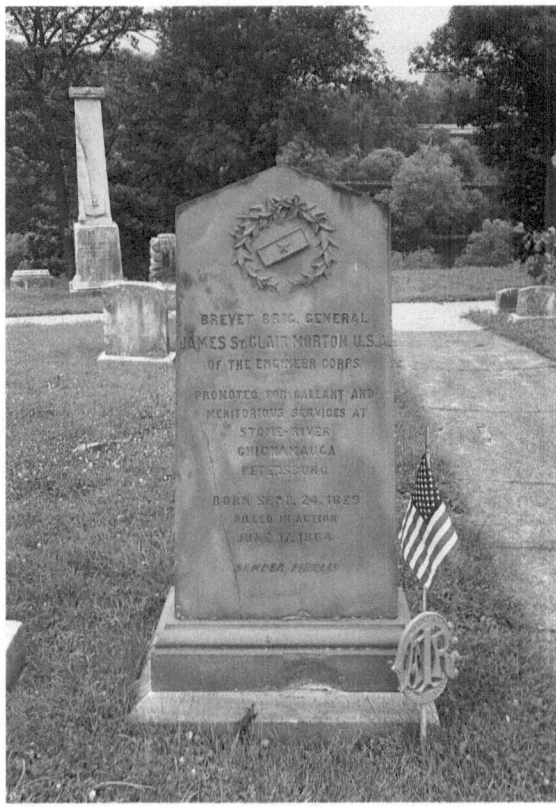

Figure 5.6. Tombstone for James St. Claire Morton. Section G, Plot 179, Laurel Hill Cemetery, Philadelphia, PA. Photograph by author.

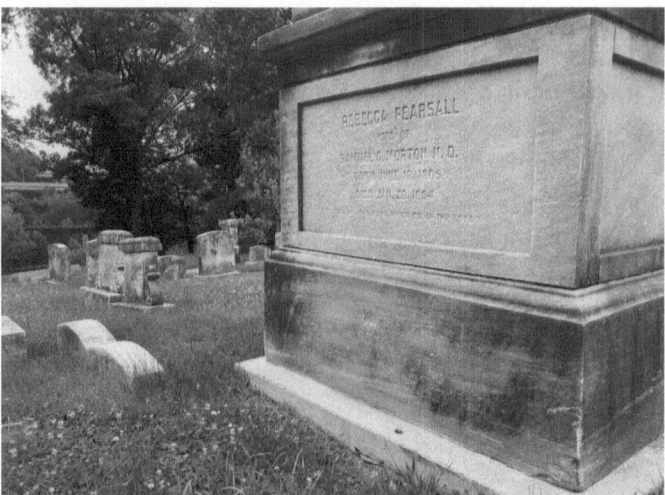

Figure 5.7. Grave markers of "Rebecca P. Morton" (*far left*) and "Samuel G. Morton" adjacent to the monument panel engraved in Rebecca's memory. Section G, Plot 179, Laurel Hill Cemetery, Philadelphia, PA. Photograph by author.

This information is wedged in between the engraved accomplishments of her husband. Despite the use of Rebecca's maiden name, her marital identity is quite clear. The verse from Revelation 14:13 attests to her Christian religiosity, which assured her eternal rest. Thus, taken together, this final resting place affirms how the regulation of women's bodies by medico-scientific practitioners gave rise to motherhood as a biopolitical reality that reinforced their second-class status.

Rebecca's grave remains undisturbed at Laurel Hill Cemetery, a pointed contrast to those of the many Indigenous females whose skulls became objects in the Morton Collection. Having not died in the Lord, they did not warrant the same sanctification. As for those decedents whose biohistorical information suggests the possibility of socio-sexual variance, they demonstrate the profound changes wrought to Indigenous sex/gender systems during European colonialism and US nation-building. To make them visible is a powerful reminder that, given their culture-historical context, such lives were socially acceptable, as well as mutable and situational in the past. Their visibility is part and parcel of a present-day decolonial project, to which I turn in this book's final chapter. As queer Indigenous writers have stressed, they offer a way forward that does not rely on assimilationist cultural tropes undergirded by racism and (hetero)sexism.

6

Legacy

Every generation confronts the task of choosing its past. Inheritances are chosen as much as they are passed on. The past depends less on "what happened then" than on the desires and discontents of the present. Strivings and failures shape the stories we tell. What we recall has as much to do with the terrible things we hope to avoid as with the good life for which we yearn. But when does one decide to stop looking to the past and instead conceive of a new order?

—Saidiya Hartman, *Lose Your Mother:*
A Journey along the Atlantic Slave Route (2007, 100)

At its base, the stone monument marking the Morton family plot contains four inset panels, one for each side. Two are dedicated to Samuel's memory. Engraved on one are the dates of his birth and death. "Physician, Naturalist, and Ethnologist" it reads (figure 6.1). Adjacent to this, a second panel elaborates:

PRESIDENT OF

THE ACADEMY OF NATURAL SCIENCES

OF PHILADELPHIA

AUTHOR OF CRANIA AMERICANA, *etc. etc.*

WHEREVER TRUTH IS LOVED OR SCIENCE

HONORED, HIS NAME WILL BE REVERED

NON MORITUR CUJUS FAMA VIVAT

In contrast to the process of becoming object, which transformed decedents, here we see Samuel becoming ancestor. His careful postmortem treatment. A grave built with grandeur and perpetuity in mind, and interment in proximity to family and friends. Reverential words set in stone. NON MORITUR CUJUS FAMA VIVAT: "He does not die whose fame may survive." The Latin phrase departs from the religious quote etched on the panel dedicated to Rebecca. Samuel's epitaph conveys a learnedness for the ages and the promise of an affecting and abiding legacy.

Legacies are handed down from one generation to the next. Transmission means that they are unlikely to remain static. Some legacies become national mythologies, shorn of their complications and nuances. For example, in portraiture, whether depicted as brave warrior or visionary president, George Washington wears a smile that never reveals the "endentured" teeth he purchased from enslaved or impoverished individuals. Alternatively, the memory of one's fame may fade altogether or turn into infamy. Such was the case for Samuel.

Just a few months prior to his death, Congress passed the first Indian Appropriations Act of many (Kladky 2013, 445–46). The 1851 version allocated funds for relocation of tribes onto reservations—to protect, manage, civilize, or disappear them, depending on who narrates that detail of American history. In two decades' time, a second version of the act prohibited the US government from brokering treaties with American Indians, which effectively negated the latter's sovereignty. Denying their status as independent nations made White settler occupation and dispossession of ancestral lands all the easier. Congress did not grant American Indians citizenship until the Indian Citizenship Act of 1924 (Barnhill 2013, 456), and the privilege to vote remained a state affair well into the mid-twentieth century. Justification for this drawn-out process is also Samuel's legacy given his hand in Indian removal. Legacies, then, can engender suffering. They are not always beneficent.

In this chapter, I reflect on the malleability of Samuel's legacy. After his death, many men scripted eulogies—he was a beloved husband, father, friend, and colleague, they all concluded. But, with time, memories about Samuel and the significance of his work morphed. His contributions to medicine were negated or forgotten, and his historic role in the inception of anthropology became outsized. Critical reflection on the discipline's colonial legacy and policies enacted to address anthropology's sins—the Native American Graves Protection and Repatriation Act (NAGPRA) of 1990 being the most notable—next changed him into a disreputable forefather. He became a cautionary tale about racism's masquerade as objective science. In the wake of the 2020 murder of George Floyd and the racial justice protests his death catalyzed, "White supremacist" now precedes Samuel's name in news coverage and social media posts. The souls of Black folk[1]—

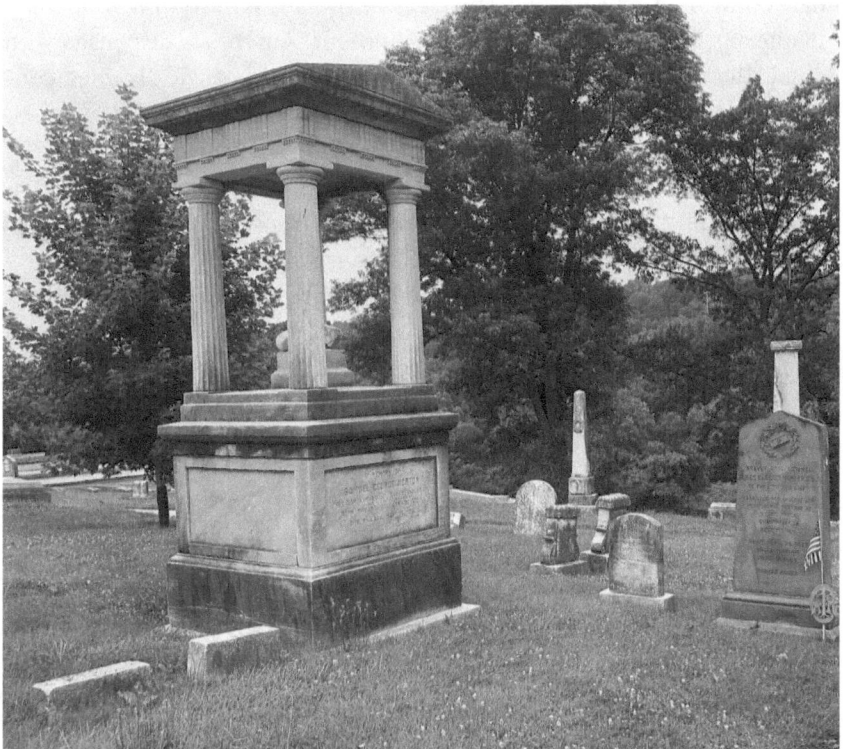

Figure 6.1. Stone monument with panels engraved in Samuel's memory overlooking the Morton family plot. Section G, Plot 179, Laurel Hill Cemetery, Philadelphia, PA. Photograph by author.

those whose skulls make up the collection, and Black Americans more generally—have become a recent priority.

Suffice it to say, Samuel's legacy is no longer regarded as beloved. It has become a burden for researchers, a shameful reminder of complicity. Which begs the question, what are we to do with the tangible remains of that legacy—"his" cranial collection?

In Memoriam

Although Samuel had suffered from poor health for years, his death, at the age of 52 on 15 May 1851, took family and friends by surprise. To determine its cause, six colleagues conducted an autopsy. The formal and respectable affair contrasted with dissections done at the almshouse in several ways (chapter 2). Samuel or his kin granted consent. Autopsists dispensed with casual dismemberment and public spectacle. Cause of death, they concluded, was "meningeal apoplexy." The physicians retained no diseased organs or specimens for their pathological cabinet. A detailed account of their findings then circulated among the medical community (Philadelphia Medical Examiner 1851; see also Fabian 2010, 9–14).

Afterward, as was then typical for White, middle-class, Christian Americans, women may have stepped in to handle Samuel's body. Female kin, friends, or hired help took up the responsibilities of "watchers" and "layers out of the dead" (Weaver 2016). Such gendered death care reiterated the religiosity and domesticity of the cult of true womanhood. This work waned in the mid-nineteenth century for several reasons, as historian Karol Weaver (2016, 45–46) has argued. Caring for the dead became increasingly commercialized and medicalized, and the enormity of loss during the Civil War created logistical and emotional changes (see also Faust 2008). The shift from female death workers to male undertakers mirrors the concomitant rise of obstetricians and demise of midwives, which I discussed in the previous chapter. Samuel's death, however, predated the profound transformation of death work, and so preparation of his autopsied corpse likely fell under the purview of women watchers and layers. A funeral was then held at Grace Church Episcopal Chapel, followed by burial at Laurel Hill Cemetery (Anonymous 1851). At each step of the way, consent from Samuel's kin and respectful treatment of his remains occurred.

Over the next few years, colleagues authored glowing memoirs to commemorate his life (Grant 1852; Meigs 1851; Patterson 1854; Wood 1853). Memoir writing was a common practice among men of medicine and science. Prestigious institutions commissioned these eulogies, which were then read aloud to members and/or published. In general, memoirists followed prescriptive norms. They outlined professional achievements while glossing over the more personal or unsavory aspects of decedents' biographies. There is an emphasis on the formative years, but minimal attention paid to personal relations cultivated as an adult. Wives are mentioned in an abbreviated capacity. Some eulogizers offered posthumous ego stroking, while others revised history. But more importantly, the discursive and performative attributes of a memoir brought nascent medical and scientific fields into being. They legitimized research foci and established best practices. In celebrating select men, memoirs spotlighted personality attributes that fostered scientific inquiry—passion in pursuit but dispassion in judgment, individual industriousness, collegiality, perseverance, and sense of duty even to the detriment of one's health. They, in brief, outlined an aspirational legacy.

In Samuel's case, colleagues extolled his myriad intellectual interests. The obstetrician Charles Meigs was among the first to pen his respects in November of 1851. He read his eulogy to members of the ANS. (Samuel had been appointed president of the academy in 1849; death cut his tenure short). Meigs (1851) remarked on Samuel's "celebrated" collection of skulls and ethnological studies. He also described *Crania Americana* (1839) in effusive terms: "sumptuous," "charming," "instructive," "grave," "full of fervency" (1851, 24–26). In time, other memoirs followed. William Grant (1852) and George Wood (1853) both spoke of Samuel's contributions to medicine—Grant to the Medical Department of Pennsylvania College and Wood the College of Physicians of Philadelphia. A fourth memoir written by Henry Patterson (1854) was included in Josiah Nott and George Gliddon's *Types of Mankind*. "What was most peculiar in him was that magnetic power by which he attracted and bound men to him, and made them glad to serve him," Patterson (1854, xviii) wrote (from his own death bed, no less). But memoirists did downplay (Patterson 1854, xxxii) or disregard (Meigs 1851; Wood 1853) entirely the role that phrenology had played in Samuel's studies of skulls. Perhaps, to salvage his intellectual legacy in the long term, they wished to distance his reputation from the pseudoscience it was becoming. Collectively, these memoirs index Samuel's influence at the time of his death. In brief, he was a gracious colleague who had advanced the practice of medicine and natural history.

Not all writers were so laudatory. Frederick Douglass roundly criticized Samuel during a speech at Western Reserve College (12 July 1854). "The Claims of the Negro Ethnologically Considered" was later published as a pamphlet and distributed widely (Douglass 1999). In it, Douglass derided Samuel and the American school of ethnology spawned by *Crania Americana* and *Crania Aegyptiaca*. (The latter text argued that "Negroes" did populate ancient Egypt but their contributions to civilization were minimal since they primarily served as slaves [Morton 1844, 66].) The scientific racism and polygenism as advanced by "the Notts, the Gliddens [sic], the Agassiz, and Mortons" were especially insidious facets of this school of thought. Douglass made clear the danger in such a position. "For, let it be once granted that the human race are of multitudinous origin, naturally different in their moral, physical, and intellectual capacities, and at once you make plausible a demand for classes, grades and conditions, for different methods of culture, different moral, political, and religious institutions, and a chance is left for slavery, as a necessary institution" (Douglass 1999, 287). Samuel and his colleagues were "pretenders of science"; because their studies were used so nakedly for insidious political ends, they did a disservice to science. But, as Douglass stressed, they did a far bigger disservice to the humanity of "Negroes."[2]

The Slow Fade

The skulls Samuel had amassed were a tangible legacy of his intellectual labor. As for the collection's fate, the terms of his will were clear:

> I wish my Anatomical Collection now deposited in the Academy of Natural Sciences of Philadelphia to be sold whenever circumstances are favorable for such sale and the proceeds to be added to the principal of my estate. But until said collection (consisting chiefly of the skulls of men and animals) can be sold I wish it to remain in the Academy of Natural Sciences in charge of such of my sons as may be of age at the time being. (Morton 1849b, 273)

There was talk of purchase by Mr. James M. Barnard on behalf of Boston's Natural History Society (Warren 1860, 230–31). He was prepared to pay $2,000. Philadelphia's medical men and natural historians were disquieted by the offer, however. Indeed, Charles Meigs had forewarned them about relocation (or removal) of the collection to a new city.

> That Museum of yours is the scientific glory of the United States; and, it is fondly to be hoped, that the wealth and the luxury of Philadelphia, its fame for letters and philosophy, shall not soon have occasion to be ashamed and penitent; as it must be, if that admirable collection, the fruit of so much toil and cares, should be greedily and pitilessly taken from you, not by the greater wealth, but by the far greater liberality and public spirit of foreign nations or individuals. (Meigs 1851, 33)

As a counterbid, in 1853, 42 of Samuel's colleagues offered Rebecca $4,000 (Academy of Natural Sciences 1854, 321–22). They then gifted the skulls—dubbed the Morton Collection—to the ANS. Their decision to do so was motivated by a desire to honor the deceased physician and maintain the museum's holdings; Samuel's collection counted for 918 of the 968 skulls housed in the ANS's south flying-gallery[3] (Patterson 1854, xxx;

Ruschenberger 1852, 31). Rebecca likely found the final purchase price far more satisfactory. Procuring skulls and publishing *Crania Americana* had placed an undue financial burden on the family from which Samuel had never fully recovered (see previous chapter).

Dr. James Aitken Meigs (no relation to Charles) took up the mantle of curating and studying the cranial collection. The ANS had originally offered the position to Dr. Joseph Leidy, but he declined. His biographer Leonard Warren suggests Leidy did so out of a desire to distance himself from scientific debates about race (1998, 193–97). The inevitable religious and social implications of such work were best avoided by serious scientists. Meigs, however, had no such qualms about publicly advancing polygenist ideas. He was fresh out of Jefferson Medical College and eager to make a name for himself. Under his aegis, the collection grew. By 1872, it numbered 1,225 skulls (Meigs 1857, 1866; Renschler and Monge 2008). But what this work ultimately did was help Meigs establish his medical career.[4] Little had changed since Samuel first sought employment. Medicine, not natural history, paid his bills. The Morton Collection provided a means for accumulating symbolic capital he then translated into paying patients and teaching positions. Eventually, Meigs became a prominent physician and was granted a professorship at his alma mater. Presumably his busy schedule curtailed involvement with the ANS and the human skulls housed there. Reflecting on Meigs's writings years later, Aleš Hrdlička noted, "They are only excellent by-products of a mind preoccupied in other though more or less related directions" (1914, 524). After Meigs's death, eulogists only briefly mentioned his involvement with the skulls amassed by Samuel, instead focusing on his contributions to medicine (e.g., Hamilton 1880; Turnbull 1881).

For anthropologists, skull collection continued unabated (Fabian 2010; Redman 2016; Roque 2010; Thomas 2000). Like their predecessors discussed in previous chapters, most researchers offered few details about the logistics of acquiring human remains. Franz Boas was an exception.[5] He wrote candidly about stealing skeletons while conducting fieldwork on the Northwest Coast. "It is most unpleasant work to steal bones from a grave, but what is the use, someone has to do it," Boas penned in his diary ([6 June 1888] in Rohner 1969, 88). He continued, "I dreamed of skulls and bones all last night. I dislike very much working with this stuff; i.e., collecting it, not having it." The diary entries suggest an ambivalence, even an anxiety about desecrating Native graves. But he was not remorseful. The scientific and financial value of skeletons was too compelling for Boas.⁶ Since Samuel had outsourced collecting activities, he never grappled with any such misgivings. Hence the facility with which decedents became objects for him.

As anthropologists began to grow institutions' collections—human remains collected by Boas found their way to the American Museum of Natural History and the US National Museum (Rohner 1969, 83)—active research on the Morton Collection ceased. Hrdlička remained loyal to Samuel's memory but did express qualms in a letter to Edward Nolan, the recording secretary and librarian at the ANS:

> The actual value of the anthropological work of Samuel G. Morton lies only in the fact that it has drawn, more than any other work, the attention of the scientists to the American man, and that it has stimulated further research. His measurements and observations are of only very little value today. He started, as you know, on the premises of phrenology, which later in the century had to be abandoned as entirely groundless. This is about all, I believe, that can be said. The American anthropologists will always have to be grateful to Morton for bringing together the great collection and making the beginnings of American anthropology. (Hrdlička, 1911)

Hrdlička reiterated this position in publications. "Physical Anthropology in the United States, speaking strictly, begins with Samuel G. Morton, in Philadelphia, in 1830," he declared (1914, 512). Yet, he saw nothing portentous in aligning the inception of the subfield with that tragic year, the year of the Indian Removal Act's passage (see chapter 3). Nor was Hrdlička critical of Samuel's opportunistic search for racially distinct skull shapes, which bolstered notions about national identity. Indeed, the two seemed to have more in common than Hrdlička was comfortable admitting. He, too, studied racial differences with a descriptive, typological approach in hand. And, as the curator of physical anthropology collections at the US National Museum (now the National Museum of Natural History), a position that he held from 1904 to 1941, Hrdlička's research contributed to a narrative about the nation's history.

In contrast, and despite the questionable tactics he used to get skeletons, Boas grappled directly with those aspects of Samuel's legacy linked to necropolitics. His consideration of hybridity in "The Half-Blood Indian: An Anthropometric Study" found no evidence that miscegenation produced sterility or degeneracy (Boas 1894). In "Changes in Bodily Form of Descendants of Immigrants" (Boas 1910, 1912), a report submitted to the US Immigration Commission, Boas tackled the effects that environmental change had on cranial plasticity. His findings—that environment and time exert small but measurable changes on head form—debunked Samuel's understanding of race as rigidly typological, fixed, and biologically discrete.[7]

Changes afoot at the ANS also played their part in Samuel's slow fade, an irony, or perhaps a betrayal, given his devotion to the institution. Ethnology and anthropology became less and less relevant with the passing years. An anthropology section, established by ANS members in 1895, was disbanded within three years (Nolan 1909, 30). Come the late-1920s, administrators refocused the institution's research agenda and displays—nonhuman natural history was spotlighted while archaeological and ethnological collections were relegated to dark corners (Mason 1964). The new managing director and president, Charles Meigs Biddle Cadwalader—who had little museum experience and even fewer scruples—attempted to secretly sell several collections to the Museum of the American Indian (MAI), Heye Foundation, of New York City. (Cadwalader also had considerable family money and Charles Meigs as his maternal great-grandfather, which perhaps explains how he acquired the position.)

Cadwalader offered the Morton Collection as an afterthought and with little concern for its continuing care. The big draw for George Heye was Clarence B. Moore's extensive collection of American Indian remains, which aligned with the museum's larger mission to preserve "everything pertaining to our American tribes."[8] Cadwalader's decision to sell, made on the cusp of the Great Depression, was a financial one that eschewed scientific importance. Accordingly, it generated much ire among the scientists associated with the ANS. Though he acquiesced to the sale, Moore referred to Cadwalader as "Mussolini" in correspondences, likening the director to Italy's fascist dictator (Peck and Stroud 2012, 208). For her part, Assistant Curator of Archaeology Harriet Newell Wardle (1929) authored scathing criticism of Cadwalader and his museum practices in *Science*. She then resigned her position.

While Heye happily purchased the Moore Collection, he passed on the Morton Collection. The MAI had established a physical anthropology department in 1915 under the direction of Dr. James B. Clemens, a New York physician (and Heye's brother-in-law). How the subfield might elaborate on "the racial problems of the American aborigines" was a primary concern of the department (Department of Physical Anthropology 1920, 12). Yet, dissimilar from Samuel's collecting practices, the MAI acquired human remains from archaeological and ethnographic expeditions sponsored by Heye and his donors. As a result, they had contextual information that most of the decedents in the Morton Collection lacked.

Their irrelevance was all but confirmed by Heye's disinterest. Accordingly, the skulls were stored in a corner of the ANS beset by leaks (Wardle 1929). The spatial demotion signaled a diminishing of legacy, the *forgetting of objects*. From 1937 until 1942, John Pim Carter, a staff member at the ANS, reexamined and sorted the collection with help from several individuals. But the project was not a priority; he did so "as time allowed." Carter's informal note-taking documented the collection's poor condition. "The collection was found in complete disorder," he observed (1937–1942). Some skulls lacked "serial" numbers. Others were so fragmentary they crumbled to bits. About 100 skulls were missing, most likely due to informal trade agreements between museum directors over the decades. Seeing that Samuel's original correspondences and the skulls were now separate entities, the necropolitical circumstances involved in the latter's collection went unrecollected.

As the twentieth century unfolded, the Morton Collection had served its purpose well enough to engender its own obsolescence. National borders had consolidated. American Indians had all but vanished or were forcibly assimilated. Emancipation had occurred, but equality remained elusive for Black Americans. Jim Crow segregation put them in their "proper" places—at the back of buses and restricted to areas for "Colored Only." The same could be said for women. The 19th Amendment may have granted them the right to vote, but little else had changed about their sociopolitical position in the body politic. Though disputed within the academy, the biological basis of racial and gender hierarchy became received popular wisdom. From the late nineteenth to the early twentieth centuries, Samuel was conjured as a disciplinary ancestor whose scientific research was primitive though by no means pernicious. In the post-WWII years, however, this assessment would change.

"Thousands of Skulls . . . No Brains at All"

"It was only a few months ago that Dr Hooton referred to me for reply a similar query concerning Morton which came to him from Victor von Hagen, who among others, is doing a piece on Morton," wrote M. F. Ashley Montagu (1946). The somewhat confusing greeting prefaced his response to J. Percy Moore, a zoology professor at Penn. Moore was conducting research on William Maclure, and Samuel had written a memoir for the geologist and former ANS president (Morton 1841). Moore attributed subsequent scholars' disdain and dismissal to Samuel's associations with phrenology (Moore 1946–1947). But Montagu added another spin. His letter continued (and is included here in its entirety):

> Physical anthropology as practiced in Morton's day was pretty idiotic activity restricted, for the most part to gentlemen of private means. It consisted in measuring and in describing skulls under the benign impression that this extraordinary activity would somehow lead to the ultimate solution of the relationships of man to one another. As a worker in this arid field Morton did excellent work; he collected, classified, measured, and sumptuously described and published. He was a man after Dr Hrdlicka's own heart . . . like Hrdlicka Morton had thousands of skulls but apparently no brains at all, and like Hrdlicka he had the complete courage of his confusion. He could not have been terribly bright, even for a pre-Mendelian naturalist. He was probably a very nice man, but I should say not an outstanding scientist, and so far as I am aware his influence upon anthropological thought in this country was neither good nor bad not very noticeable. I have somewhere, somehow picked up a warm feeling for the man, and I have rather definitely held him in some respect, but I don't quite know why. Possibly because as a youth I may have been impressed with his Crania Americana, but I now think that he should have known a little better than that. I have never heard the name of Morton mentioned among contemporary anthropologists, and certainly he is entirely without influence upon them. Doubtless some of his theories were discussed by mid-19th century anthropologists, but not for long, they seem to have made no great impress upon the world. At any rate, this is my impression, but I may be entirely wrong. Someone ought to do a thorough study of the man, who from his portrait would seem to have been a very charming man.

While Montagu agreed with Moore that Samuel was a bit player in the history of science, his reflections about the man are an interesting mix of condemnation and affection. (His snide remarks about Hrdlička also contrast with the effusive obituary he authored—"America's most distinguished physical anthropologist," he concluded [Montagu 1944]). Montagu reiterated earlier sentiments about the nineteenth-century physician's amicability. But he disagreed with Hrdlička about Samuel's contribution to anthropology, alluding to the deficiency of his polygenist ideas about human races as separate species. Such beliefs undercut his academic legacy. Montagu is strangely incurious, however, about the cultural evolutionary ideas (i.e., racist, sexist, nationalist tenets) furthered by Samuel's study of skulls. As to why, a brief pause on the biography of Montagu reveals the pliancy of Samuel's legacy. Researchers at the midpoint of the twentieth century may have quickly dismissed him, but Samuel's imprint on anthropological practice is discernible under close inspection.

Born Israel Ehrenberg on 28 June 1905, the future Montagu spent his childhood in London's East End.[9] He was the son of Jewish working-class parents who had emigrated from eastern Europe. Like many Jews living in Russia and Poland during this period, oppressive and violent antisemitism forced westward migration. In the year of Montagu's birth, the British Parliament sought to restrict the increasing flow of such "undesirable" immigrants by passing the Aliens Act (Rubenstein 1996). While England may have granted Jewish immigrants protection from physical harm and a modicum of financial stability, the reactive legislation speaks to a structural, commonsensical variant of racism more difficult to identify and address.

To avoid antisemitism and class bias, Ehrenberg changed his name to Montague Francis Ashley-Montagu a year after enrolling at the University College London (Shipman 1994, 159–60). Several friends had adopted the strategy and Ehrenberg took note. When Montagu immigrated to the United States in 1931, he carried the formal moniker with him across the ocean. After becoming a US citizen in 1940, he dropped the hyphen and added initials. His 1946 letter to Moore, for instance, bore the signature "M. F. Ashley Montagu." Along with his name, he acquired an "upper-class British accent and manner" that belied his humble, Semitic beginnings (Shipman 1994, 160). Dissimilar from the rechristenings we have seen in other chapters—Dimick's signals celebration and Rebecca's effacement—Montagu's chosen alias is an agentive, calculated decision that allowed him to find a foothold in a body politic, first among his British compatriots and later as a US citizen. The creation of a fictive "native" White identity was a form of passing, of border crossing, that yielded professional rewards and personal anxiety (Ginsberg 1996). As a result, Montagu possessed "a heightened sensitivity to possible racism" throughout his life (Shipman 1994, 160). On the latter issue, he proved to be a prolific and eloquent authority (e.g., Montagu 1942, 1964, 1965, 1970, 1975, 1997).

Given his interests in physical anthropology and race, Montagu looked to Boas as a mentor. The latter's complicated relationship with his Jewish heritage may have also been a draw.[10] Boas, a German Jew, had emigrated to escape antisemitism, but, as Leonard Glick (1982, 546) has argued, he then "advocated assimilation to the point of literal disappearance for Jews." Nevertheless, his identity as a Jew surfaced in the research he pursued. For instance, included among the eastern European immigrants Boas sampled in his study of cranial plasticity were Jews from Germany, Lithuania, Poland, Galicia, Russia, Ruthenia, Hungary, and Romania. But Boas also recognized that despite being a Jew he could pass as White (and white) with ease. "I should not go quite so far as to ascribe all racial antagonism to economic factors," he advised Montagu. "When religions happy to be distributed among different types you get the same result, with the difference, of course, that if one party adopts the religion of the others the complication disappears, while a Negro cannot adopt the skin color of the White" (Boas 1939). His words evoke the idea of boundary shifting, a changing understanding of Whiteness at the twentieth century's midpoint.

Montagu was awarded his PhD from Columbia University in 1937. At this early stage in his career, he identified as a "craniologist" (Lieberman et al. 1995, 835). During graduate training and several years after conferral of his degree, he found positions teaching anatomy, first at New York University's College of Dentistry (1931–1938) and then Hahnemann Medical College in Philadelphia (1939–1949). Montagu pursued these jobs after failing to find a physical anthropology position. He even beseeched Boas for employment, but the latter was unable to help. "I hardly know what to answer because there are so many well equipped anthropologists in this country looking for positions," Boas (1931) replied.

As it had for Samuel, teaching anatomy afforded Montagu intellectual opportunities. While he may not have sought to emulate the nineteenth-century physician, it was hard to escape the "common sense" of disciplinary practices established by him and his colleagues. Montagu's study of porion, for instance, is demonstrative (Ashley-Montagu 1939). Experiments and observations about this cranial landmark, located at the upper margin of the ear canal, occurred in the dissecting rooms where he trained medical students. Who were the cadavers that Montagu and his students dissected? By his count, the sample, from NYU and Hahnemann, included 36 White males, 7 White females, 10 "negro" males, 3 "negro" females, and 1 Chinese male (Ashley-Montagu 1939, 284, 292). The likelihood that these individuals were indigent is great. As Ann Garment and colleagues (2007, 1000) explain, "By the early 1900s, nearly all dissected cadavers were unclaimed bodies made available to medical schools through state statutes."

The Pennsylvania legislature first grappled with indigent and unclaimed bodies in the Armstrong Act of 1867 (Forbes 1898; Sappol 2002, 123).[11] The act aimed to deter the dubious acquisition of bodies for dissection, from graveyards and almshouse hospitals, which Samuel and his medical colleagues had normalized (but did not deign to dig up themselves). More stringent measures came in 1883 with passage of the Anatomy Act.[12] The law required public officials to notify a "board of distribution" about the recently deceased in their care. Unless claimed within 36 hours of death, decedents' bodies could "be used within the State for the advancement of medical science." This legislation was crafted by Dr. William S. Forbes (1898) along with William J. McKnight—a rural doctor, convicted grave robber, and state senator—and Dr. William H. Pancoast, a professor of anatomy at Jefferson (Wright 2016). Forbes's professorship of anatomy at Jefferson Medical College seemed to present no conflict of interest. (He was also an alumnus of Penn's Medical Department, class of 1866). Implementation of the policy had several results. It hindered the illicit traffic in cadavers and regulated legal access to unclaimed bodies. The public no longer had to incur the cost of burying indigents, who, in turn, acquired postmortem social value via dissection. Medical school students now had an adequate number of specimens to study. Professors of anatomy no longer feared being accused of colluding with grave robbers. This last outcome was especially important to Forbes who had been arrested and charged with hiring men to steal corpses from Lebanon Cemetery (Forbes 1898).[13] Resurrectionists had long robbed this Black cemetery, much to the distress of Philadelphia's Black community. But up to this point, few men had been held accountable. Unsurprisingly, then, racial tensions flared during Forbes's 1883 trial (Wright 2016). His acquittal, based on insufficient evidence of direct involvement, came at the relief of the medical community and consternation of Black Philadelphians.

Several decades later, the Anatomy Act, with its utilitarian justification for dissecting disenfranchised decedents, was still germane to the work of anatomists. But the moral quandary raised by commonsensical practices may have begun to dawn on Montagu. Starting in the 1930s, economic, social, and political factors were shifting relations between medico-scientists and dead bodies. The Great Depression swelled the numbers of impoverished US citizens. And so, after the public demanded a decent burial for all, state governments began to subsidize funerary costs (Garment et al., 2007, 1002). This welfare legislation also meant that the number of cadavers available for dissection dwindled.

The other prime mover impelling change was World War II. In the mid-1940s, as the horrors of Nazi science came to light, few could ignore the genocidal outcomes wrought from racializing bodies. Natural historians desecrated Jewish cemeteries and collected skulls to study racial differences (Berner 2010; Steinweis 2006). Doctors experimented on the bodies of prisoners, living and dead, in the death camps (Hildebrandt 2016; Proctor 1988). Just two days before Montagu typed his letter to Moore (on 28 January 1946), Marie Claude Vaillant-Couturier, a Gentile and French resistance fighter, testified at Nuremberg. She had survived Auschwitz and Ravensbrück. In painstaking detail, she spoke of gassing, unchecked disease, starvation, daily dehumanization, and medical research.[14] Vaillant-Couturier also described how her treatment had differed from that of Jewish victims.

Though a lapsed Jew, Montagu likely found these revelations grim and galvanizing. His concern for race, which had germinated under Boas's tutelage, only deepened with the onset of World War II. In 1942, he published his first edition of *Man's Most Dangerous Myth: The Fallacy of Race* (1942). The book, in which he argued that race was a social construct, was a direct rejoinder to the White supremacy that had flourished during the American eugenics movement and culminated in the Nazis' Final Solution. (The latter had taken inspiration from homegrown ideologues like Madison Grant [1916].) Montagu's book was widely read and well received. He did have a few critics, however. Wilton Krogman (1943), for instance, found little that was new in the book and much that was confusing, per his review in *American Anthropologist*. Undeterred, Montagu joined an international panel in 1950 tasked with crafting UNESCO's first two Statements on Race. These debunked several cultural evolutionary tenets advanced by Samuel's nineteenth-century studies: there is but one human race; race involves social mythmaking not biological facts; classification of human differences is arbitrary and dynamic but should not be hierarchical or concerned with intelligence; hybridization, that is, race mixing, does not produce deficient offspring.

As for changes in practice, the mid-twentieth century saw the consolidation of bioethics. To guide them during the Nuremberg Doctors' Trial, prosecutors drafted a 10-point code in 1947. This Nuremberg Code brought ethical concepts like non-maleficence and utilitarian justification to the fore, but voluntary consent was its crux. For the first time in history, consent was formalized as a prerequisite for medical research on the living. By the mid-1950s, the ethicality of dissecting the unclaimed and indigent, *those who did not consent*, began to be questioned. "Formal body donation programs," Susan Lederer and Susan Lawrence (2022, 152) explain, "had begun to supplant the decades-long reliance on the anatomy acts that made the bodies of the indigent and unclaimed available for medical education and research." Voluntary donation entailed a "participatory citizenship" of the wider body politic that departed from prior centuries (Lederer and Lawrence 2022, 165). As for legacy collections composed of skeletal remains, however, the issue of consent did not arise for several decades.

Legacy Collection

The histories of legacy collections[15] are rarely conflict-free, as previous chapters in this book have made clear. Myriad types of violences—interpersonal, structural, or institutional—often preceded their consolidation. Though individual initiative was the catalyst for collection, such efforts were usually undertaken in association with an educational or medico-scientific institution. Disenfranchised and vulnerable peoples who did not consent to their inclusion in them constitute most legacy collections. The fragmentation and mobility of these decedents' body parts triggered a process of becoming object, a shift from corporeal subjects to scientific specimens.

Once assembled, a legacy collection necessitates maintaining object, a preservation that belies its continuing dynamism. Because institutions or researchers inherit legacy collections, materials may go missing over time. Biographical or contextualizing records may be lost or archived separately and language rescinded or adopted. "Specimens" may be renumbered and curation standards amended. Institutions may also forsake their inheritance by loaning or deaccessioning a legacy collection. In the past, administrators and curators informally traded select specimens to fill gaps in their holdings. While legacy collections have a contemporary salience (intellectual or methodological), it need not align with the original collector's intent. Etic categories, for instance, may no longer be useful or culturally sensitive as has increasingly become the case for Samuel's racial taxonomy. Because of the circumstances that begot legacy collections—often unsavory or nefarious and certainly unethical by today's standards—researchers now approach them with ambivalence.

There is little to suggest that the Morton Collection saw the light of day for the first half of the twentieth century. Scientists continued to send the ANS skulls, which staff added to the collection, but few researchers referenced it for analytical purposes. In 1966, the ANS arranged to loan the collection to Penn Museum. It was a welcome inheritance. (When the collection was formally accessioned to the museum in 1997, it included approximately 1,300 decedents.) Dr. Wilton (Bill) Marion Krogman was responsible for its stewardship; in addition to serving as curator and professor of physical anthropology, he held an appointment in the Graduate School of Medicine and the School of Dental Medicine. There are multiple reasons Krogman may have found access to the Morton Collection advantageous. From his mentor T. Wingate Todd, he had learned that sizeable skeletal collections benefited teaching and advanced scholastic pursuits.

Todd, who was affiliated with Western Reserve University (later Case Western Reserve), was one of the two physicians responsible for the Hamann-Todd Osteological Collection.[16] Like Samuel, Carl Hamann trained at the University of Pennsylvania's School of Medicine, class of 1890 (University of Pennsylvania 1891, 278). And, like Samuel, he taught comparative anatomy, a field of study he sought to advance by building "an anatomical teaching museum" (Cobb 1959, 234). Hamann started these efforts in 1893, recruiting Todd, a Scottish physician, to replace him in 1912. Under Todd's aegis, the number of skeletons in the collection grew 30-fold. To facilitate collecting, Todd lobbied to rewrite legislation that regulated access to cadavers. As Carlina de la Cova (2021, 158) has documented, decedents were culled from "Cleveland's charity and public hospitals, the city poor farm (including the City Infirmary/Poorhouse, prison workhouse, and the tuberculosis clinic), and Cleveland State Hospital, the city's mental asylum." These institutions were to notify Todd when bodies went unclaimed. Once Todd staked his claim on those destined for the potter's field, the process of becoming object was set in motion. When Todd died in 1936, collecting activities ceased (Muller et al. 2017, 189, 192). His death coincided with shifting public opinions about unclaimed bodies and lack of consent that led to the creation of new policies.

Who are the decedents that make up the Hamann-Todd Collection? Collectively, about 65.5 percent are White and 34.5 percent Black (Muller et al. 2017, table 9.2). Like most unclaimed bodies, precarity contributed to all their deaths. Poverty is surely to blame, but we can also not discount racism. In comparison to Cleveland's total population, the 1920 Census lists Whites' representation at 95.6 percent, while Negroes accounted for 4.3 percent. (The category of "Whites" was further divided into "Native White" [65.6 percent] and "Foreign-born White" [30.1 percent], a distinction laden with significance about the shifting notion of Whiteness during this time.)[17] Hence, while Blacks were a minority population in Cleveland during the early twentieth century, they are overrepresented in the Hamann-Todd Collection (Geller 2021, 108–9). W. Montague Cobb—a student of Todd's who went on to be the first African American PhD in anthropology, a board-certified physician, and eminent physical anthropologist in his own right—explained: "The highest seven causes of death in the cadavera, reveals that the diseases of poverty and exposure—tuberculosis, pneumonia and external causes—have produced more casualties in this group than in the general population" (1935, 161; see also de la Cova 2014). The prevalence of respiratory disease in the collection's Black decedents, he noted, mirrored their high mortality rates in the broader United States.

Cobb went on to establish his own legacy collection at Howard University in 1932, the W. Montague Cobb Human Skeletal Collection (Watkins and Muller 2015). Dissimilar from his colleagues, however, Cobb's collecting was motivated by a research interest in socioeconomic inequity and underpinned by an anti-racist agenda (1935; see also Blakey and Watkins 2022; Watkins 2008).

From Todd and Cobb, Krogman may have recognized the importance of securing a sizeable collection of human remains for comparative anatomical studies. Given his research interests, the Morton Collection seemed to fit the bill. As an associate professor of anatomy and physical anthropology at Western Reserve, he conducted craniological research well into the 1940s (Haviland 1994, 298–99). During this period, he also published several papers about the Seminole Indians and their "race mixture" with Whites and Blacks (e.g., Krogman 1934, 1935a, 1935b, 1936, 1948). In these studies, we can hear echoes of Samuel's work on hybridity though shorn of its opposition to miscegenation (see chapter 4). Once the Morton Collection was ensconced at Penn Museum, however, Krogman does not seem to have actively researched or published on it.[18] It is likely that he found the nonsystematic ways by which Samuel went about collecting skulls—calculated solicitations that produced arbitrary ends—and scant information about biography or provenience as incompatible with the more standardized efforts of colleagues like Todd and Cobb.

Nor did Stephen Jay Gould examine the Morton Collection when he visited Penn Museum to reassess Samuel's findings in the 1970s. At the time, Gould was a professor of geology and a member of the biology and history of science departments at Harvard University. Rather than an inquiry about anthropology, he was interested in the implicit biases that inform objective scientific work more generally. To this end, Gould (1978,

1981) reassessed the "hard" craniometric data included in Samuel's *Crania Americana* (1839), *Crania Aegyptiaca* (1844), and *Catalogue of Skulls of Man and the Inferior Animals* (1849a). Based on his findings, he argued that the good doctor had finagled data to better support a priori ideas about racial ranking. That he did so unconsciously made him no less a racist. Ultimately, Gould's study served to conjoin the name Samuel G. Morton with scientific racism.[19]

Many subsequent scholars have discussed the heavy hand that racism had in making and naturalizing race for Samuel and his medico-scientific colleagues (e.g., Blakey 1987; Fabian 2010; Thomas 2000; Redman 2016; Willoughby 2022). Though, like Gould, few have directly examined the Morton Collection. Instead, they have relied on archival materials and secondary sources.

Researchers who have revisited the skulls have focused on the methodological implications of Samuel's work rather than the ideological ones. Jason Lewis and colleagues (2011), for instance, reanalyzed a portion of the cranial collection (n=308). Their findings indicate that Samuel's scientific methods were "sound" (a suggestion John S. Michael [1988] advanced some two decades earlier). Such technical accuracy, they claim, demonstrates that personal biases did not skew Samuel's results, though it may have done so for Gould. In response, other scholars have found several of their assessments illogical or at least in need of debate (Marks 2011; Tattersall 2013; Weisberg 2014).

More recent methods-focused work has applied technological advances. One initiative, the Open Research Scan Archive (or ORSA), involved the creation of a virtual archive using high-resolution, three-dimensional (3D) computed tomography (CT) imaging. This project, which received funding from the National Science Foundation,[20] was a collaborative effort between then Penn anthropology faculty (Thomas Schoenemann and Janet Monge) and physicians at the Department of Radiology at the Hospital of the University of Pennsylvania.[21] While access to CT scans is contingent on the submission of a clear research proposal, a searchable online database contains information and photographs of the 4,000 plus "specimens" in the archive, inclusive of the Morton Collection. Images of skulls from North America are no longer viewable. The absence of these photographs signals an ethical decision motivated by federal legislation, to which I return shortly. As of fall 2023, all other skulls were still displayed on ORSA (though the site's weblink was disabled come the beginning of 2024). Since creation of the database, researchers have used these CT scans as the basis for additional analyses (e.g., Bastir et al. 2008; Butaric et al. 2010; Schoenemann et al. 2007). But it has become increasingly evident that the sustained utility of the collection neither cancels out Samuel's complicity in necropolitics nor excuses researchers' inattention to this sordid history.

By his own admission, Gould selected Samuel because he presented an obvious and uncontroversial case study of finagling. "Since contemporary examples may be too threatening to inspire a general acknowledgment of the phenomenon," he explained, "I present Morton on cranial capacity—an excellent example because the case is so distant and the controlling a priori so clear" (1978, 505). Passage of NAGPRA in 1990 would prove Gould mistaken. The federal law sought to redress the interpersonal violence of colonial expansionism that begot collections like the one amassed by Samuel. (Legal practice sometimes aspires to be ethical praxis.) But the law also stressed that the past was prologue—not distant, not obvious, and certainly not undisputed. That is, sustained analysis or "ownership" of decedents could result in ontological insecurity for living descendants, as well as maintain the power imbalances that perpetuate structural violence.

Descendants

In 1997, the ANS transferred formal ownership of the Morton Collection to Penn Museum. Penn faculty had long used the collection for teaching purposes, and now the responsibility of complying with NAGPRA became a priority.[22] As I discuss in the book's preface, I first interacted with the Morton Collection in the early 1990s while an undergraduate anthropology major at Penn. My classroom's cabinets housed its skulls. Into the aughts, and now a doctoral student, I was hired as a NAGPRA project assistant tasked with inventorying the legacy collection. With the passing years, my ambivalence has grown, a consequence of several factors. My increasing knowledge about the violent settler colonialism and necropolitics that yielded scientific opportunity for Samuel is one reason. Extended deliberation about the ethics of studying human remains has also come to inform my thinking, as well my own positionality and privileges.

I am a White scholar. But my Jewish ancestors' experiences align more with those of Boas and Montagu than they do with Samuel. Antisemitism impelled their emigration from Poland and Russia in the early twentieth century. My great-grandparents and grandparents disembarked in Baltimore and Philadelphia as "aliens" and became naturalized US citizens within the decade (figure 6.2). Their racial categorization as Caucasian

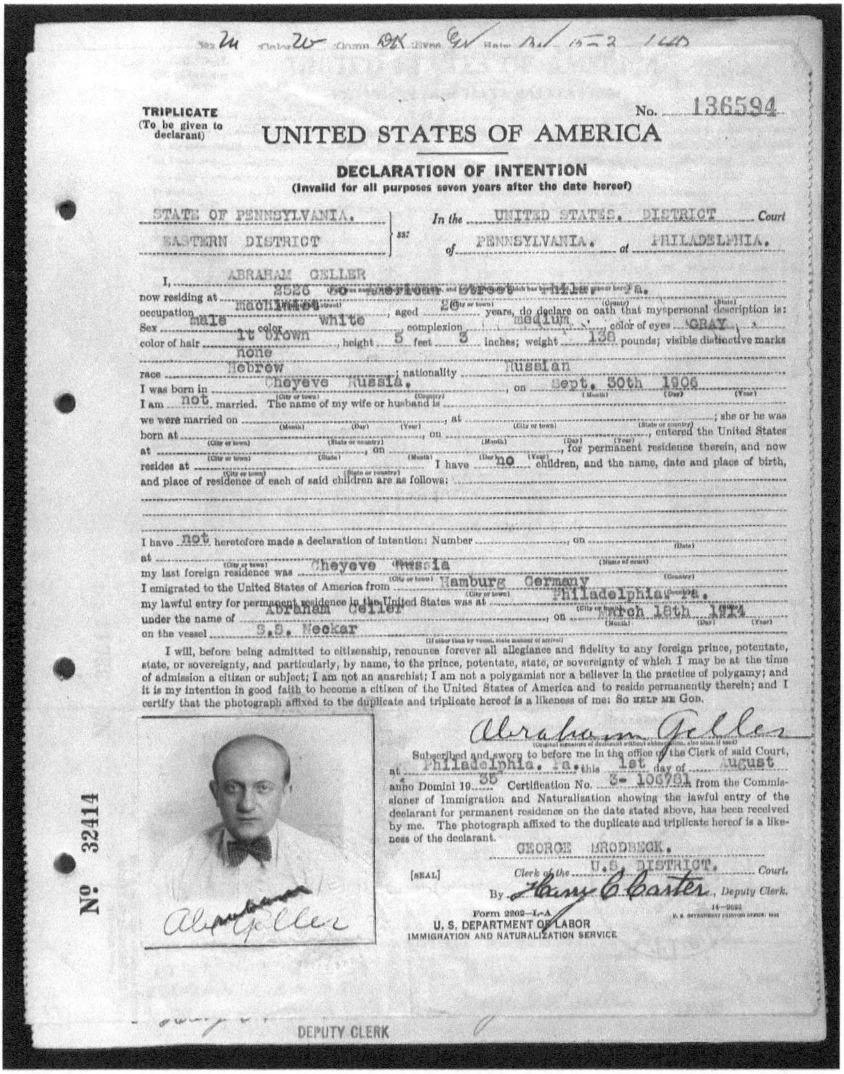

Figure 6.2. The naturalization papers of the author's paternal grandfather, Abraham Geller. Note that race is listed as "Hebrew." Photograph by author.

may have expedited this process, but they remained a part of a community apart. They spoke Yiddish at home, maintained a separate religious calendar, and occupied redlined neighborhoods. But they also embraced their national identity. My maternal grandfather fought in World War II, pulling the dead bodies of his fellow soldiers from Italian battlefields. Around his neck were dog tags embossed with an H for Hebrew, distinguishing him

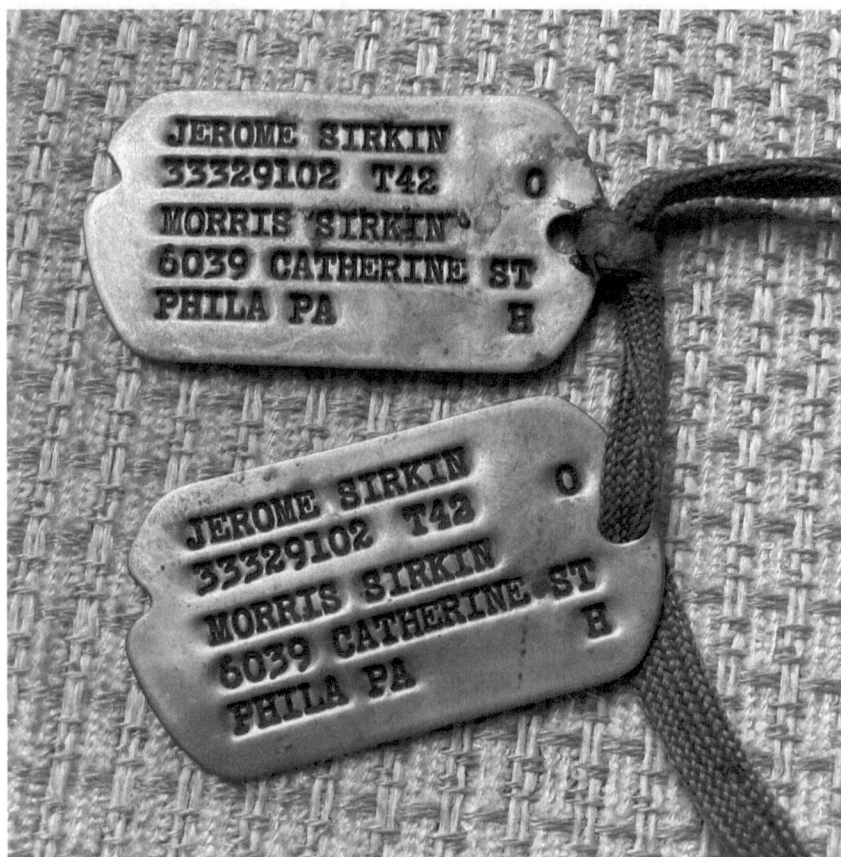

Figure 6.3. World War II dog tags for the author's maternal grandfather, Jerome Sirkin. Note the H in the righthand corner for Hebrew. Photograph by author.

from the Ps for Protestants and Cs for Catholics (the only three religions recognized by the US military at the time) (figure 6.3). Should one die in the line of duty, religious information ensured the proper performance of funerary rites and handling of remains.

Near the war's conclusion, the Polish jurist Raphael Lemkin coined the term *genocide*: "New conceptions require new terms. By 'genocide' we mean the destruction of a nation or of an ethnic group. This new word, coined by the author to denote an old practice in its modern development, is made from the ancient Greek word *genos* (race, tribe) and the Latin *cide* (killing)" (Lemkin 1944, 79). A hitherto inexpressibility, a crime without a name in the words of Winston Churchill, that intertwined power, violence, and identity. Both of my parents were born into a world forced to grapple—existentially, intellectually, punitively—with the repercussions of genocide. Five days after my mother's birth the International Medical Tribunal at Nuremberg (on 19 August 1947), referencing the 10-point code it had drafted, found Nazi doctors guilty of war crimes and crimes against humanity. Their actions, which had been alchemized from American eugenics, Jim Crow segregation, and Nazi political ideology, predominantly targeted European Jews. In the wake of World War II, many Holocaust survivors came to the United States; the Miami Beach neighborhood where I have lived since 2009 had the third-largest population in the world. Jews in America, like my family in Philadelphia and transplants to South Florida, gradually assimilated. Racially, they identified or passed as White and thereby accrued middle-class privileges. But antisemitism was and is still a thing, and so their history and culture made them all too cognizant of the dangers of White supremacist ideology.

This story, my history, has imparted a deeper understanding of nationalism and necropolitics. A desire to conduct research that does no harm—research that does good. Of course, I also recognize that when you study legacy collections—often composed of decedents who did not consent and whose descendants grapple with their own legacy of trauma and survival—that such a desire may be naïve. That concessions must occur, humility is necessary, and a good death should be forthcoming.

When I returned to the Morton Collection in the 2010s, I did not come with questions about genocide in hand. Lemkin coined the term to understand European phenomena though envisioned a broader applicability. Yet, in response to a 1951 petition advanced by the Civil Rights Congress to the United Nations that charged the US government with committing genocide against Black Americans (Patterson 1951), Lemkin (1953) wrote a pointed letter to the *New York Times*. Discrimination, he averred, should not be confused for genocide. Nor might he have found the concept germane to American Indians' experiences of settler colonialism, forced relocations and reservations, assimilation protocols like boarding schools, and so forth. Nevertheless, many subsequent writers have evoked genocide to qualify the US government's historic treatment of American Indians (e.g., Churchill 1997; King 2019; Lindsay 2012; Mato Nunpa 2013; Woolford et al. 2014). After studying the Morton Collection, I concur with them. Traces of genocide are what I found.

I saw violences in decedents' gunshot wounds and marks of malnourishment. The presence of children in the collection revealed a special kind of tragedy. Notations on skulls tracked the distance from the almshouse hospital and ancestral homeland to Samuel's display cabinets. Removal and alienation of a decedent was measurable in miles as well as degrees of separation from one's humanity. I saw normative practices develop in personal letters between Samuel and his colleagues, as they casually conferred about their methods of collecting and curating. Beliefs naturalized in their scientific publications supported racialized assessments of diseases, behaviors, and intelligence. Historic retellings celebrated White, Christian, heroic masculinity, and little else. I documented the erasure of names and persons whose biographic information could not be contained within census categories and simplistic, analytical classifications of race or gender. And in that erasure, an effective exclusion from the American body politic and historic annals occurred.

Decolonial Work

During my research the central part that Samuel and his colleagues played in the necropolitics of nation-building became clear. But so did the presence of individuals who challenged official history and national mythologizing. To access those stories, Saidiya Hartman's method of critical fabulation is useful. "It is a narrative of what might have been or could have been," she explains (2008, 12); "it is a history written with and against the archive." There are limits to what the archive gives up, Hartman stresses; it is stubbornly silent about "disposable lives" (2008, 11). The archives I visited revealed little about decedents in the Morton Collection aside from their dead-end names and violations, and narratives about Black Indians and Two-Spirits were omitted altogether. But to critically fabulate—to bring together archival and historic materials, skeletal data, and speculative arguments—presents the possibility of crafting counter-histories. These narratives, while not definitive, are worth imagining for they are disruptive. They disrupt the linearity and surety of traditional historic accounts. They disrupt temporal connections; the past is not cordoned off but "inseparable from writing a history of present," Hartman (2008, 4) says (taking up Foucault's earlier efforts). From such ruptures, a new world order may arise, as her quote at the beginning of this chapter anticipates. Critical fabulation then is a tool for doing decolonial work.

In the case of Two-Spirits, for instance, their acknowledgment and acceptance, in the past and present, aids in decolonizing Native communities, as queer Indigenous writers and activists have voiced (e.g., Driskill

2004, 2016; Driskill et al. 2011; Finley 2011; Gilley 2006; Morgensen 2011; Smithers 2022). Historically, such socio-sexual variance was antithetical to western heteropatriarchy and Christian beliefs, they explain. With cultural and religious assimilation, a violent disruption, Native communities came to stigmatize two-spiritedness. To write a history of the present is to reveal these processes of intolerance and erasure, as well as the complex perceptions of contemporary Native communities.

The experiences of Michael Red Earth (1997), a queer-identified Sisseton Dakota, are a poignant and salient example. His family lived on the Lake Traverse Reservation of the Sisseton-Wahpeton Dakota Tribe,[23] making him a descendant of the Sioux that Samuel had described in *Crania Americana* as a "warrior of bad character" (Morton 1839, 198; see chapter 5). As an activist and writer, Red Earth has discussed his conflicted identification as *winkte*, a male-bodied person who performed women's gender roles. Tribal members who maintained more traditionalist views about gender and sexuality accepted his identity, while those who articulated assimilationist beliefs responded with homophobia. About his coming out, Red Earth (1997, 216) wrote, "The difficulty of my family came when they tried to incorporate their indoctrinated feelings from assimilation with our cultural legacy." Hence, queer Indigenous scholars and activists read homophobia and heteronormativity as a type of symbolic violence, the maintenance of colonial oppression by Native communities. At the same time, reclamation of two-spiritedness by Indigenous actors demonstrates the resilience and dynamism of cultural traditions. Embracing two-spiritedness then has the potential to be part of a larger decolonial project, sexual sovereignty being "a vital part of Native sovereignty" (Smithers 2022, 248; see also Driskill 2004, 2016; Morgensen 2011).

Repatriation of the unnamed Sioux decedent in the Morton Collection—identified by the Penn Museum's Registrar as 97-606-605, a catalogue number that is a legacy of its contingent ownership—echoes this historic tension, resilience, and decolonial promise. In August 2006, a delegation from the Sisseton-Wahpeton Oyate of the Lake Traverse Reservation, with the support of other affiliated groups, traveled to Philadelphia. According to the Penn Museum's website, "Members of Kitt-Fox Society performed a ceremony in the Warden Garden prior to the groups [*sic*] departure that day."[24] For this society, which is one of several traditional warrior societies among the Plains tribes (Kessel and Wooster 2005, 182), the sex or two-spiritedness of the decedent was not acknowledged. Rather, more important was the decedent's identity as a warrior. Ancestor and descendants then returned to South Dakota, where the former was laid to rest. While repatriation as a decolonial process is an imperfect one, in this instance it did ameliorate some of the suffering set in motion by settler colonialism.

If we continue to only use NAGPRA as a guide, however, we will certainly shortchange those whose historic disenfranchisement extends beyond its purview. Here Hartman's critical fabulation allows us to explore the possibility of a Black Seminole in the Morton Collection. Granted, we will never know if this decedent, labeled 730 by Samuel and discussed in chapter 4, had been enslaved, a tributary ally, or the offspring of a miscegenetic union, but his presence is evocative of the intimate relationships between Blacks and Americans Indians. NAGPRA says nothing explicitly about such hybridity, however. It only deals in the illusion of purity and immutability (Liebmann 2008). Of course, the federal law's silence on hybridity may be beside the point. The concept presupposes purity, as critical considerations have teased out (e.g., Liebmann 2015; Palmié 2013; Silliman 2013). Hence, hybridity is also a product of "the operation of classificatory regimes," in the words of Palmié, (2013, 465). Which means that affirming hybrid identities may serve to uphold rather than subvert asymmetrical power dynamics.

These complications were magnified when the Seminole Tribe of Florida (STOF) submitted a repatriation claim in 2013. Because institutions receiving federal funds are only obligated to consult with or repatriate to federally recognized Native American tribes in the United States, Penn Museum was under no obligation to contact contemporary Black Seminole communities, which are currently located in Oklahoma, Texas, Mexico, and the Bahamas (Mock 2010; Mulroy 2007). Nor do these groups have official recourse to repatriate decedents identified as their ancestors. The issue is made more contentious by the Seminole Indians' stance on Black Seminoles.[25] Some writers have soft-pedaled Seminole enslavement of Blacks (e.g., Miller 2003, 2005; Porter 1996). "The status of Seminole slaves was far less onerous than the status of American, Muscogee, or Cherokee slaves," Susan Miller has remarked (2005, 26). A statement that makes Miller sound like an apologist at worst or a historical amnesiac at best. No matter how "less onerous" the Seminoles' enslavement of Blacks may have been, it remained slavery.

The representation of slavery as practiced by the Seminoles—unique, more indulgent, less peculiar though still suggestive of separate and unequal—has served as justification for contemporary disenfranchisement. In 2000, the Seminole Nation of Oklahoma voted to restrict tribal citizenship to members who had one-eighth quantum of Seminole blood. Much of what drove the tribe's decision, as Melinda Micco (2006) has argued, was money and blood. In 1990, the US government awarded the Seminole Nation $56 million in reparations for forced removal and lands stolen during the Seminole Wars. But the tribe refused to allot any funds to Black Seminoles, adamant that they had an insufficient amount of Native blood and one drop too much of Black blood (hypodescent ruled). Though the Black Seminoles contested their exclusion in court, the US Supreme Court refused to intervene, citing the Seminole Nation's sovereign immunity (Mulroy 2007, 318–20).[26]

Similarly, in March 2007, the Cherokee Nation of Oklahoma voted to limit tribal membership to those with "Indian blood." The decision resulted in the disenrollment of 2,800 Cherokee Freedmen, the descendants of historically enslaved Blacks. "The Cherokee who voted to disenfranchise the Freedmen," Jodi Byrd (2011, 141) has observed, "are in the process of mirroring the colonial racisms embedded within discourses of multiculturalism as a means to deny their own immoral and racist disenfranchisement of a group of people because they are descendants of their forbears' slaves." In this case, disenrollment effaced historic complicity in enslavement, exacerbated socioeconomic disadvantages and ontological insecurity, and created animosity among tribal members. Tribal sovereignty was also compromised when a US federal judge intervened and ordered the reinstatement of Freedmen in August 2017 (an outcome that contrasted with the Seminole case). More recently, in a 2021 ruling, the Cherokee Nation Supreme Court mandated that the tribe strike "by blood" from its constitution and other tribal laws (Kelly and Eltohamy 2021).

The analysis of blood to determine membership is a double-edged sword, as the court's ruling hints at and Kimberly TallBear (2003, 2013) has recognized. It can create a biopolitical sense of being for tribal members. But it can also devolve into necropolitics, the maintenance of nonbeing, when used to disenroll the descendants of enslaved Blacks. A narrative that relies on a preponderance of biological evidence and is inattentive to shared history also replicates hoary scientific logic about classifying "racial" differences. That is, the biologizing of race resurrects scientific racism emergent with Linnaean classification and advanced with nineteenth-century physicians' studies of diseases and skulls. Native communities may reiterate ideas about race that legitimated the cruelties of colonialism while obscuring its complexities. In so doing, they run the risk of derailing a decolonial project.

These charged sociopolitical circumstances—defined by dispossession and an increasing reliance by tribes on analyses of biological data to determine affiliation—were the backdrop for repatriation of the Morton Collection's possible Black Seminole. In total, the STOF repatriated 21 skulls from Penn Museum on 12 October 2015.[27] Four days later these remains were buried at Okeechobee Battlefield Historic State Park. Interment was overseen by the funeral director who donated the burial vault, a city commissioner, and members of the Tribal Historic Preservation Office. In keeping with their cultural beliefs about dead bodies, tribal members were not present save for Tribal Court Chief Justice Willie Johns (Gallagher 2015). Given the Okeechobee Battlefield's pivotal role in the Seminole Wars, or White Wars as the Seminoles refer to them (Shire 2016, 103), the burial location is a fitting one. The possible Black Seminole warrior also comes full circle—to the site of his death and unceremonious beheading at the hands of US Army surgeon Dr. Eugene Abadie. It is a suitable resolution in lieu of direct involvement from contemporary Black Seminole descendants.

For their part, scholars have grappled with semantics. More than a gratuitous intellectual exercise, this work recognizes that language can make visible what power structures have long disappeared. To this end, writers draw a distinction between decoloniality and decolonization (e.g., Lyons et al. 2017; Maldonado-Torres 2016; Mignolo and Walsh 2018). Decoloniality, they explain, indicates a type of praxis, the undoing of colonial legacies. Decolonization, on the other hand, refers to the political independence (i.e., sovereignty) or formation of nation-states that were formerly colonized. Frantz Fanon envisioned this process as a violent one: "In its bare reality, decolonization reeks of red-hot cannonballs and bloody knives" (1961, 3). Naming him here is a reminder that a decolonial project has deeper intellectual and political roots than recent movements, though most contemporary efforts do not seek to emulate Fanon's call for violence.

In the case of legacy collections liable to be subjected to repatriation, I see both decoloniality and decolonization as germane. The praxis, or theoretically informed action, involved in decoloniality (ideally) brings researchers and disenfranchised communities into partnership or collaboration. The decolonization of institutions requires their deference to sovereign entities. Repatriation means that independent tribal nations or descendant communities can exercise autonomy over their ancestors. But repatriation is not enough.

Since the passage of NAGPRA in 1990, many anthropologists have assessed the law's impact.[28] They have found it to be productive and paradigm-shifting for anthropology. But writers, Indigenous or otherwise, have also expressed discontent with institutional responses—the glacial pace of progress, foot-dragging, or outright flouting of tribes' requests (e.g., Colwell 2017; Cryne 2009; Dumont, 2011; Starn 2004; Wheeler et al. 2022). Hence, while legislation like NAGPRA is one facet of a decolonial agenda, it is not the only one or always the most effective one. To extend beyond the letter of the law, institutions will have to further amend their policies and procedures. As one moral and creative corrective that honors the spirit of the law, Elizabeth Moore (2010) has discussed the propatriation of Tlingit totem poles. Propatriation—"the sending forth of an object from its country or lineage of origin in acknowledgment of an object returned" (Moore 2010, 126)—is a tangible facet of the undoing involved in decolonial work. It is arguable that such a response is more challenging to implement when human remains are at issue. Though the need to think creatively and beyond NAGPRA is certainly applicable.

In the case of the Morton Collection, Penn Museum has transferred the cranial remains of 126 American Indians to affiliated tribes; for an additional 19 decedents the regulatory process has been completed and their transfer is pending (Stacey Espenlaub, personal communication, September 2022). Consultation and repatriation, more generally, is done as a collaborative effort between pertinent Native tribes and staff from Penn Museum's NAGPRA Office and Physical Anthropology Section.[29] From my personal experiences as a NAGPRA project assistant at the institution, practitioners exercised procedural flexibility so as to honor tribal requests. I am reminded of a consultation visit from the Little Traverse Bay Band of Odawa Indians of Michigan, in which I was permitted to take part. In May 2002, two members of the tribe, a religious leader and NAGPRA representative, visited Penn Museum to consult with repatriation staff about five skulls in the Morton Collection. Dr. George Leib exhumed four of these skulls, describing his activities in an 1841 letter to Samuel. He neither identified the decedents as ancestors, nor recognized his actions as disruptive to their afterlives. The Odawa regarded his actions as a desecration and consultation with the tribe provided an opportunity to reestablish decedents' ontological security and by association their descendants.

During the visit, I took photographs as staff and tribal members toured the museum and reviewed its culturally affiliated holdings; the Odawa religious leader had consented. He and the NAGPRA representative then performed a Calumet Ceremony in the museum's Main Garden, inviting repatriation staff to participate. As the ceremony got underway, the religious leader requested that I stop taking photographs. And so, I did. The ritual continued. Sage smoke "washed" the living and the dead of negative forces. Purification meant that Odawa ancestors, represented by decedents' skulls, could safely continue their journey to the land of the dead. Wafting smoke also offered a channel for communicating with spiritual forces. Ceremony completed, Odawa tribal members asked that human remains be stored in containers with colored cloth and special medicines. Their requests were in keeping with tribal protocols the Little Traverse Bay Band of Odawa later outlined in an online handbook (Hemenway et al. 2012, 24). For now, these Odawa ancestors continue to be housed at Penn Museum. When I returned to the museum in 2011 to conduct research on the Morton Collection, the skulls were wrapped in the same muslin and accompanied by the medicinal bundles, plastic bins functioning as burial spaces. Their presence signals an institutional commitment to hold and care for these decedents until the tribe chooses to take them home. And now, in the wake of our own interesting times, their repatriation may be imminent.

Interesting Times

> Decolonization, which sets out to change the order of the world, is clearly an agenda for total disorder.
> —Frantz Fanon, *The Wretched of the Earth* (1961, 2)

In 2020, "decolonization" became a buzzword, circulating far beyond the academy. In larger part, the term's ubiquity had to do with the "total disorder" (as Fanon anticipated) in which we currently live. Racialized epidemics. Scientific research undertaken in the name of nation. Partisan debates about settler colonialism and White supremacy. Corporeal violence that targets the vulnerable, becomes spectacle, or propels sociopolitical change. There is a striking relationality between Samuel's interesting times and our own. But there are also important differences. Those White men of science and medicine found opportunism in nineteenth-century settler colonialism and the necropolitics of US nation-building. Today's popularization of the term decolonization reflects a commitment to dismantle their colonial legacy. Twenty-first-century technological advances in communication have also driven these efforts. Specifically, in the wake of George Floyd's brutal murder by four Minneapolis police officers on 25 May 2020, social media activism snowballed. Local protests against racial injustice, situated under the umbrella of the Black Lives Matter (BLM) movement, mobilized into global events.³⁰ Calls to decolonize spread as rapidly online as the video footage documenting the final 9 minutes and 29 seconds of Floyd's life.

At this critical moment in the nation's history, the Morton Collection once again erupted into the public consciousness. Attention turned to its decedents of African descent.³¹ As early as 2017, an undergraduate initiative at the University of Pennsylvania, the Penn & Slavery Project, had sought information about enslaved individuals in the collection. But the Sturm und Drang of BLM protests in summer 2020 motivated Penn students to press for its complete dissolution and repatriation. In July 2020, Penn Museum responded by moving the collection's skulls from a classroom in the Center for the Analysis of Archaeological Materials (CAAM 190)—designed specifically to teach Penn students skeletal analysis and inaugurated in 2014 (Almanac 2014)—to a closed storage room. Access for research or teaching purposes was then halted. Prior to this, skulls filled wooden cabinets running the perimeter of CAAM 190. And, like classrooms in the Department of Anthropology where I first encountered the Morton Collection, skulls were visible through the cabinets' glass doors. NAGPRA ensured that none of these skulls were Native American. Nevertheless, and according to Stephanie Mach (2021), many people of color who frequented the classroom found the storage and ongoing use of these "specimens" anxiety-inducing.

Information about the Morton Collection was disseminated via assorted mediascapes. Online news sources offered reports. Their varying levels of journalistic integrity meant that some stories explained adequately, others sensationalized, and still others distorted. Ironically enough, photographs of the skulls appeared in articles that also decried the unethical treatment of the collection's decedents.³² Stories in the popular press, in turn, generated shares, comments, likes, posts, and tweets in social media. Rather than contemplative, such virality often produced reductive, kneejerk responses and lazy public intellectualism. While social media initially raised awareness, it inevitably exacerbated tensions and obfuscated the complex history of the Morton Collection.

For their part, Penn Museum formed the Morton Collection Committee and tasked its members with drafting a report and plan of action. The report was publicly disseminated in April 2021.³³ Skulls of Black Philadelphians were identified as a primary concern. In summer 2021, a new committee was established, the Morton Cranial Collection Community Advisory Group, which brought local community members into the fold.³⁴

After deliberating, the group recommended that 13 Black decedents be reburied at Eden Cemetery, a historic Black cemetery in Philadelphia. They then petitioned the Philadelphia Orphans' Court to proceed. In February 2023, the court, with Judge Sheila Woods-Skipper presiding, granted the museum's request to rebury (Jones 2023).[35] Reburial of these 13 decedents and the crania of an additional seven individuals is set to occur at the beginning of February 2024 (as of the writing of this book). Additionally, Penn has committed to establishing a permanent marker of remembrance on campus to be dedicated with a commemoration ceremony. The university will also organize a community-led public forum. (Penn Museum outlines this sequence of events on several of its website's pages and updates the timeline as necessary.)[36]

In many ways, the Morton Cranial Collection Community Advisory Group is establishing an important precedent. While the House and the Senate have introduced federal legislation that identifies, documents, and preserves Black American burial grounds, nothing like NAGPRA currently exists.[37] For this reason, many now call for an African American Graves Protection and Repatriation Act (AAGPRA). Such legislation would address anti-Black racism as it has informed the treatment (or disregard and destruction) of human remains, not just at Penn but more broadly. As Justin Dunnavant, Delande Justinvil, and Chip Colwell (2021) have commented, collections in American institutions need to be inventoried to catalogue the remains of Black Americans, research paused, and descendants consulted. But federal legislation could do so much more. "Such a law would protect graves and provide guidance on the care and repatriation of human remains in scientific collections," they write. "It could do so in a manner that also addresses a growing interest in genetic samples, both for genealogical testing services and for medical and historical research" (Dunnavant et al. 2021, 338). It would make reparations for historic wrongs. It would prioritize care, collaboration, consent, and dignity. And it would anticipate future ethical transgressions that may result from scientific advances and biobanking.

"Return Them All"

Into the spring of 2021, Penn students and West Philadelphia community members continued with their protests and calls to "Return Them All." While this response is well intentioned, I do see it as reactionary and unnuanced. "Return Them All" is a one-size-fits-all solution. It presumes that all descendant communities desire the return of remains in an institution's care. It also implies that context does not matter. That the historic specificities of imperialism are unnecessary to track. That we do not need to account for today's geopolitics when seeking to consult about or repatriate skulls whose original proveniences are located beyond the borders of the United States. "Return Them All" elides concerns about modern nation-states characterized by instability or authoritarianism, which can impede collaborative efforts, or nationalist agendas that do not prioritize the repatriation of human remains. As an example of how "Return Them All" will fall short, we can look to skulls in the Morton Collection from Egypt and Cuba.

The collection's Egyptian skulls were gifted to Samuel by George Gliddon. The politics and economics of imperialism expedited their collection. Gliddon was born in England (b. 1809, d. 1857) but moved to Egypt in 1818 where his father John was appointed US consul in Alexandria. Gliddon followed in his footsteps, first as the US vice-consul in Cairo in 1833 and, four years later, with a promotion to consul. Throughout the 1830s and 1840s, both men oversaw American commercial interests and the wellbeing of American travelers, the majority of whom were state officials, wealthy tourists, or archaeologists (Finnie 1967, 153–54, 281–85). As consul, Gliddon procured and shipped 137 skulls to Samuel. Inferences he drew from these skulls, which advanced a hierarchical understanding of race first articulated in *Crania Americana*, formed the crux of *Crania Aegyptiaca*. To show his gratitude, Samuel dedicated the book to Gliddon (Morton 1844, 1–2). Knowing that the Morton Collection's Egyptian skulls are a legacy of British and American imperialism and White supremacist ideology, however, does not mean that returning them all is the obvious course of action. Presently, the challenges of identifying a specific descendant community are multitude. Besides, the Egyptian government has yet to call for repatriation of the skulls; artifacts or royal decedents are more often the focus of their efforts.

Comparable measured consideration must also inform handling of the collection's Cuban skulls. Samuel acquired these skulls from José Rodriguez Cisneros in 1840. The Cuban physician's letter described them as "50 pure rare African crania." Additional information provided by Cisneros suggests that the skulls belonged to enslaved individuals whose deaths occurred soon after arriving on the island. "I myself have searched for and found in the sandy soil of the Vedado Farm, where more *negros bozales* are buried," he (1840) wrote. At the time, El Vedado was a farmed area where the bodies of unbaptized and enslaved Africans were buried (Martínez-Fernández 2002, 43). And Cisneros's use of *bozales* (singular *bozal*) confirms these decedents' African origins (Zeuske 2002). While he promised to send Samuel details about their tribe and country, he does not seem to have done so. Here the archives offer silences that make it challenging to flesh out stories. So to whom do we return them? The Department of Anthropology at the University of Havana, which Cuban researchers—many of whom were scientific racists in their own right—established in 1900 with the support of the US military during their occupation (Bronfman 2004, 16; Geller 2021)? The Cuban government (or its Ministry of Culture), which continues to crack down on its citizens who protest in the name of *patria y vida*? Or perhaps, some place in West Africa given historians' tracings of origins (though, undeniably, this region is geographically sizeable and culturally diverse)? While genetic testing may help narrow down this provenience, the technique raises further ethical concerns, about consent, destruction during analysis, and biobanking.

I present these challenges to repatriation not to be contrarian or undercut reparative justice efforts. But, if we are sincere about realizing a decolonial project that is thoughtful, effective in the long-term, and healing for descendant communities, we must first acknowledge that this work at the scale of the global will be difficult, complicated, and protracted. Colonialism and imperialism were extended processes, not single events. And because European and American states adapted to exploit local conditions, a one-size-fits-all solution is untenable. How then to foster international collaborations that acknowledge the specifics of historical relations and present-day turmoil?

As far as ethical practices and legislative policies, NAGPRA can guide us whether remains are culturally affiliated or unidentified. But this American law may not be the best model since it does not cover international repatriations. A better example may come from France. This nation-state enacted legislation to repatriate Saartjie Baartman's remains to South Africa, as well as *mokomokai*, Māori preserved heads, to descendants in New Zealand (Paterson 2010). Additionally, we can turn to the "Vienna Protocol," a document that guides decisions about the human remains of Holocaust victims, whether housed in historic collections or disinterred in situ (Polak et al. 2021; Seidelman et al. 2017). These protocols were crafted collaboratively by international scholars and Jewish religious leaders. Their recommendations will help us grapple with collections that were made possible by and justified necropolitics, which targeted certain racial or ethnic groups. Regardless of what we use, the crux of any guidelines should be respect for human dignity, attention to histories, and compassion as praxis.

Prelude as a Coda

It is the summer of 2021. I am in Philadelphia, spending time with my family after a long COVID-induced separation. I am also multitasking, undertaking some final research on Samuel and his cranial collection. So four days after the nation has celebrated its declaration of independence from the British Empire, I find myself at Laurel Hill Cemetery. Despite having grown up in the Philadelphia suburbs, attended college and graduate school in the city, and returned seasonally, I have never visited the cemetery where Samuel is buried. The day is slightly overcast and humid—the one constant of July in Philadelphia. My mother is accompanying me, humoring me, and together we meander through Laurel Hill. We encounter no one, save a lone red fox that pauses amid the tombstones to observe our passage. There is a hushed quiet, interrupted by sporadic bird chatter and car honks. The once rural cemetery has long since been folded into the city's urban grid and grit.

In many ways, I have come full circle. But more than a decade after beginning my research, social, political, economic, and epidemiological forces have changed Philadelphia. It is a city humbled by pandemic deaths and quarantines, rocked by BLM protests and riots. The quiet of the cemetery belies this tumultuous and interesting time in the nation's history. Historical amnesia is no longer condonable. Yet responses to critical alternatives about national history have run the gamut—from urgent activism to shrugs of resignation for those who have long known about structural inequities to first encounters and good intentions to vehement opposition.

As it pertains to the Morton Collection, contemporary sociopolitics demonstrate how a utilitarian position—that the use of this legacy collection serves a higher scientific purpose—is hard to justify.[38] But how to proceed scholastically with such affective and politically charged human remains? How to decolonize a legacy collection? How to foster ethics of compassion and care, which, if done habitually and collectively, becomes an ethos that guides ongoing actions and interactions?

For my part, as I stressed in these pages, I have sought to recognize the power of storytelling. "Power is the ability not just to tell the story of another person, but to make it the definitive story of that person," Chimamanda Ngozi Adichie has stated.[39] She warns of the dangers in narrating a single story. In telling Samuel's story, I have aimed not to represent him as a caricature but to communicate how he was complicated, fallible, and protean . . . which makes him human. But some humans, because of their actions and the marks they make upon their worlds, are less deserving of forgiveness than others. For this reason, in Samuel's story, I have shown his central involvement in larger-scale processes—those which consolidated fields of study (i.e., medicine, anthropology), national borders, and the body politic. This narrative thread allows us to understand the complicity and callousness of historic actors as they benefited from and legitimated necropolitical interventions in nineteenth-century America.

Instead, Adichie urges us, "Start the story with the arrows of the Native Americans, and not with the arrival of the British, and you have an entirely different story." In telling alternative stories about decedents associated with or in the Morton Collection, I have sought to subvert dominant narratives. Flipping the script—to include stories about named individuals, Black Indians, and Beloved women—aims to contest deeply entrenched power structures. Or, when this proved too difficult empirically (as Hartman recognized it would), I endeavored to expose the process of silencing, the becoming object, the total erasure of biographies.

Aside from the power of storytelling, I see practicing humility as essential for decolonizing legacy collections. Even more so for White academics like myself, whose privilege has historically made it easier to conduct our work with human remains. The Morton Collection teaches us that while specialized scientific knowledge is important, we must also let others speak and we must actively listen (not just hear). To do so gives equal (or greater) weight to living descendants. Humility also prods us to acknowledge what we do not know, what we may never know. Descendant communities may be reticent to share information about their cultural practices, beliefs, and ancestors. Archives may fall silent on certain subjects or persons. Humility also invites flexibility, a useful quality for when the ground shifts. Policies will be implemented, ethical framings fine-tuned, sociopolitical events catalyzing. As this book draws to a close, I am aware that my words here will likely need amending at some future juncture.

Knowing that words are prone to revision or deletion, I also see the need for tangible reminders. If the whole Morton Collection were to be returned or reburied eventually, I suggest keeping one skull to display centrally—not relegated to a cabinet or forgotten in a storage drawer. It would materialize Samuel's legacy, which does tell us about the life and work of one man but is far more informative about the larger-scale, historic processes involved in scientific advancement and American nation-building. A single skull to conjure those who have benefited or strategized or suffered or were silenced. Ideally, for the interesting times in which we live, that skull should belong to one who offered consent, though the unlikelihood of finding someone who did speaks more about the interesting times in which Samuel lived. Placing the onus of consent on living descendants also seems cruel, given many groups' historic suffering and disenfranchisement. An alternative solution is to exhume Samuel's skull for use as a pedagogical specimen and talisman against historical amnesia. Justice would then be reparative and poetic.

NOTES

Introduction

1 The Academy of Natural Sciences of Philadelphia was founded in 1812. In 2011, "Philadelphia" was dropped from the name. "Drexel University" was added to indicate its new affiliation with the ANS.
2 Of course, the same could now be said for Audubon, who maintained White supremist views and bought and sold enslaved Black people. The organization that bears his name, the National Audubon Society, is now reckoning with these ignominious aspects of his legacy. See https://www.audubon.org/news/the-myth-john-james-audubon.
3 See the preface, where I explain why I use Samuel's first name.
4 Skulls in the Morton Collection come from globally disparate places, and roughly 25 percent—or 250–300 decedents—are from various locations in the United States.
5 Morton's Spanish-speaking colleagues signed off with "Q.S.B.M.," an acronym for "que beso su mano." The translation, "who kisses your hand," also belies the formalness of the farewell (e.g., Cisneros 1840).
6 Foucault originally hyphenated the terms bio-history, bio-power, and bio-politics. His frequent hyphenation of concepts, power-knowledge being another good example, was done to emphasize interconnection not interchangeability of words.
7 Mbembe's 2003 journal publication "Necropolitics" appears as a slightly revised chapter 3 in his 2019 book *Necropolitics*. I quote from the most recent version.
8 Many medical institutions that continue to use "Pernkopf's Atlas" now detail its sordid history while imparting humanity and dignity to the victims who appear in its pages. For example, see the Amara Yad Project affiliated with UCLA, which publishes open-access anatomic atlases (https://www.uclahealth.org/medical-services/heart/arrhythmia/about-us/amara-yad-project). Such a position is in keeping with recommendations made in the "Vienna Protocol" (Polak et al. 2021). This Responsum (a rabbinical reply to a query about Jewish law)—authored by Joseph Polak, a Holocaust survivor and Rabbinical Court judge rabbi, with input from medical ethicist Michael Grodin—works to reconcile the evil that underpinned the atlas's creation and its use to save human lives, a Jewish concept known as "pikuach nefesh."
9 The exact number of skulls is difficult to pin down. Samuel's recording methods often involved a logic known only to the physician. In his eulogy for Samuel, Henry Patterson (1854, xxx) put the number of human skulls at 918.

10 For a history of the Ridgway Library and its connection to the Library Company of Philadelphia, see https://librarycompany.org/2017/06/09/treasures-from-the-library-company-of-philadelphia-7/.

11 Sex estimations were assessed based on cranial variation following Buikstra and Ubelaker (1994). Tooth wear (Miles 2001) and ectocranial suture closure (Meindl and Lovejoy 1985) were used to estimate age. I measured skulls using traditional landmark-based measurements following the protocol of Howells (1989) and Martin (1928). Recognizing that critics may regard my use of craniometrics as disingenuous and futile—the master's tools will never dismantle the master's house, to paraphrase Audre Lorde—I refer the reader to Geller and Stojanowski (2017) for further explanation. In brief, my aim is to document a *process* of racialization, or the making of race during a pivotal historic and sociopolitical moment. Seeing value in craniometrics is not an admission that race has a biological basis.

12 These tribes are the Cherokee, Choctaw, Chickasaw, Creek, and Seminole. White settlers designated them "civilized" because they adopted Christianity, entered into economic relations, and embraced Euro-American cultural practices (e.g., enslavement of Africans).

13 There are two major collections of papers associated with Samuel Morton. Technically owned by the Library Company of Philadelphia, papers compiled by Samuel's son Thomas and granddaughter Helen Kirkbride Morton are housed at the Historical Society of Pennsylvania (HSP). At the American Philosophical Society (APS) are the Samuel George Morton Papers. Arthur V. Morton and Mrs. John Story Jenks (née Isabella Fitzgerald Morton) gifted these materials in 1943; these siblings are also Samuel's grandchildren (their father was Thomas, and their sister was Helen). The papers at APS include correspondences to Samuel, a diary penned by him in 1833, and craniological sketches for *Crania Americana*. There is also a separate series of microfilmed letters, the originals of which were owned by Dr. Hugh Montgomery, Samuel's great-grandson. In addition to these institutions, in-person archival research occurred at the following institutions (listed in alphabetical order): Academy of Natural Sciences; Ah-Tah-Thi-Ki Museum; College of Physicians of Philadelphia; National Archives in Washington, DC; Penn Museum; University of Miami's Special Collections at Richter Library; and Wistar Institute. I also conducted in-depth online research at the University of North Carolina–Chapel Hill's Wilson Library; Florida State University's Strozier Library; Medical University of South Carolina's Waring Historical Library; and Library of Congress. Archivists at Bowdoin College Library's George J. Mitchell Department of Special Collections + Archives, the Germantown Historical Society, and National Library of Medicine also provided information or sent along germane documents.

14 Whereas I am invested intellectually and politically in a decolonial project, I have neither personal (nor ancestral) connections to decedents comprising the Morton Collection. Nor did their descendants consent to the inclusion of photographs in this book. Hence, I have opted to not include them here.

15 Or gender ... at this time, biological determinism underpinned analyses. Hence, physicians and natural historians did not distinguish between sex and gender (though they only used the former term).
16 Porotic hyperostosis is spongy or porous bone tissue that develops on the surface of the cranium. Cribra orbitalia refers to porous skeletal lesions that form on the roof of the orbits, or eye sockets; these can be in healed or active stages.
17 Conversations during the NSF Research Team Seminar *Excavating Bodies in the Archives: Generating New Methods and Collaborations*, which convened at the School for Advanced Research from 2–4 May 2023, deepened my thinking about foot/endnotes. I am exceedingly grateful to seminar participants: cochair Shannon Novak, Meredith Ellis, Maura Finkelstein (whose seminar paper was the catalyst for these conversations), Zeynep Devrim Gürsel, Lucy Mulroney, Heather Law-Pezzarossi, Andrew Roddick, Paul White, and cochair Alanna Warner-Smith (who, after reading a draft of *Becoming Object*, guided my thinking about the salience of those discussions to this book).

Chapter 1. The Friend

1 Here I transcribe spelling, capitalization, and punctuation as they appeared in Thomas's original letter.
2 Per Thomas's original letter to his son: "Your Choise of A young woman whose Agreeable Accomplishments & the family Connextions adds much to the Sattisfaction I find in having my Children Agreeably Settled. In my time nor shale I Omitt any thing in my power to forwd there happiness I heartily Congrualte you on the Occasion may you by frugall Industry Injoy the Social Comforts of this life and Raise Afamily that wile be an Honor to you at your decline."
3 Monthly minutes of Friends of Philadelphia for the Southern District, p. 129, 25 May 1785, US, Quaker Meeting Records, 1681–1935, Ancestry.com.
4 "A Register of Burials for the Year 1795, 1796, 1797, 1798, 1799, 1800, by the Reverend Doctor Nicholas Collin," *Marriages, Baptisms, and Burials, 1789–1795*, pp. 74a–74b, Gloria Dei Church, https://philadelphiacongregations.org/records/items/show/381 #?c=&m=&s=&cv=189&xywh=-366%2C-2339%2C10892%2C12670.
5 To do this, she would have first had to request a certificate of removal from the Quaker congregation in Philadelphia, as described in *Rules of Discipline and Christian Advices of the Yearly Meeting of Friends for Pennsylvania and New Jersey*; this certificate provided the new congregation with requisite information (e.g., family members' names, reason for removal) (Philadelphia Yearly Meeting of the Religious Society of Friends 1797, 18–21).
6 Quaker Marriages, Purchase Monthly Meeting, Westchester County, New York, p. 43, https://archive.org/details/quakermarriagesp00frie/page/n91/mode/2up.
7 Philadelphia Monthly Meeting, Minutes 1804–1818, 13 and 27 February 1812, p. 190, US Quaker Meeting Records, 1681–1994, Ancestry.com.
8 The Female Medical College of Pennsylvania (renamed the Woman's Medical College of Pennsylvania in 1867) is not to be confused with the Pennsylvania Medical College where Samuel taught from 1839 to 1843 (see chapter 2). Sarah also attended

classes at the short-lived Ladies Institute of Pennsylvania Medical University in 1855, 1857, and 1858 (Bacon 2001, 30; Lerner 1972, 85–86; Lindhorst 1995, 174).

9 After the opening of Penn's Medical Department, medical practitioners living elsewhere—in other colonies and then states in a new nation—soon followed suit: New York (King's College, later Columbia University); New Jersey (Queen's College, later Rutgers University); Massachusetts (Harvard University); Virginia (William and Mary College); New Hampshire (Dartmouth College); and Kentucky (Transylvania University in Lexington) (Norwood 1970, 472).

10 Foucault's critical commentary about the medical gaze is equally applicable to Eakins's exploitative photographs of young girls, which have further tainted his legacy. One titled *African-American girl nude, reclining on couch* has come under fire recently and is no longer accessible digitally on the Pennsylvania Academy of Fine Arts's website (https://www.theartnewspaper.com/2021/12/17/thomas-eakins-reckoning-philadelphia). For an analysis of this photo, see Saidiya Hartman (2019, 24–29); she offers commentary about the violence of the archive and consent (or lack thereof), which, for those whose race (Black), sex (female), and economic status (impoverished) imparted vulnerability, was given rarely and/or constrained by history and circumstances.

11 This source is a handwritten note that appears in genealogical documents currently housed at the HSP. The note explains: "It has occurred to Dr. [Thomas George] Morton as well as to myself that these [previous biographical sketches] could be drawn upon and condensed—some perhaps amplified—in the preparation of a sketch for preservation by the family." The note's author goes unnamed. While Samuel's son Thomas George compiled the documents, the use of "Dr. Morton" suggests he is not the source. John Phillips, Samuel's technical assistant, seems a possible candidate given the inclusion of personal details and deference for the subject at hand. Helen Kirkbride Morton, Samuel's granddaughter, is also listed as a contributor to the compilation.

12 Perhaps this is the reason that the Mütter Museum of the College of Physicians of Philadelphia has experienced backlash more recently. The museum, which began as the private collection of Dr. Thomas Dent Mütter (b. 1811, d. 1859), long functioned as a large-scale pathological cabinet, accessible to medical practitioners and nonspecialists alike. (Cristin O'Keefe Aptowicz's [2014] book length treatment of Mütter, though comprehensive, is overly flattering. That is, like Samuel, Mütter invites critical attention.) While today's entrance fee is considerably more expensive than in the nineteenth century, visitors can still view its myriad holdings. Warts, tumors, cysts, and stillborn fetuses float in glass jars. Dozens of skulls decorate gallery walls. Obsolete medical instruments share space with anatomical models crafted from wax. Proponents argue that such displays offer a glimpse into the annals of medicine's history. Critics, however, level charges of insensitivity and amorality, or even immorality given the absence of consent in many instances. (My inclination is to concur with the latter, as I explain in this book's final chapter. But, in my opinion, I find that both supporters and opponents like screaming into the black void that is social media.) In response, the Mütter Museum temporarily removed its online

content and halted researchers' access to collections in May 2023. At the writing of this book, the institution was reevaluating how to proceed ethically with the handling and display of human remains—6,500 "specimens" in total, according to an online news source (Pérez Ortega 2023).
13. Philadelphia Monthly Meeting, Western District, Minutes 1814–1830, US Quaker Meeting Records, 1681–1994, p. 157, Ancestry.com.
14. The Samuel George Morton Papers at the American Philosophical Society contains 11 letters from Hodgkin, which he penned from 1822 to 1842.
15. Spencer (1983, 336) translated much of Samuel's thesis from Latin, including the passage quoted here.
16. As recorded in minutes from 1824, the society changed its name to the Phrenological Society of Philadelphia within two years of its founding. Philadelphian physicians' interest in phrenology abated as quickly as it had emerged, however; the society disbanded by 1827. In George Combe's correspondences to Samuel, now housed at the APS, he noted that the Phrenological Society's president Dr. John Bell retained the society's collection.
17. Central Phrenological Society of Philadelphia Constitution and Minutes 1822–1827, Historical Society of Pennsylvania, Philadelphia, PA.
18. *Registers of Vessels Arriving at the Port of New York from Foreign Ports, 1789–1919*, Microfilm Publication M237, rolls 1–95, National Archives, Washington, DC.

Chapter 2. "Licence to Kill and Cure"

1. Samuel resided at 411 Mulberry Street from 1825 to 1828 according to *The Philadelphia Directory and Stranger's Guide, for 1825* (Wilson 1825) and *Desilver's Philadelphia Directory and Stranger's Guide, for 1828* (Desilver 1828). Mulberry Street would later be renamed Arch Street.
2. To become a new member of the ANS, one had to be nominated by two current members and then elected by the ANS's remaining members. Correspondents, on the other hand, did not live in Philadelphia, though in some exceptional cases one could be elected as a nonresident member. Such was the case for Colonel J. J. Abert (Academy of Natural Sciences of Philadelphia 1877, 3), who is discussed in chapter 4.
3. At the time of Samuel's appointment, the almshouse was located on the corner of 11th and Spruce Streets (Desilver 1833). After much delay, its new facilities opened on the west side of the Schuylkill River in Blockley Township—"on the 28th day of July, 1834, four years, two months and two days from the time of laying the corner stone" (Lawrence 1905, 132). (Today this area, at 34th Street and University Avenue, is the southeastern corner of the University of Pennsylvania.) In time, the institution became known as Blockley Almshouse, or, more familiarly, Old Blockley. Within a few months of the new building's opening, however, Samuel resigned from the almshouse's medical staff.
4. *Mania à potu* is a type of alcoholic insanity, a madness derived from habitual alcohol consumption. Physicians also called the condition *delirium tremens*. Ric Caric (2007, 471) attributes its increase in the 1830s to anxiety induced by the "more com-

plex, difficult, and demanding economic environment" that early industrialization generated. See chapter 5 for the gendered aspects of *mania à potu*.

5   When quoting from the *Catalogue*, I have tried to replicate the style of the original entry (e.g., small caps, italics) to make clear Samuel's editorial choices.

6   These individuals include: "9. Negro Idiot. S. G. M."; "17. Mulatto Lunatic. *Died of Religious Mania, 1831, aged 22 years. S. G. M.*"; "24. Anglo-American Female; a fille-de-joie, aged 26. Died of mania à potu."; "36. Anglo-American Idiot. S. G. M."; "55. Negro Lunatic. S. G. M."; "57. Lunatic Irishman. S. G. M."; "58. German Lunatic, A.D. 1833. S. G. M."; "62. Lunatic Englishman, aged 30 years. 1832. S. G. M."; and "64. Mulatto Lunatic, female. S. G. M." The handwritten annotation for this last individual reads, "64. Died of the Cholera, 1832, aged 18 years" (Morton 1840a). There is also one other individual associated with the Almshouse. His *Catalogue* entry is a detailed one:

> 1319 Skull of John Voorhees, a Mulatto porter, born in Chester county, Pennsylvania, and died of consumption in the Blockley Hospital, November 5, 1846, aged 35 years. About an hour before his death, he called the nurse to him, and confessed as follows: That eighteen or twenty years before, having a hatred against another boy of his own color, two years younger than himself, he strangled and killed him. After committing the murder he became alarmed, and placed the dead body in a chair near the window, hoping to revive it. He then fled; and not having been seen to enter the house was never suspected of the murder; and the boy, being found dead in the chair, was supposed to have died of apoplexy. I have these facts and the skull from my friend Dr. Adolphus L. Heerman. (Morton 1849a)

Samuel did not personally acquire this decedent's skull, seeing that his tenure at the institution had ended by 1835. His acquisition of the skull hints at practices that solidified into formal policy come the late-nineteenth century, the transferring of unclaimed bodies to scientists and physicians.

7   Contributions in Nystrom's (2017) edited volume *The Bioarchaeology of Dissection and Autopsy in the United States* might be of interest to bioarchaeologists who wish to further explore the distinction between dissection and autopsy.

8   In 1829, the Irish resurrectionists William Burke and William Hare were accused of selling their murder victims to Dr. Robert Knox. (This anatomist, as discussed in chapter 1, was likely an acquaintance of Samuel's.) Hare confessed to the crime and, as a result, received immunity from prosecution. Burke was convicted, hanged, and dissected. The punishment, as Ruth Richardson (1987, 143–44), has pointed was fitting but did little to dispel the general public's loathing of dissection. As for Knox, he had purchased corpses from Burke and Hare but claimed ignorance of their grisly misdeeds. A committee of enquiry only censured him for being "incautious," though his name thereafter was linked with illicit activities and postmortem violations (Richardson 1987, 140). The scandal became the stuff of urban legends

and linguistic coinage. Thenceforth, "burking" referred to an act of murder, as by suffocation, that leaves no or few marks of violence on a body.
9 The Pennsylvania Statute was Title 35 P.S.—Health and Safety, chapter 11: "Disposition of Dead Human Bodies" (Section 1092)—"Notice to board of bodies in institutions; claims of relatives or friends; bodies of soldiers, sailors, and marines; burial of paupers." See chapter 6 for additional information about the Anatomy Act.
10 Exceptions to this rule included bodies "unfit for anatomical purposes" or military men, "a soldier, sailor, or marine of the United States or of the militia of the State of Pennsylvania."
11 Samuel formally became an APS member on 18 January 1828.
12 See note 10 of chapter 1 for information about this source.
13 It was the English physician John Snow who, in 1854, first observed that cholera has a waterborne transmission. Where drainage and water purification systems are lacking, sewage can contaminate water supply systems (Tulchinsky 2018, 77–99). The consequences of contagion can be severe and quite sudden. Symptoms of cholera are always painful and often fatal where medical intervention is inadequate. Excessive diarrhea and vomiting induce extreme dehydration. Poor circulation or inadequate oxygenation of the blood signaled by skin discoloration, or cyanosis, may also result. While we now know that cholera, or *Vibrio cholerae*, is an infectious disease caused by a toxigenic bacterium (Clemens et al. 2017), outbreaks are still quite disruptive. The bacterium's comma-like shape then seems appropriate; a cholera pandemic produces a pause in normal routines and interactions.
14 Today, the distinction between epidemic and endemic cholera is not so clear cut. Physicians and epidemiologists note that these terms "represent two ends of a spectrum, and large outbreaks termed as epidemics can occur in populations with endemic cholera" (Clemens et al. 2017, 1540).
15 Those physicians present included Drs. Benjamin Neill, Hugh Hodge, William Horner, John Rhea Barton, and Jacob Randolph (Lawrence 1905, 117).
16 The other twelve physicians were Drs. Chapman, Otto, Parrish, Horner, Jackson, Lukens, Harris, Meigs, Mitchell, Emerson, Hodge, and Taylor.
17 Of course, established medical institutions, like the one at Penn, also sought profit. On average, about one-third of a medical department's student body received diplomas at the conclusion of an academic year. The low graduation rate was not seen as a negative. "The number of graduates," medical faculty at Penn (1839, 96) noted, "cannot be taken as a just measure of the prosperity of the school; for it does not by any means bear the same relation to the number of students attending the lectures at different periods." Men who did not complete their degrees still paid to attend lectures. Hence, financial solvency was as important a goal for institutions as physicians' training.
18 To be clear, Samuel never taught at Penn, though he did serve as a preceptor and take students who attended its medical school under his tutelage.
19 There are various locations listed for the Pennsylvania Medical College. In 1846, this organization's address appears to be 365 Walnut Street (Stillé 1846, 7). In 1854, the school is reported as occupying Filbert Street above 12th Street (Hayward 1854,

518). Hexamer and Locher's map of the city, which dates from 1858 to 1860, places it on the west side of Ninth Street below Locust Street (https://libwww.freelibrary.org/digital/item/11767). Movement may have signaled its institutional instability.

20 John Jay Smith's version of the recollections, titled *Recollections of John Jay Smith*, is stored at the Library Company and consists of three volumes in total. His daughter Elizabeth Pearsall Smith later published a two-volume edition.
21 Dewees was also an alumna of the Medical Department at Penn (class of 1806).
22 The first and second reports of the Aborigines Protection Society do not use an apostrophe, but the third one does (i.e., Aborigines' Protection Society).
23 Prichard also became a correspondent in the ANS in 1838 (Academy of Natural Sciences of Philadelphia 1877, 31); presumably Samuel nominated him.

Chapter 3. "Your Obedient Servant"

1 "Andrew Jackson: First Annual Message to Congress Excerpts," December 8, 1829, https://billofrightsinstitute.org/activities/handout-c-andrew-jackson-first-annual-message-to-congress-excerpts, accessed 19 January 2021.
2 Jackson's entire speech to Congress on Indian removal can be found here: https://www.nps.gov/museum/tmc/manz/handouts/andrew_jackson_annual_message.pdf.
3 Later the Supreme Court, in the 1832 ruling *Worcester v. Georgia*, also found that it was unconstitutional for states to impose laws on American Indians' lands (in this case, those belonging to the Cherokee Nation) (Sundquist 2010). Jackson disregarded this decision outright and soldiered ahead with Indian removal.
4 The *Army and Navy Chronicle* are a good resource for tracking the whereabouts of medical officers during this time. Mentions of Walker appear in vol. 6 (p. 120), vol. 8, vol. 10 ([20 Feb 1840], n. 8, p. 128), vol. 11 ([23 July 1840], n. 4, p. 56), and vol. 12 (no. 1, p. 7). In addition to the rationalizing of letting American Indians die, Walker was also very supportive of Black Americans' enslavement. So supportive, in fact, that it got him killed. After resigning from the army in 1849, he settled in Platte County, Missouri, and continued to practice medicine. The pro-slavery group with which he was affiliated threatened to kill any Northern Methodist ministers who continued to sermonize about abolition. One defiant anti-slavery minister, Reverend Charles Morris, met his untimely fate in July 1864 at the group's hands. Morris's kin then shot and killed Walker in retaliation (Paxton 1897, 372).
5 Cave burial may signal a more longstanding precarity that tracks back to an early colonial juncture. According to Martin (1838a), interment of decedents in this setting was a response to a prior wave of epidemics:

> There is a tradition in relation to these caves among the Cherokees that serves to account for the very large collection of bones found in them. Near a century since, the small pox broke out among this people, it is said, which destroyed great numbers of them, tho' the custom of committing their dead bodies to these natural cemeteries had over time begun to decline, yet such was the great

mortality from this scourge or pestilence that they were compelled to bring them to these caves, and into which they were thrown in promiscuous heaps.

6 Age assessments for the four Cherokee individuals were based primarily on dental development. In the case of 632, the right and left maxillary (upper) third molars were just beginning to erupt but remained within their crypts, and the roots were only one-quarter formed. For 633, the left maxillary third molar was still a tooth germ visible in the socket though not fully formed or erupted. The individual labeled 634 has an erupted left maxillary third molar with no dental wear but slight polish, and a CT scan indicated that the roots were no longer open. Additionally, this individual's basilar suture had not yet fused completely (this suture is located at the base of the skull and joins the occipital bone to the sphenoid). In the case of 635, neither maxillary third molars erupted but tooth buds had formed in the sockets. This individual also displayed parietal bossing (or a marked prominence in the parietal region).
7 Florida became a US territory in 1821 and officially joined the Union as the twenty-seventh state on 3 March 1845.
8 Here he is citing Clay MacCauley (1887), Unitarian minister and amateur anthropologist. Clay, at the request of the Smithsonian Institute's Bureau of American Ethnology, conducted ethnographic work among the Seminole during the winter of 1880–1881. See also Missall and Missall 2004, 7; Perdue and Green 2001, 92; Sturtevant and Cattelino 2004, 431; and Weisman 2007, 200.
9 Many scholars have treated these events in detail (e.g., Baptist 2002; Covington 1993; Garbarino 1989; Lancaster 1994; Missall and Missall 2004; Mulroy 2007; Perdue and Green 2001; Porter 1996; Sturtevant and Cattelino 2004; Weisman 1989, 1999, 2007). Additional information, which extends the narratives of Euro-American writers, can be found on the Seminole Tribe of Florida's website: https://www.semtribe.com/history/introduction. For information about the Second Seminole War specifically, see Bemrose 1966; Mahon 1967; Potter 1836; and Sprague 1848.
10 Although Abadie obtained three skulls, only two, 726 and 727, are in the Morton Collection. Abadie also misspelled the fort's name. The correct spelling is "Fort Gardiner," which is located along the Kissimmee River in Polk County. It was established in 1837 during General Zachary Taylor's campaign against the Seminole. The fort was named after George Washington Gardiner, a captain who died under the command of Major Dade. The fort also served as a hospital for US soldiers wounded in battle.
11 Interestingly, Seminole mortuary practices point to Euro-American acculturation (coffins made from local woods) and cultural resilience ("the burial of food containers with the dead, the hammering and perforation of silver coins, the use and contents . . . of pouches, and the traditional adornments of beads, earbobs, bodice pieces, and pendants") (Piper et al. 1982, 127).
12 The child's skull contained a handwritten notation; on the left parietal appeared "Fort Gardner December 30th" and along the squamous suture was the word "Seminole."

13 To confuse the matter, the *Catalogue* includes the following information: "729. Seminole Girl, of the Fuke-luste-Hadjo tribe. *Dr. Abadie, U.S.A*" (1840a, 22). Abadie appears to have based his identification on grave goods, while it is unclear what criteria Samuel used to estimate sex.
14 Abadie phoneticized Coacoochee as Cow-a-gee. Alternative spellings also include Kowakochi, Cowacoochee, or Coa-cuchee.
15 Archaeologists successfully documented the location of Taylor's camp but were unable to detect the soldiers' mass grave (Carr et al. 1989).
16 Mbembe connects becoming-object to consumptive practices under late capitalism. In a November 2013 interview, he remarked: "If we look carefully at the operations of consumption world-wide today, we might observe that, many people want to become objects, or be treated as such, if only because becoming an object one might end up being treated better than as a human." He seems to suggest that individuals today choose this objectification, while recognizing that choice is circumscribed by social, economic, and political circumstances. In my nineteenth-century case study, choice is not at issue but certainly transformation is. Interview dated 20 November 2013; accessible on https://africasacountry.com/2013/11/africa-and-the-future-an-interview-with-achille-mbembe/.
17 Of the Caucasian race, Samuel (1839, 5) wrote, the "skull is large and oval, and its anterior portion full and elevated . . . , [and it] is distinguished for the facility with which it attains the highest intellectual endowments." In comparison, the American race was characterized by a skull that "is small, wide between the parietal protuberances, prominent at the vertex, and flat on the occiput." He continued, Americans were "slow in acquiring knowledge; restless, revengeful, and fond of war, and wholly destitute of maritime adventure" (ibid., 6). He also acknowledged that the Ethiopian race does "present a singular diversity of intellectual character . . . [but] the far extreme is the lowest grade of humanity" (ibid., 6–7).
18 Like Samuel, Barnes was also born in Philadelphia (b. 21 July 1817, d. 5 April 1884). Additional information about his biography comes from the 1883 death noticed circulated by the US Surgeon General's Office.
19 Today the Army Medical Museum is known as the National Museum of Health and Medicine (NMHM) and is in Silver Spring, Maryland (https://armymedicalmuseum.org/about/#history). See Elise Juzda (2009) for a discussion of the museum's creation and abandonment of its cranial collection. The latter, Juzda argues, was a consequence of museum administrators' disenchantment with craniology by the end of the nineteenth century.
20 One year after Otis's presentation, Congress passed the Indian Appropriations Act, a piece of legislation that in retrospect demonstrates the subtlety of necropolitics in nation-building. Whereas the 1851 version of this law established the reservation system, the Indian Appropriations Act of 1871 stipulated: "That hereafter no Indian nation or tribe within the territory of the United States shall be acknowledged or recognized as an independent nation, tribe, or power with whom the United States may contract by treaty." Treaties, to clarify, are formal agreements between foreign nations. As stated in the Constitution, the president "shall have Power, by and with

the Advice and Consent of the Senate, to make Treaties." Prior to 1871, the US government had entered into many treaties with American Indians, thereby affirming the latter's status as independent nations. But when Indian sovereignty was refuted, the US government did not need to broker treaties, thereby more easily dispossessing Natives of their ancestral land.

Chapter 4. Border Making, Border Crossing

1 Tiffany Lethabo King's (2019) analysis of "1757 Map of South Carolina and Parts of Georgia" extends a critique of "White cartography" even further back in time, to the mid-eighteenth century. She argues that the map created by William Gerard de Brahm—he was a German-born cartographer who served the British Empire and, coincidently, died the year (1799) of Samuel's birth—was a product of "White settlers' ongoing anxiety about resistance by Black fugitives and Cherokees" (2019, 75). As a technology of conquest, King explains, mapmaking carved out a physical space for Anglo-Americans, while dehumanizing and disappearing enslaved Africans and Indigenous inhabitants. For her part, she introduces the "shoal," an in-between or liminal zone that functions as a geographic disruption. Because shoals are difficult to map, they call to mind the dissolution of borders rather than their cartographic consolidation. King also sees the metaphor as germane for framing the historic and contemporary relations of Blacks and Indigenous peoples.
2 Initially, Corinna thought the stories were exaggerated. She wrote to her brother in 1836, "As for the abominable tough tales in circulation respecting the Seminoles—all I can say is turn a deaf ear to them—some are true but more false" (Denham and Huneycutt 2004, 41).
3 In 1828, Abert's family lived at 6 N. 11th Street and then relocated to 5. N 11th Street from 1829 to 1833. At the time, Samuel was living at 411 Mulberry Street, which today is Arch Street. Given his professional responsibilities, Abert's primary residence was in Washington, DC, however. The two enslaved peoples he owned made it easy to maintain a household there in his wife's absence; the 1830 US Federal Census lists a male slave (10–24 years of age) and a female slave (24–36 years of age) who resided at the Abert home in Washington Ward 1. The 1850 Census also lists two Black people living with the family. David Copeland (25 years old) and Christina Anderson (55 years old); given their ages, they are likely the same unnamed slaves listed 20 years prior. According to the census document, both individuals were born in Virginia, and neither could read nor write.
4 As the head of the corps, Abert was stationed in Washington, DC (Anonymous 1839, 208). From this home base, Abert was also instrumental in founding the National Institute of Science, which eventually was folded into the Smithsonian Institution (Wilson and Fiske 1887, 8).
5 Later Abert sent Samuel the skull of a "POTAWATOMIE of Michigan"; he was around 70 years of age at the time of death. In the *Catalogue*, this decedent is labeled 737 (Morton 1840a).
6 I confirmed sex estimations based on cranial variation following standards established by Buikstra and Ubelaker (1994). Many of the cranial traits observed were

intermediary (e.g., orbital ridges, gracility/robusticity, mastoid process). Both the nuchal ridge and supraorbital ridges were moderate. The zygomatic processes extended as a crest past the external auditory meatus (EAM) and the mandible was square in shape, which are more typical male attributes. With regard to age, dental wear on the first and second molars was moderate with some dentin exposure. The third molars had erupted but were missing so they could not be evaluated.

7   Throughout his military career, Dimick waged war against Florida's Indians three times: 1835–1838, 1849–1850; and 1856–1857 (Wilson and Fiske 1888, 179).

8   Primary source information was housed at the Historical Society of Pennsylvania (Emerson 1837). On one side of a single page is written "Dr. Emerson" atop "57 South 5th St." The other side recounts Dimick's slaying of the decedent Samuel labeled 604. Dissimilar from a letter, the document starts mid-sentence and contains neither a greeting nor a closing. At the bottom of the excerpt, written in pencil and what appears to be Samuel's handwriting, is "From G. Emerson." The left top corner contains an impressed stamp of a dove on a branch with another branch in its beak. The word "AMIES" arches above and "PHILADELPHIA" below. This watermark was created by Thomas Amies, who operated Dove Mill, a paper mill located in Lower Merion Township, Pennsylvania (Barker 1926, 11). Rather than rewrite the passage, Emerson ripped it directly from his medical notebook and sent it along to Samuel. The notebook is housed at College of Physicians of Philadelphia's Historical Medical Library and contains missing pages (Emerson n.d.).

9   Sex estimations were confirmed based on cranial variation following Buikstra and Ubelaker (1994). The skull was large overall but appeared to be lightly muscled. Typical male traits included rounded orbital rims, pronounced mastoid processes, zygomatic processes that extend as crests past EAM, and a square mandible. More intermediary traits were a moderate nuchal ridge area, and supraorbital ridges. Age was indicated by the lack of ecto- or endocranial suture fusion. Additionally, the right and left maxillary third molars had erupted but displayed no wear. Minimal wear appeared on the first and second molars.

10 Here it may be useful to refer back to my preface where I lay out my ambivalence about using Samuel's first name. It does emphasize the distance between his humanity and "specimens" stripped of personhood, names, and kinship ties. But to do so—to be on a first name basis with Samuel while continuing to use catalogue numbers for the individuals whose skulls he collected—does run the risk of "replicating the grammar of violence," to borrow from Hartman (2008, 4). Such an end is not my intent, whereas bringing these individuals back into historical narratives is. And so, I reiterate, as well as make transparent, my qualms and inadequacies. Thank you to Alanna Warner-Smith for holding me accountable here.

11 Based on Toomey's (1917) analysis of proper names from the Muskhogean language, Eoklo may translate as "yellow." He (1917, 13, 15) translates Ocklokonee (or Oklokonee), which refers to a river originating in Georgia and running through Florida, as "yellow water."

12 Like Samuel, Wilson was more interested in being a naturalist than a professional medical practitioner; he gravitated to geology, ornithology, and entomology. He served in various administrative roles at the ANS, including president (1863–1864). All told, he donated more than 12,000 texts to the institution's library and 26,000 specimens (floral, faunal, and human) to its museum (Ennis et al. 1865, 8, 10).

13 The following individuals—listed here by number and racial designation as they appear in the *Catalogue* (1849a)—fall under the umbrella of "Mixed Races": 17 MULATTO, 64 MULATTO, 61 CHOLO, 636 SAMBO, 690 Mixed Indian and Spaniard?, 982 MIXED NEGRO AND INDIAN?, 1294 mixed Negro and Egyptian, 1234 MULATTO?, 1319 Mulatto.

14 In subsequent censuses, the preoccupation with nativity and race only grew more complex. In the 1870 census, for instance, place of birth inquired about one's "Parentage." Additionally, "Color" was expanded; it came to include White, Black, Mulatto, Chinese, and Indian. There was also a query about "Constitutional Relations": If a male citizen aged 21 or older, had the right to vote been denied or abridged? By the 1880 census, "Nativity" replaced "Parentage." And come 1890, there were queries about one's ability to speak English, naturalization status, and racial gradations. Per the latter, "Color" now differentiated between White, Black, Mulatto, Quadroon, Octoroon, Chinese, Japanese, and Indian. Analysis of these shifts over time surely has something to tell us about immigration, the process of racialization, and legislative policy making, among other issues.

15 For an insightful analysis of the foldout and narrative by Jim Cusick, a curator of the P. K. Yonge Library of Florida History, see https://ufsasc.domains.uflib.ufl.edu/hidden-meanings-second-seminole-war-pamphlet-florida/.

16 For this biohistorical study, our concern was understanding the development of social race during the nineteenth century. To this end, we started with craniometric measurements from the seven Seminole warriors in the Morton Collection. These data were then compared to samples from appropriate geographic provenances and time periods: from nineteenth-century Florida (soldiers identified as White from the Fort St. Marks Military Cemetery); the Howells database (Blacks, Whites, and Native groups from the nineteenth century); and the Forensic Data Bank (identified as twentieth-century White, Black, and "Amerind" males). To assess craniometric affinity between the select individuals in the Morton Collection and these historic samples, i.e., to allocate the former, we used Fordisc 3.1, a statistics-based software program. Temporal and geographical contextualization served two interrelated purposes: to recognize data as a biocultural product; and to avoid reifying racial taxonomies, like those created by Samuel, while teasing out racialization processes. Robust archival sources then deepened the inferences drawn from craniometric data.

17 Writing on this skull is variably preserved. Based on the inked letters that have not faded, "Talokc . . . Hatchee" is likely "Talakchopco Hatchee," translated as "River of the Long Peas" and alternatively known as Peas Creek or Peace River (Rivers and Brown 1997, 2). There is also a word written below "Lake" that is not legible.

Chapter 5. The Beloved Woman

1. This obituary was adapted from a eulogy authored by Charles Meigs (1851, 41).
2. Quaker Meeting Records from 4 February 1827 note that the family was brought into the fold of the Philadelphia Quaker community soon after they moved to the city (Anonymous 1827a).
3. According to Philadelphia's city directories, the family initially resided at 11th and Arch Streets in 1833 but relocated to 431 Arch Street by 1835 (Desilver 1833, 151, 1835–1836, 132; McElroy 1844, 226). (Arch Street was originally known as Mulberry Street.) At the time of Samuel's death, the family lived at 387 Arch Street (McElroy 1849, 269, 1852, 320).
4. Pediatrics did not become a separate specialty until the early twentieth century (Zipursky 2002).
5. This condition involves the displacement of the uterus from its normal position, usually following childbirth.
6. This biologization of women's passivity sustained well into the twentieth century. As Emily Martin (1991) has argued, the narrative (or "scientific fairy tale") used to describe the reproductive process—in medical textbooks and clinical training—represented sperm as "strong," "heroic," and "invariably active," while the egg is "passive," "rescued," "fragile," and "caught" (by a sperm who "assaults" it). Menstruation was framed as a failure whereas the egg's fertilization was a success. The truth of (in) the matter, Martin stressed, is that eggs are active, as well as engaged in more equitable interactions, not hierarchical relations, with sperm.
7. Meigs presented this skull in May 1852 to Dr. James Aitken Meigs (no relation), who continued to curate and study the Morton Collection after Samuel's death. In the *Catalogue* revised by James Aitken Meigs, he labeled the skull 1556 (1857, 67). But there are some categorical complications. In an annotated version of the *Catalogue*, someone had crossed out the published 1556 number and handwritten 753 in the margins. On the actual skull, someone has crossed out 753, which appears on the right frontal bone, and written the number 1840 in several areas of the cranium. Inked notations (e.g., "Coronal Suture," "Sagittal") also indicate that Charles Meigs used the skull for teaching purposes.
8. The envelopes of numerous letters attest that the Morton house was located at 431 Arch Street, and Mott resided at 338 Arch Street (Palmer 2002).
9. On 2 March 1846, Lucretia wrote to the Combes: "The true grandeur of Nations she [Anne D. Morrison] would send by Mr. whom you had introduced to her, was left with the letter at Dr. Morton's. But he, supposing it was sent to him to read, did not hand it to the gentleman with the letter" (Palmer 2002, 141). Beverly Wilson Palmer (2002, 142n9), the editor of *Selected Letters of Lucretia Coffin Mott*, does argue that the Dr. Morton referenced in Lucretia's letter was William Thomas Green Morton. But this identification makes little sense for several reasons. She and Samuel were both friends with Combe. Samuel was a practicing physician in Philadelphia and neighbor of the Motts, whereas William Thomas Green Morton, the dentist and physician who introduced ether as an anesthetic, was based in Massachusetts.

10 Though, after *Romeo and Juliet* debuted in Britain, George Combe did write Charlotte to express concern about the incestuous implications of two sisters playing the lead roles (Cushman 1845a, 1845b).
11 For sex estimation of skulls in the Morton Collection, standards outlined in Buikstra and Ubelaker (1994) were referenced. Assessing cranial features to estimate sex is accurate in 85 percent to 90 percent of the time (Mays and Cox 2000, 119–20; Meindl et al. 1985; Walker 1995).
12 Brokenleg (2006, 5–6) regards terms like *wingkte*, "would-be woman," or *winkte*, "kill-woman," as the result of linguistic changes made by non-Lakota speakers during colonization and Christianization. Will Roscoe also identified alternate spellings that relate to group differences; the Santee and Western Dakota, for instance, use the term *wingkta* (Roscoe 1998, 216).
13 Per Buikstra and Ubelaker (1994), this skull was intermediary to gracile and had rounded orbital rims, unmarked supraorbital ridges, an intermediary nuchal ridge area, zygomatic processes that did not extend as crests past the external auditory meatus, and a mastoid process of moderate size. I could not evaluate the mental eminence because the mandible was missing.
14 In time, Shoemaker Lane was rechristened East Penn Street.

Chapter 6. Legacy

1 Here I invoke W.E.B. Du Bois. While much about the Black American experience has changed since Du Bois first authored the groundbreaking *The Souls of Black Folk* in 1903, few would argue that a double consciousness for Black Americans, "this sense of always looking at one's self through the eyes of others" ([1903] 2007, 3), is irrelevant today. Yet, as Henry Louis Gates Jr. stresses in the introduction to a more recent edition of the book, "Double consciousness, once a disorder, is now the cure" (2007, xv).
2 For a more extended discussion of Douglass's speech, see Fabian (2010, 116–19).
3 Three flying galleries, located on the north and south sides of the ANS's main hall, were raised above the main floor and "supported by graceful iron columns" (Ruschenberger 1852, 16).
4 Aside from Meigs, the physician Harrison Allen (1867, 173) assessed lower jaws from "the very fine Morton Cabinet in the Museum of the Academy of Natural Sciences" to determine the antiquity of a specimen discovered at Moulin Quignon, France.
5 Ann Fabian also documents how Boas borrowed skulls from the Morton Collection in the 1890s for evidence of culture's impact on cranial morphology (2010, 44, 231n75).
6 His diary entry from 12 June 1888 notes, "Besides having scientific value these skeletons are worth money" (Boas in Rohner 1969, 90).
7 Boas's research on cranial plasticity remained a topical concern well into the twenty-first century. Some have verified his findings with slight revision (Gravlee et al. 2003a, 2003b), while others have taken issue with his findings about environment's impact (Sparks and Jantz 2002, 2003).

8   In 1989, Heye's collections were transferred to the Smithsonian Institution and became a branch of the National Museum of the American Indian. For a history of the collection see https://americanindian.si.edu/explore/collections/history.
9   To cure an unspecified childhood disease, Moses was added as a forename (Shipman 1994, 159).
10 Columbia, like Penn, was also more amenable to admitting Jews during the first half of the twentieth century. As sociologist Jerome Karabel (2005) has found, most prestigious universities—the Ivy League schools, Stanford, Johns Hopkins, University of Chicago, and so forth—normalized casual antisemitism, and eventually they formalized it in their admission policies. For instance, starting in 1922, Harvard posed the following question to applicants: "What change, if any, has been made since birth in your own name or that of your father? (Explain fully.)" (Karabel 2005, 94). This query, along with information solicited about religion, birthplace, race, and color, was designed to weed out Jews.
11 Massachusetts was the first state in the United States to pass an anatomy act, legalizing cadaver acquisition in 1831 (Sappol 2002, 123).
12 Over the years, the Pennsylvania legislature has amended—in 1919, 1921, and 1925—but never repealed the state's Anatomy Act. Philadelphia's unclaimed bodies no longer end up on dissecting tables, however. Today, ironically enough, its Medical Examiner's Office cremates unclaimed bodies, stores the remains for up to 10 years, inters them in a mass grave at Laurel Hill Cemetery (where Samuel is buried), and marks the spot with an inscribed gravestone (Allyn 2016).
13 This cemetery was condemned by the city in 1899 and closed in 1903. All the bodies were exhumed and moved to Eden Cemetery (Wright 2016, 444), one of the oldest continually active Black owned cemeteries in the United States.
14 *Trial of the Major War Criminals before the International Military Tribunal, Nuremberg, 14 November 1945–1 October 1946*, Vol. 6, http://avalon.law.yale.edu/imt/01-28-46.asp. Live video feed can be found at https://www.ushmm.org/online/film/display/detail.php?file_num=2972. Both web links were accessed 27 July 2017.
15 Allen and colleagues (2019, xv) define the concept as it pertains to archaeology: "Legacy collections can be described as previously curated collections that are the result of planned and research-sponsored archaeological activities, whether originating from university, government agency, or cultural resource management activities." While a useful conceptual starting point, I think legacy collections composed of human remains raise issues that extend beyond the purview of archaeological materials (see also MacFarland and Vokes 2016). I draw on some of Allen et al.'s insights with adaptations given the subject matter at hand.
16 The collection was transferred to the Cleveland Museum of Natural History in the 1950s. It currently consists of more than 3,100 human skeletons. For information, see https://www.cmnh.org/biological-anthropology and https://www.cmnh.org/cmnh/media/cmnh_media/pdfs/policiesandguidelines.pdf.
17 Hamann and Todd acquired skeletons from 1893 to 1938. I selected the 1920 Census to gauge Cleveland's demographics because it falls within the midpoint of the physicians' collecting activities. Per the census data, Cleveland in 1920 had a total

population of 796,841. "Native" Whites accounted for 522,448, while "foreign-born" Whites represented 239,538 individuals. The number of "Negro" males and females living in Cleveland during this time were 34,451. "Indian, Chinese, Japanese, and all other" account for an even smaller fraction of Cleveland's total population, less than .05 percent. See https://www2.census.gov/prod2/decennial/documents/06229686v32-37ch3.pdf, accessed on 25 August 2020.
18 At Penn, Krogman contributed to the nascent subfield of forensic anthropology and understandings of human growth and development.
19 Gould's writings are perhaps the best known during this period, though several other scholars also explored Samuel's scientific racism (e.g., Horsman 1975; Stanton 1960).
20 See Award Abstract #0447271, Expansion and Improvement of the Penn Cranial CT Database, US National Science Foundation, https://www.nsf.gov/awardsearch/showAward?AWD_ID=0447271&HistoricalAwards=false.
21 Initially the Penn Cranial CT Database, the archive was later renamed the Open Research Scan Archive (or ORSA). See Monge and Schoenemann (2011) and Monge (2008).
22 At the time of NAGPRA's passage Dr. Alan E. Mann was the curator in charge of the Physical Anthropology Section at Penn Museum. In 2001, Mann retired from Penn and joined the faculty at Princeton. The curatorship then transferred to Dr. Janet Monge, who held the position until 2023.
23 According to their website, the tribe passed a measure in 2002 that changed "Sioux Tribe to the traditional Dakota word 'Oyate,' meaning people or nation" (https://www.swo-nsn.gov/tribal-history/).
24 See https://www.penn.museum/about-collections/statements-and-policies/nagpra-compliance/repatriations#17 and Fowler Williams and colleagues (2016, 36).
25 For individuals of African ancestry who interacted with Seminole communities, there have been multiple referents—Black Seminoles, Seminole Blacks, Seminole Negroes, Seminole Freedmen, freedmans, Afro-Seminoles, Seminole maroons, or Black Muscogulges. In Muskogee, *estelusti* means "black man" (Micco 2006, 143), while an alternative spelling in Creek is *isti-lásti* (Mulroy 2007, xxiii–iv). These designations hint at the dynamism and complexity of identity, whether self-selected or imposed by others. Contemporary selection of a term may also indicate one's political stance on the relations between a federally recognized tribe and a group with African ancestry. According to the STOF, for instance, they see Black Seminole as a "misnomer" because it confuses more than it explains (https://www.semtribe.com/helpful-linksmain/helpful-links).
26 For a defense of this position, see Susan Miller (2005), and for a criticism of it see Micco (2006), Kevin Noble Maillard (2008), and Kim TallBear (2003, 95–98). More recently, the pandemic laid bare the necropolitical implications of disenrollment when Indian Health Service facilities denied Black Seminoles medical care and COVID vaccines (Walker and Cameron 2021).
27 In September 2013, the Eastern Band of Cherokee Indians, the Cherokee Nation, and the United Keetoowah Band of Cherokee Indians repatriated the six skulls

Drs. Hardy and Martin had procured for Samuel's collection (https://www.penn.museum/about-collections/statements-and-policies/nagpra-compliance). To date, the four skulls identified as Creek have not been repatriated and remain under the care of Penn Museum staff.

28 While not an exhaustive list, recommended readings include the following: Bruning (2006), Burke et al. (2008), Fine-Dare (2002), Gould (2017), Kakaliouras (2008, 2017), Nash and Colwell (2020), Rose et al. (1996), and Watkins (2004).

29 The NAGPRA Office operates under the aegis of the American Section, and Stacey Espenlaub has served as the Kamensky NAGPRA project coordinator since 2002. See Fowler Williams et al. (2016) and https://www.penn.museum/about-collections/statements-and-policies/nagpra-compliance/repatriations.

30 BLM is a larger response to violence experienced by Black communities at the hands of state actors (i.e., police brutality) and individuals who go unpunished by the state. Its inception occurred after the 2013 acquittal of Trayvon Martin's murderer, George Zimmerman, and the movement consolidated with the 2014 murder of Mike Brown by Ferguson police officer Darren Wilson (https://blacklivesmatter.com/herstory/).

31 The Penn & Slavery Project aims to investigate the institution's ties to enslavement (https://pennandslaveryproject.org/); the project is an undergraduate research endeavor, which is under the advisement of Penn faculty and fellows. Making complicity visible and narrating Others' stories are crucial first steps in remedying past institutional failings and structural violence, and for these efforts the project should be commended. I do, however, have some qualms about the accuracy of research conducted. Information included in the Augmented Reality Mobile App about Samuel Morton and his relationship to Penn, for instance, contains several mistakes (https://pennandslaveryproject.org/exhibits/show/mededucation/southerndoctors/samuelmorton). To clarify, while Samuel graduated from Penn's Medical Department in 1820 and later served as a physician preceptor for students enrolled there, he never did teach at the university (see chapter 2).

32 For example, see Johnny Diaz, "Penn Museum to Relocate Skull Collection of Enslaved People," *New York Times*, July 27, 2020, https://www.nytimes.com/2020/07/27/us/Penn-museum-slavery-skulls-Morton-cranial.html.

33 Also in April 2021, news broke that Penn Museum retained the human remains of two children killed in the 1985 MOVE bombing (e.g., Ayers 2021; McCoy 2021). To properly address what transpired would require considerable attention and word count (i.e., a book project). But, here, it is worth noting that while the events surrounding this case are distinct from the sociopolitics of the Morton Collection (we should take care not to conflate the two), both raise concerns about the connection between necropolitics and scientific inquiry. The MOVE case also underscores that, if the discipline is committed to furthering a decolonial ethos, we must continue to hold institutions and individual practitioners accountable, as well as assess and change disciplinary norms.

34 Reporters and well-intentioned scholars have claimed, mistakenly I believe, that consultation has not occurred with the descendant community (e.g., Stantis et al. 2023; Tumin 2022). Their confusion may stem from the complexities of demarcating

a descendant community. That is, heterogeneity has long characterized Black life in Philadelphia, an observation first made by W.E.B. Du Bois (1899) in *The Philadelphia Negro*, a study of Black residents in the Seventh Ward. For a more recent discussion see Hartman (2019). Without homogeneity, then, what does a descendant community look like?

35 It is also worth noting, per the prior note's discussion about the heterogeneity of Philadelphia's Black community, that Judge Sheila Woods-Skipper likely qualifies as a member; she is a Black Philadelphian with roots in the city, as well as an alumnus of the University of Pennsylvania. See https://alumni.temple.edu/s/705/alumni/16/interior_1col_breadcrumb_nav_nosocial.aspx?sid=705&gid=1&pgid=12942 and "Honorable Shiela Woods-Skipper," Girls Inc., https://girlsincpa-nj.org/honorable-sheila-woods-skipper/.

36 For information about Penn Museum's ethical practices and ongoing reparation efforts, see "Morton Cranial Collection," Penn Museum, https://www.penn.museum/sites/morton/ (last updated December 21, 2023).

37 While nothing has been signed into law (as of September 2023), members of both the House and Senate have introduced legislation that directs the National Park Service (NPS) to identify, interpret, and preserve African American burial grounds. On 13 February 2019, Representatives Alma Adams (D-NC), Donald McEachin (D-VA), and 48 other cosponsors introduced the African-American Burial Grounds Network Act (see https://www.congress.gov/bill/116th-congress/house-bill/1179/text). In the Senate, Senator Sherrod Brown (D-OH) introduced the African American Burial Grounds Study Act on 7 November 2019, which passed in December 2020. The act then went to the House, where it is being held at the desk (see https://www.congress.gov/bill/116th-congress/senate-bill/2827). In February 2022, Representatives Adams, McEachin (D-VA), and Brian Fitzpatrick (R-PA) and Senators Sherrod Brown (D-OH) and Mitt Romney (R-UT) introduced the African American Burial Grounds Preservation Act in the House and Senate, respectively (https://www.congress.gov/bill/117th-congress/house-bill/6805; https://www.congress.gov/bill/117th-congress/senate-bill/3667).

38 As a comparative, see Alanna Warner-Smith's (2022) analysis of the Huntington Anatomical Collection and the utilitarian position that underpinned its assemblage and study.

39 See Chimamanda Ngozi Adichie, "The Danger of a Single Story," TEDGlobal, July 2009, https://www.ted.com/talks/chimamanda_ngozi_adichie_the_danger_of_a_single_story. In this same vein, James Flexner (2020, 166) reiterates that "in post-normative science, *storytelling matters*." In our publications, he suggests, it behooves us to slow down the creation of these stories, seek out input from an array of people, and deliberate about the impact they may have on different audiences.

REFERENCES

Abadie, Eugene H. 1836. Creek (Emigration) Letters from Dr. E H Abadie. Letter to General George Gibson, 20 October 1836. Indian Removal to the West, 1832–1840, Files of the Office of the Commissary General of Subsistence. National Archives, Washington, DC.
———. 1838a. Letter to Samuel G. Morton, 3 February 1838. Samuel George Morton Papers. American Philosophical Society, Philadelphia.
———. 1838b. Letter to Samuel G. Morton, 24 August 1838. Samuel George Morton Papers. American Philosophical Society, Philadelphia.
Abbot, George Maurice. 1913. *A Short History of the Library Company of Philadelphia: Compiled from the Minutes, Together with Some Personal Reminiscences.* Philadelphia, PA: The Board of Directors.
Abert, John J. 1832. Letter to Franklin Bache, 2 May 1832. American Philosophical Society Archives. Record Group IIc. American Philosophical Society, Philadelphia.
Abert, S. Thayer. 1890. Application for Membership. Sons of the American Revolution Membership Applications, 1889–1970. National Society of the Sons of the American Revolution, National Society of the Sons of the American Revolution, Louisville, KY.
Aborigines Protection Society. 1838. *The First Annual Report of the Aborigines Protection Society: Presented at the Meeting in Exeter Hall, May 16th, 1838, with List of Officers, Subscribers, and Benefactors.* London: P. White & Son.
———. 1839. *The Second Annual Report of the Aborigines Protection Society: Presented at the Meeting in Exeter Hall, May 21st, 1839, with List of Officers, Subscribers, and Benefactors.* London: P. White & Son.
Aborigines' Protection Society. 1840. *The Third Annual Report of the Aborigines' Protection Society: Presented at the Meeting in Exeter Hall, June 3rd, 1840, with List of Officers, Subscribers, Benefactors, and Honorary Members.* London: P. White & Son.
Academy of Natural Sciences of Philadelphia. 1877. *Members and Correspondents of the Academy of Natural Sciences of Philadelphia.* Philadelphia: The Academy.
Adair, James. 1775. *The History of the American Indians.* London: Edward and Charles Dilly.
Adjutant General's Office. 1838. Edward S. Aldrich. Compiled Service Records of Volunteer Soldiers Who Served in Organizations from the State of Florida during the

Florida Indian Wars, 1835–1858. Records of the Adjutant General's Office, 1780's–1917. National Archives, National Archives, Washington, DC.

Agassiz, Elizabeth Cary, ed. 1893. *Louis Agassiz: His Life and Correspondence*. Boston: Houghton Mifflin.

Agnew, Brad. 1980. *Fort Gibson: Terminal on the Trail of Tears*. Norman: University of Oklahoma Press.

Agnew, D. Hayes, Alfred Stillé, Lewis Bush, Charles Mills, and Roland Curtin. 1890. *History and Reminiscences of the Philadelphia Almshouse and Philadelphia Hospital*. Philadelphia: Detre & Blackburn.

Allen, Harrison. 1867. "The Jaw of Moulin Quignon." *Dental Cosmos* 9(4): 169–80.

Allen, Rebecca, Ben Ford, and J. Ryan Kennedy. 2019. "Introduction: Reclaiming the Research Potential of Archaeological Collections." In *New Life for Archaeological Collection*, edited by Rebecca Allen and Ben Ford, xiii–xxxix. Lincoln: University of Nebraska Press and the Society for Historical Archaeology.

Allyn, Bobby. 2016. "In Philadelphia, Finding Dignity for Bodies Left Unclaimed." *WHYY PBS NPR*, 25 May 2016. Accessed 11 September 2023. https://whyy.org/segments/in-philadelphia-finding-dignity-for-bodies-left-unclaimed/.

Almanac. 2014. "New Center for the Analysis of Archaeological Materials (CAAM), in Penn Museum's Renovated Conservation and Teaching Labs." *Almanac* 61(7). Accessed 11 September 2023. https://almanac.upenn.edu/archive/volumes/v61/n07/museum-caam.html.

Alsheh, Yehonatan. 2014. "The Biopolitics of Corpses of Mass Violence and Genocide." In *Human Remains and Mass Violence: Methodological Approaches*, edited by Jean-Marc Dreyfus and Élisabeth Anstett, 12–43. Manchester, UK: Manchester University Press.

American Psychological Association. 2019. "Racial and Ethnic Identity." Accessed 11 September 2023. https://apastyle.apa.org/style-grammar-guidelines/bias-free-language/racial-ethnic-minorities.

Amos, Alcione M. 1977. "Captain Hugh Young's Map of Jackson's 1818 Seminole Campaign in Florida." *Florida Historical Quarterly* 55(3): 336–46.

Andrews, Lori, Nancy Buenger, Jennifer Bridge, Laurie Rosenow, David Stoney, R. E. Gaensslen, Theodore Karamanski, Russell Lewis, Jordan Paradise, and Amy Inlander. 2004. "Constructing Ethical Guidelines for Biohistory." *Science* 304(5668): 215–16.

Angelino, Henry, and Charles L. Shedd. 1955. "A Note on Berdache." *American Anthropologist* 57: 121–26.

Anonymous. 1827a. At a Monthly Meeting of Friends of Philadelphia for the Western District Held 2 Mo 4th 1827, Minutes, 1814–1830. US, Quaker Meeting Records, 1681–1935. Ancestry.com, Swarthmore College Friends Historical Library, Swarthmore, PA.

———. 1827b. At a Monthly Meeting of Friends of Philadelphia for the Western District Held 12 Mo 19th 1827. Women's Minutes, 1831–50. US, Quaker Meeting Records, 1681–1935. Ancestry.com, Swarthmore College Friends Historical Library, Swarthmore, PA.

———. 1833. "Presentation to the Cholera Physicians." *Journal of Health and Recreation* IV(7): 204–6.

———. 1839. "List of Officers Now in the Army who Were Brevetted during the Late War." *Army and Navy Chronicle* 8(13): 207–8.

———. 1843. At a Monthly Meeting of Friends of Philadelphia for the Western District Held 8 Mo 6th 1843. US, Quaker Meeting Records, 1681–1935. Ancestry.com, Haverford College, Haverford, PA.

———. 1851. Funerals Continued, Dr. Samuel George Morton, Pennsylvania and New Jersey, US, Church and Town Records, 1669–2013. Grace Church Episcopal Chapel, Historic Pennsylvania Church and Town Records. Pennsylvania and New Jersey, US, Church and Town Records, 1669–2013, Ancestry.com, Historical Society of Pennsylvania, Philadelphia, PA.

———. 1864. Burials, Rebecca P. Morton, Pennsylvania and New Jersey, US, Church and Town Records, 1669–2013. St Luke's Church, Historic Pennsylvania Church and Town Records. Pennsylvania and New Jersey, US, Church and Town Records, 1669–2013, Ancestry.com, Historical Society of Pennsylvania, Philadelphia, PA.

———. 1904. Encyclopedia of Genealogy and Biography of the State of Pennsylvania. New York: Lewis.

———. 1908. *The Annual Monitor for 1909: Being an Obituary of Members of the Society of Friends in Great Britain and Ireland, from October 1, 1907, to September 30, 1908*. Vol. 96. London: Headley Brothers.

———. 1919. *Catalogue of the University of Pennsylvania, 1918–1919*. Philadelphia: For the University of Pennsylvania.

———. n.d. a. Genealogical Notes. Morton and Allied Families includes Langstaffe, Latham, Morton, Moore and Others, Surnames L–M; Contributor Helen Kirkbride Morton. Historical Society of Pennsylvania, Philadelphia, PA.

———. n.d. b. Newspaper clippings re. Dr. Morton's death. Samuel George Morton Papers. American Philosophical Society, American Philosophical Society, Philadelphia, PA.

Anzaldúa, Gloria. 1987. *Borderlands / La Frontera: The New Mestiza*. San Francisco: Aunt Lute Books.

Appiah, Kwame Anthony. 2020. "The Case for Capitalizing the B in Black." *Atlantic*, 18 June 2020. Accessed 11 September 2023. https://www.theatlantic.com/ideas/archive/2020/06/time-to-capitalize-blackand-white/613159/.

Aptowicz, Cristin O'Keefe. 2014. *Dr. Mütter's Marvels: A True Tale of Intrigue and Innovation at the Dawn of Modern Medicine*. New York: Penguin.

Ashley Montagu, M. F. 1946. Letter to J. Percy Moore, 30 January 1946. J. Percy Moore Papers, 1850–1856 [Biography Correspondence Notes: Maclure-Morton, 1946–1947]. Academy of Natural Sciences of Philadelphia, Philadelphia, PA.

Ashley-Montagu, M. F. 1939. "Location of Porion in the Living." *American Journal of Physical Anthropology* 25(2): 281–95.

Atlas, Michel C. 2001. "Ethics and Access to Teaching Materials in the Medical Library: The Case of the Pernkopf Atlas." *Bulletin of the Medical Library Association* 89(1): 51–58.

Ayers, Elaine. 2021. "The Grim Open Secret of College Bone Collections." *Slate*, 30 April 2021, 2021. Accessed 11 September 2023. https://slate.com/news-and-politics/2021/04/move-bombing-victims-princeton-penn-museum-history-anthropology.html.

Bachman, John. 1850. *The Doctrine of the Unity of the Human Race Examined on the Principles of Science*. Charleston, SC: C. Canning.

Bacon, Margaret Hope. 2001. "New Light on Sarah Mapps Douglass and Her Reconciliation with Friends." *Quaker History* 90(1): 28–49.

Baer, Hans A. 2001. *Biomedicine and Alternative Healing Systems in America: Issues of Class, Race, Ethnicity, and Gender*. Madison: University of Wisconsin Press.

Baltrusis, Sam. 2016. *Haunted Boston Harbor*. Charleston, SC: The History Press.

Baptist, Edward E. 2002 *Creating an Old South: Middle Florida's Plantation Frontier before the Civil War*. Chapel Hill: University of North Carolina Press.

Barker, Charles R. 1926. "Old Mills of Mill Creek, Lower Merion." *Pennsylvania Magazine of History and Biography* 50(1): 1–22.

Barnes, Joseph K. 1867–1868. "Circular No. 2." *The Medical Record, A Semi-Monthly Journal of Medicine and Surgery* 2: 167.

Barnhill, John H. 2013. "Indian Civil Rights." In *Encyclopedia of American Indian Issues Today, Volume 2*, edited by Russell M. Lawson, 454–63. Santa Barbara, CA: Greenwood.

Barratt, John Perkins. 1846. Letter to Samuel G. Morton, 2 September 1846. Samuel George Morton Papers, 1832–1862. Historical Society of Pennsylvania, Philadelphia, PA.

Bastir, Markus, Antonio Rosas, Daniel Lieberman, and Paul O'Higgins. 2008. "Middle Cranial Fossa Anatomy and the Origin of Modern Humans." *Anatomical Record* 291(2): 130–40.

Bates, Alan 2010. *The Anatomy of Robert Knox: Murder, Mad Science and Medical Regulation in Nineteenth-Century Edinburgh*. Thornhill, Ontario: Sussex Academic Press.

Beers, Henry P. 1942. "A History of the U.S. Topographical Engineers, 1813–1863." *Military Engineer* 34(200): 287–91.

Bell, John. 1873. "Obituary Notice of Charles D. Meigs, MD." *Proceedings of the American Philosophical Society* 13(90): 170–79.

Bell, Whitfield J. 1943. "Philadelphia Medical Students in Europe, 1750–1800." *Pennsylvania Magazine of History and Biography* 67(1): 1–29.

Bemrose, John. 1966. *Reminiscences of the Second Seminole War*. Gainesville: University of Florida Press.

Berner, Margit. 2010. "Race and Physical Anthropology in Interwar Austria." *Focaal* 2010(58): 16–31.

Bhabha, Homi K. 1985. "Signs Taken for Wonders: Questions of Ambivalence and Authority under a Tree outside Delhi, May 1817." *Critical Inquiry* 12: 144–65.

———. 1994. *The Location of Culture*. New York: Routledge.

Biddle, Clement. 1833. Letter to the Hon. Louis M. Late, Secretary of State, 29 December 1833, passport application for Samuel G. Morton. US, Passport Applications,

1795–1925. National Archives and Records Administration (NARA), Washington, DC.

Bieder, Robert E. 1986. *Science Encounters the Indian, 1820–1880: The Early Years of American Ethnology.* Norman: University of Oklahoma Press.

Bilson, Geoffrey. 1980. *A Darkened House: Cholera in Nineteenth-Century Canada.* Toronto, Canada: University of Toronto Press.

Blakey, Michael L. 1987. "Skull Doctors: Intrinsic Social and Political Bias in the History of American Physical Anthropology." *Critique of Anthropology* 7(2): 7–35.

———. 2001. "Bioarchaeology of the African Diaspora in the Americas: Its Origins and Scope." *Annual Review of Anthropology* 30(1): 387–422.

Blakey, Michael L., and Rachel Watkins. 2022. "William Montague Cobb: Near the African Diasporic Origins of Activist and Biocultural Anthropology." *Anatomical Record* 305(4): 838–48.

Blanton, DeAnne, and Lauren Cook. 2002. *They Fought Like Demons: Women Soldiers in the American Civil War.* Baton Rouge: Louisiana State University Press.

Blumenbach, Johann Friedrich. 1865. *The Anthropological Treatises of Johann Friedrich Blumenbach.* Translated by Thomas Bendyshe. London: Longman, Green, Longman, Egberts, & Green.

Boas, Franz. 1894. "The Half-Blood Indian." *Popular Science Monthly* 45: 761–70.

———. 1910. *Changes in Bodily Form of Descendants of Immigrants (Final Report, United States Immigration Commission, Senate Document 208).* Washington, DC: Government Printing Office.

———. 1912. "Changes in Bodily Form of Descendants of Immigrants." *American Anthropologist* 14(3): 530–62.

———. 1931. Letter to M. F. Ashley-Montagu, 9 February 1931. Franz Boas Papers. American Philosophical Society, Philadelphia.

———. 1939. Letter to M. F. Ashley-Montagu, 26 October 1939. Franz Boas Papers. American Philosophical Society, Philadelphia.

Bonaparte, Alicia. 2015. "Physicians' Discourse for Establishing Authoritative Knowledge in Birthing Work and Reducing the Presence of the Granny Midwife." *Journal of Historical Sociology* 28(2): 168–94.

Booth, Benjamin. 1774. Letter to George Morton, 18 March 1774. Morton and Allied Families includes Langstaffe, Latham, Morton, Moore and Others, Surnames L–M; Contributor Helen Kirkbride Morton. Historical Society of Pennsylvania, Philadelphia, PA.

Boston Courier. 1836. "Captain Dimick and Captain Dimmock." 7 November, 1836.

Bourdieu, Pierre. 1990. *The Logic of Practice.* Translated by Richard Nice. Stanford, CA: Stanford University Press.

Braund, Kathryn E. Holland. 1990. "Guardians of Tradition and Handmaidens to Change: Women's Roles in Creek Economic and Social Life during the Eighteenth Century." *American Indian Quarterly* 14(3): 239–58. https://doi.org/10.2307/1185653.

Breidenbough, E. S. 1882. *The Pennsylvania College: 1832–1882.* Philadelphia: Lutheran Publication Society.

Brokenleg, Martin. 2006. "Lakota Hca." In *Other Voices, Other Worlds: The Global Church Speaks Out on Homosexuality*, edited by Terry Brown, 5–14. New York: Church Publishing.

Bronfman, Alejandra. 2004. *Measures of Equality: Social Science, Citizenship, and Race in Cuba, 1902–1940*. Chapel Hill: University of North Carolina Press.

Brown, Matthew, and Donald J. Ortner. 2011. "Childhood Scurvy in a Medieval Burial from Mačvanska Mitrovica, Serbia." *International Journal of Osteoarchaeology* 21(2): 197–207.

Bruning, Susan. 2006. "Complex Legal Legacies: The Native American Graves Protection and Repatriation Act, Scientific Study, and Kennewick Man." *American Antiquity* 71(3): 501–21.

Bry, Theodor De, Editor, Charles De L' Ecluse, and Jacques Le Moyne De Morgues. 1591. *Narrative of Le Moyne, an Artist Who Accompanied the French Expedition to Florida under Laudonnière*. Frankfurt am Main: Theodor de Bry.

Buchanan, Robert C. 1950. "A Journal of Lt. Robert C. Buchanan during the Seminole War." *Florida Historical Quarterly* 29(2): 132–51.

Buikstra Jane E., and Douglas Ubelaker. 1994. *Standards for Data Collection from Human Skeletal Remains*. Fayetteville, AR: Arkansas Archaeological Survey Research.

Bureau of the Census. 1830. Fifth Census of the United States, 1830. Records of the Bureau of the Census. National Archives, National Archives, Washington, DC.

———. 1850. Seventh Census of the United States, 1850. Records of the Bureau of the Census. National Archives, National Archives, Washington, DC.

Burke, Heather, Claire Smith, Dorothy Lippert, Joe Watkins, and Larry Zimmerman, eds. 2008. *Kennewick Man: Perspectives on the Ancient One*. New York: Routledge.

Butaric, Lauren, Robert McCarthy, and Douglas Broadfield. 2010. "A Preliminary 3D Computed Tomography Study of the Human Maxillary Sinus and Nasal Cavity." *American Journal of Physical Anthropology* 143(3): 426–36.

Butler, Judith. 1997. *Excitable Speech: A Politics of the Performative*. New York: Routledge.

———. 2009. *Frames of War: When Is Life Grievable?* London: Verso.

Bynum, W. F. 1994. *Science and the Practice of Medicine in the Nineteenth Century*. Cambridge: Cambridge University Press.

Byrd, Jodi. 2011. *The Transit of Empire: Indigenous Critiques of Colonialism*. Minneapolis: University of Minnesota Press.

Cain, Daniel, James Cahusac, and Francis Peyre Porcher. 1850. Letters to Samuel G. Morton, 25 March–28 December 1850. Samuel George Morton Papers, 1832–1862. Historical Society of Pennsylvania, Philadelphia, PA.

Canguilhem, Georges. 1951. "Le Normal et le Pathologique." In *Somme de Médecine Contemporaine*, edited by René Leriche, 27–32. Paris, France: Editions de la Diane Française.

Canny, Nicholas P. 1973. "The Ideology of English Colonization: From Ireland to America." *William and Mary Quarterly* 30(4): 575–98.

Cantor, Geoffrey. 2005. *Quakers, Jews, and Science*. Oxford: Oxford University Press.

———. 2013. "Quakers and Science." In *The Oxford Handbook of Quaker Studies*, edited by Stephen W. Angell and Pink Dandelion, 520–34. Oxford: Oxford University Press.

Card, Jeb J., ed. 2013. *The Archaeology of Hybrid Material Culture*. Carbondale: Southern Illinois University Press.

Caric, Ric N. 2007. "The Man with the Poker Enters the Room: Delirium Tremens and Popular Culture in Philadelphia, 1828–1850." *Pennsylvania History: A Journal of Mid-Atlantic Studies* 74(4): 452–91.

Carr, Robert, Marilyn Masson, and Willard Steele. 1989. "Archaeological Investigations at the Okeechobee Battlefield." *Florida Anthropologist* 42(3): 205–36.

Carson, Joseph. 1869. *A History of the Medical Department of the University of Pennsylvania from Its Foundation in 1765*. Philadelphia: Lindsay and Blakiston.

Carter, John Pim. 1937–1942. Work and Notes of Morton Collection of Human Crania. Academy of Natural Sciences of Philadelphia, Philadelphia.

Cave, Alfred A. 2003. "Abuse of Power: Andrew Jackson and the Indian Removal Act of 1830." *Historian* 65(6): 1330–53.

Cazden, Elizabeth. 2013. "Quakers, Slavery, Anti-Slavery, and Race." In *The Oxford Handbook of Quaker Studies*, edited by Stephen W. Angell and Pink Dandelion, 347–62. Oxford: Oxford University Press.

Chaloner, John. 1823. Letter to Samuel G. Morton, 7 July 1823. Samuel George Morton Papers, Series I—Correspondences 1819–1850. American Philosophical Society, Philadelphia, PA.

Chapman, Nathaniel. 1822. "Medical and Philosophical Intelligence." *Philadelphia Journal of the Medical and Physical Sciences* IV: 204–28.

Churchill, Ward. 1997. *A Little Matter of Genocide: Holocaust and Denial in the Americas 1492 to the Present*. San Francisco: City Lights Books.

Cisneros, José Rodriguez. 1840. Letter to Samuel G. Morton, 27 July 1840. Samuel George Morton Papers. American Philosophical Society, Philadelphia, PA.

Cleaveland, Parker. 1839. Letter to Samuel G. Morton, 7 March 1839. Samuel George Morton Papers. American Philosophical Society, Philadelphia, PA.

Clemens, John D., G. Balakrish Nair, Tahmeed Ahmed, Firdausi Qadri, and Jan Holmgren. 2017. "Cholera." *Lancet* 390(10101): 1539–49.

Clement, Priscilla Ferguson. 1985. *Welfare and the Poor in the Nineteenth-Century City: Philadelphia, 1800–1854*. Cranbury, NJ: Associated University Presses.

Cobb, W. Montague. 1935. "Municipal History from Anatomical Records." *Scientific Monthly* 40(2): 157–62.

———. 1959. "Thomas Wingate Todd, MB, Ch. B., FRCS (Eng.), 1885–1938." *Journal of the National Medical Association* 51(3): 233–46.

College of Physicians of Philadelphia. 1799. *Facts and Observations Relative to the Nature and Origin of the Pestilential Fever, which Prevailed in the City of Philadelphia, in 1793, 1797, and 1798*. Philadelphia: George Yard.

Colwell, Chip. 2017. *Plundered Skulls and Stolen Spirits: Inside the Fight to Reclaim Native America's Culture*. Chicago: University of Chicago Press.

Combe, George. 1819. *Essays on Phrenology, or an Inquiry into the Principles and Utility of the System of Drs. Gall and Spurzheim and into the Objections Made against it.* Edinburgh, Scotland: Bell & Bradfute.

———. 1824. "(Preliminary Dissertation.) On the Progress and Application of Phrenology." *Transactions of the Phrenological Society*, 1–62.

———. 1825. *A System of Phrenology.* Edinburgh: John Anderson.

———. 1830. *A System of Phrenology.* Edinburgh: John Anderson.

———. 1835. *The Constitution of Man Considered in Relation to External Objects.* Boston: William D. Ticknor.

———. 1840a. Letter to Samuel G. Morton, 13 March 1840. Samuel George Morton Papers, Series I—Correspondences 1819–1850. American Philosophical Society, Philadelphia, PA.

———. 1840b. Letter to Samuel G. Morton, 27 March 1840. Samuel George Morton Papers, Series I—Correspondences 1819–1850. American Philosophical Society, Philadelphia, PA.

———. 1840c. Letter to Samuel G. Morton, 20 August 1840. Samuel George Morton Papers, Series I—Correspondences 1819–1850. American Philosophical Society, Philadelphia, PA.

———. 1841. Letter to Lucretia Mott, 8 February 1841. Mott Manuscript. Swarthmore College Friends Historical Library, Swarthmore College, Swarthmore, PA.

———. 1845. Letter to Samuel Morton, 29 January 1845. Historical Medical Library, College of Physicians of Philadelphia, Philadelphia, PA.

———. 1852. Letter to Lucretia Mott, 22 October 1852. Mott Manuscripts, SFHL-MSS-035, In Her Own Right, Swarthmore College. Swarthmore College Friends Historical Library, Swarthmore College, Swarthmore, PA.

Commissary General of Subsistence. 1834. *Document 512. Correspondence on the Subject of the Emigration of Indians, between the 30th November 1831 and 27 December 1833, with Abstracts of Expenditures by Disbursing Agents in the Removal and Subsistence of Indians, &c. &c.* Vol. 1. Washington, DC: Duff Green.

———. 1835. *Document 512. Correspondence on the Subject of the Emigration of Indians, between the 30th November, 1831 and 27th December, 1833, with Abstracts of Expenditures by Disbursing Agents in the Removal and Subsistence of Indians, &c. &c.* Vol. 3. Washington, DC: Duff Green.

Conway, Jill K. 1982. *The Female Experience in Eighteenth- and Nineteenth-Century America: A Guide to the History of American Women.* New York: Garland.

Corkran, David H. 1967. *The Creek Frontier, 1540–1783.* Norman: University of Oklahoma Press.

Cott, Nancy. 1977. *The Bonds of Womanhood: "Woman's Sphere" in New England, 1780–1835.* New Haven, CT: Yale University Press.

Cotter, John L. 1992. *The Buried Past: An Archaeological History of Philadelphia.* Philadelphia: University of Pennsylvania Press.

Covington, James W. 1993. *The Seminoles of Florida.* Gainesville: University Press of Florida.

Croom, Hardy B. 1834–1837. Letter to John Torrey, 22 May 1836. John Torrey Papers (PP), Hardy Bryan Croom and John Torrey correspondence, 1834–1837. The New York Botanical Garden, New York.
Croom, William W. 1836. Letter to Hardy B. Croom, 1 July 1836. Florida Documents Collection, 1777–1979. University of Miami Libraries, Special Collections, University of Miami, Coral Gables, FL.
Crossland, Zoë. 2009. "Acts of Estrangement. The Post-Mortem Making of Self and Other." *Archaeological Dialogues* 16(1): 102–25.
Cryne, Julia A. 2009. "NAGPRA Revisited: A Twenty-Year Review of Repatriation Efforts." *American Indian Law Review* 34(1): 99–122.
Cullum, George W. 1891. *Biographical Register of the Officers and Graduates of the US Military Academy at West Point, N.Y. from its Establishment, in 1802, to 1867 with the Early History of the United States Military Academy*. 3rd revised and expanded ed. New York: Houghton, Mifflin and Company.
Currie, William. 1800. *A Sketch of the Rise and Progress of the Yellow Fever, and of the Proceedings of the Board of Health, in Philadelphia, in the Year 1799: To Which is Added, a Collection of Facts and Observations Respecting the Origin of the Yellow Fever in This Country; and a Review of the Different Modes of Treating It*. Philadelphia: Budd and Bartram.
Cushman, Charlotte. 1845a. Letter to George Combe, 21 November 1845. National Library of Scotland, Edinburgh, Scotland.
———. 1845b. Letter to George Combe, 23 November 1845. National Library of Scotland, Edinburgh, Scotland.
Cutter, Barbara. 2003. *Domestic Devils, Battlefield Angels: The Radicalism of American Womanhood, 1830–1865*. DeKalb: Northern Illinois University Press.
Daniel, Thomas. 2000. *Pioneers of Medicine and Their Impact on Tuberculosis*. Rochester: University of Rochester Press.
D'Antonio, Patricia. 2006. *Founding Friends: Families, Staff, and Patients at the Friends Asylum in Early Nineteenth-Century Philadelphia*. Bethlehem, PA: Lehigh University Press.
Darlington, William. 1891. "Pennsylvania Weather Records, 1644–1835." *Pennsylvania Magazine of History and Biography* 15(1): 109–21.
Darwin, Charles. 1847. Letter to Charles Lyell, 2 June 1847. Charles Darwin Papers, 1831–1882. American Philosophical Society, American Philosophical Society, Philadelphia.
———. 1859. *On the Origin of Species by Means of Natural Selection: Or the Preservation of Favoured Races in the Struggle for Life*. London: John Murray.
———. 1871. *The Descent of Man, and Selection in Relation to Sex.* London: John Murray.
Darwin, Francis, ed. (1887) 2010. *The Autobiography of Charles Darwin*. London: Bibliolis Books.
Davis, David Brion. 1986. *From Homicide to Slavery: Studies in American Culture*. Oxford: Oxford University Press.
de la Cova, Carlina. 2014. "The Biological Effects of Urbanization and In-Migration on 19th-Century-Born African Americans and Euro-Americans of Low Socioeco-

nomic Status: An Anthropological and Historical Approach." In *Modern Environments and Human Health: Revisiting the Second Epidemiological Transition*, edited by Molly K. Zuckerman, 243–64. Hoboken, NJ: John Wiley & Sons.

———. 2019. "Marginalized Bodies and the Construction of the Robert J. Terry Anatomical Skeletal Collection: A Promised Land Lost." In *Bioarchaeology of Marginalized People*, edited by Madeleine L. Mant and Alyson Jaagumägi Holland, 133–55. London: Elsevier.

———. 2021. "Making Silenced Voices Speak: Restoring Neglected and Ignored Identities in Anatomical Collections." In *Theoretical Approaches in Bioarchaeology*, edited by Colleen M. Cheverko, Julia R. Prince-Buitenhuys, and Mark Hubbe, 150–69. New York: Routledge.

Deloria, Philip Joseph. 1998. *Playing Indian*. New Haven, CT: Yale University Press.

Denham, James M. 1991. "'Some Prefer the Seminoles': Violence and Disorder among Soldiers and Settlers in the Second Seminole War, 1835–1842." *Florida Historical Quarterly* 70(1): 38–54.

Denham, James M., and Keith L. Huneycutt, eds. 2004. *Echoes from a Distant Frontier: The Brown Sisters' Correspondence from Antebellum Florida*. Columbia: University of South Carolina Press.

Department of Physical Anthropology. 1920. *Annual Report for the Period from April 1, 1919, to April 1, 1920 of the Board of Trustees of the Museum of the American Indian, Heye Foundation to George G. Heye, Grantor*. New York: The Museum of the American Indian, Heye Foundation.

Desilver, Robert. 1828. *Desilver's Philadelphia Directory and Stranger's Guide, for 1828*. Philadelphia: Robert Desilver, 110 Walnut Street.

———. 1829. *Desilver's Philadelphia Directory and Stranger's Guide, 1829*. Philadelphia: Robert Desilver, 110 Walnut Street.

———. 1831. *Desilver's Philadelphia Directory and Stranger's Guide, 1831*. Philadelphia: Robert Desilver, 110 Walnut Street.

———. 1833. *Desilver's Philadelphia Directory and Stranger's Guide, for 1833*. Philadelphia: Robert Desilver, 110 Walnut Street.

———. 1835–1836. *Desilver's Philadelphia Directory and Stranger's Guide, for 1835 & 36*. Philadelphia: Robert Desilver, 110 Walnut Street.

Desmond, Adrian J., and James Moore. 2009. *Darwin's Sacred Cause: How a Hatred of Slavery Shaped Darwin's Views on Human Evolution*. London: Penguin Group.

Dewees, William Potts. 1833. *A Practice of Physic, Comprising Most of the Diseases Not Treated of in "Diseases of Females," and "Diseases of Children."* Philadelphia: Carey, Lea & Blanchard.

Dixon, Anthony E. 2007. "Black Seminole Involvement and Leadership during the Second Seminole War, 1835–1842." PhD dissertation, Department of History, Indiana University.

Donaldson, Thomas. 1886. "Appendix (Part V).—The George Catlin Indian Gallery in the U.S. National Museum (Smithsonian Institution) with Memoir and Statistics." In *Annual Report of the Board of Regents of the Smithsonian Institution,*

Showing the Operations, Expenditures, and Condition of the Institution to July, 1885. Part II, edited by George Goode, 1–939. Washington, DC: US Government Printing Office.

Dorsey, John Syng. 1818. Letter to John Sergeant, 10 June 1818. Archives General Collection of the University of Pennsylvania, 1740–1820. Archives of the University of Pennsylvania, Philadelphia.

Douglass, Frederick. 1882. *The Life and Times of Frederick Douglass, from 1817–1882*. London: Christian Age Office.

———. (1854) 1999. "The Claims of the Negro Ethnologically Considered, address delivered at Western Reserve College, July 12, 1854." In *Frederick Douglass: Selected Speeches and Writings*, edited by Philip S. Foner and Yuval Taylor, 282–97. Repr., Chicago: Lawrence Hill Books.

Drake, Samuel G. 1854. *The Aboriginal Races of North America*. Boston: Higgins and Bradley.

Driskill, Qwo-Li. 2004. "Stolen from Our Bodies: First Nations Two-Spirits/Queers and the Journey to a Sovereign Erotic." *Studies in American Indian Literatures* 16(2): 50–64.

———. 2016. *Asegi Stories: Cherokee Queer and Two-Spirit Memory*. Tucson: University of Arizona Press.

Driskill, Qwo-Li, Chris Finley, Brian Joseph Gilley, and Scott Lauria Morgensen. 2011. "Introduction." In *Queer Indigenous Studies: Critical Interventions in Theory, Politics, and Literature*, edited by Qwo-Li Driskill, Chris Finley, Brian Joseph Gilley and Scott Lauria Morgensen, 1–28. Tucson: University of Arizona Press.

———, eds. 2011. *Queer Indigenous Studies: Critical Interventions in Theory, Politics, and Literature*. Tucson: University of Arizona Press.

Du Bois, W.E.B. 1899. *The Philadelphia Negro: A Social Study*. Vol. 14. Philadelphia: University of Pennsylvania.

———. 1903. *The Souls of Black Folk: Essays and Sketches*. Chicago: A. C. McClurg.

Dumont, Clayton W., Jr. 2011. "Contesting Scientists' Narrations of NAGPRA's Legislative History: Rule 10.11 and the Recovery of 'Culturally Unidentifiable' Ancestors." *Wicazo Sa Review* 26(1): 5–41.

Dunbar, Erica Armstrong. 2008. *A Fragile Freedom: African American Women and Emancipation in the Antebellum City*. New Haven, CT: Yale University Press.

Duncan, William, and Christopher Stojanowski. 2016. "Criminality, Narrative and the Expert Witness in American Biohistory." *Mortality* 21(3): 263–78.

Dunnavant, Justin, Delande Justinvil, and Chip Colwell. 2021. "Craft an African American Graves Protection and Repatriation Act." *Nature* 593: 337–40.

Ecker, Alexander. 1868. "On a Characteristic Peculiarity in the Form of the Female Skull, and Its Significance for Comparative Anthropology." *Anthropological Review* 6(23): 350–56.

Edgar, Heather J. H. 2009. "Biohistorical Approaches to 'Race' in the United States: Biological Distances among African Americans, European Americans, and their Ancestors." *American Journal of Physical Anthropology* 139(1): 58–67. http://dx.doi.org/10.1002/ajpa.20961.

Ellis, Howard. 2001. *A History of Surgery*. London: Greenwich Medical Media Limited.
Emerson, Gouverneur. 1837. Note to Samuel G. Morton, 7 October 1837. Samuel George Morton Papers, 1832–1862. Historical Society of Pennsylvania, Philadelphia, PA.
———. n.d. G. Emerson medical notebook. The Historical Medical Library, The College of Physicians of Philadelphia, Philadelphia, PA.
Ennis, Jacob, James H. B Bland, and J. Frank Knight. 1865. *A Memoir of Thomas Bellerby Wilson, M.D.* Philadelphia: American Entomological Society.
Epps, Charles H., Jr., Davis G. Johnson, and Audrey L. Vaughan. 1993. "Black Medical Pioneers: African-American 'Firsts' in Academic and Organized Medicine. Part One." *Journal of the National Medical Association* 85(8): 629–44.
Fabian, Ann. 2010. *The Skull Collectors: Race, Science, and America's Unburied Dead*. Chicago: University of Chicago Press.
Fanon, Frantz. 1961. *The Wretched of the Earth*. New York: Grove Press.
Faulkner, Carol. 2011. *Lucretia Mott's Heresy: Abolition and Women's Rights in Nineteenth-Century America*. Philadelphia: University of Pennsylvania Press.
———. 2019. *Unfaithful: Love, Adultery, and Marriage Reform in Nineteenth-Century America*. Philadelphia: University of Pennsylvania Press.
Faust, Drew Gilpin. 2008. *This Republic of Suffering: Death and the American Civil War*. New York: Vintage Books.
Fausto-Sterling, Anne. 1995. "Gender, Race, and Nation: The Comparative Anatomy of 'Hottentot' Women in Europe, 1815–1817." In *Deviant Bodies: Critical Perspectives on Difference in Science and Popular Culture*, edited by Jennifer Terry and Jacqueline Urla, 19–48. Bloomington: Indiana University Press.
Federici, Silvia. 2004. *Caliban and the Witch: Women, the Body and Primitive Accumulation*. Brooklyn, NY: Autonomedia.
Fine-Dare, Kathleen Sue. 2002. *Grave Injustice: The American Indian Repatriation Movement and NAGPRA*. Lincoln: University of Nebraska Press.
Finley, Chris. 2011. "Decolonizing the Queer Native Body (and Recovering the Native Bull-Dyke): Bringing 'Sexy Back' and Out of Native Studies' Closet." In *Queer Indigenous Studies: Critical Interventions in Theory, Politics, and Literature*, edited by Qwo-Li Driskill, Chris Finley, Brian Joseph Gilley, and Scott Lauria Morgensen, 31–42. Tucson: University of Arizona Press.
Finnie, David H. 1967. *Pioneers East: The Early American Experience in the Middle East*. Cambridge, MA: Harvard University Press.
Fitzgerald, G. 1823. Letter to Samuel G. Morton, 13 April 1823. Samuel George Morton Papers. American Philosophical Society. Philadelphia, PA.
Flexner, Abraham. 1910. *Medical Education in the United States and Canada: A Report to the Carnegie Foundation for the Advancement of Teaching*. New York: The Carnegie Foundation for the Advancement of Teaching.
Flexner, James. 2020. "Degrowth and a Sustainable Future for Archaeology." *Archaeological Dialogues* 27(2): 159–71.
Forbes, Jack D. 1993. *Africans and Native Americans: The Language of Race and the Evolution of Red-Black Peoples*. Urbana: University of Illinois Press.

Forbes, William Smith. 1898. *History of the Anatomy Act of Pennsylvania*. Philadelphia: Philadelphia Medical Publishing.
Foreman, Grant. 1972. *Indian Removal: The Emigration of the Five Civilized Tribes of Indians*. Norman: University of Oklahoma Press.
Foreman, Grant, and Carolyn Thomas Foreman. 2015. *Fort Gibson: A Brief History*. Norman: University of Oklahoma Press.
Forry, Samuel. 1928. "Letters of Samuel Forry, Surgeon U.S. Army, 1837–1838: Part III." *Florida Historical Society Quarterly* 6(3): 88–105.
Foucault, Michel. (1963) 1973. *The Birth of the Clinic: An Archaeology of Medical Perception*. Repr., New York: Vintage Books.
———. 1977. *Discipline and Punish: The Birth of the Prison*. Translated by Robert Hurley. New York: Pantheon.
———. 1978. *The History of Sexuality, Volume 1: An Introduction*. Translated by Robert Hurley. New York: Pantheon.
———. 2000. "The Birth of Social Medicine" (1974). In *Power*, edited by James D. Faubion, 134–56. New York: New Press.
———. 2003. *"Society Must Be Defended": Lectures at the Collège de France, 1975–1976*. Translated by David Macey. New York: Picador.
Fraser, Rebecca. 2013. *Gender, Race and Family in Nineteenth Century America: From Northern Woman to Plantation Mistress*. New York: Palgrave Macmillan.
French, Stanley. 1974. "The Cemetery as Cultural Institution: The Establishment of Mount Auburn and the 'Rural Cemetery' Movement." *American Quarterly* 26(1): 37–59. https://doi.org/10.2307/2711566.
Gagnon, Gregory O. 2011. *Culture and Customs of the Sioux Indians*. Santa Barbara, CA: Greenwood.
Gallagher, Peter. 2015. "Seminole Indian Remains Complete Circle of Life." *Seminole Tribune*, 30 October 2015, Community section. Accessed 11 September 2023. https://seminoletribune.org/seminole-indian-remains-complete-circle-of-life/.
Gannal, Jean-Nicolas. 1840. *History of Embalming, and of Preparations in Anatomy, Pathology, and Natural History; Including an Account of a New Process for Embalming*. Translated by R. Harlan. Philadelphia: Judah Dobson.
Garbarino, Merwyn S. 1989. *The Seminoles*. New York: Chelsea House Publishers.
Garment, Ann, Susan Lederer, Naomi Rogers, and Lisa Boult. 2007. "Let the Dead Teach the Living: The Rise of Body Bequeathal in 20th-Century America." *Academic Medicine* 82(10): 1000–5.
Gates, Henry Louis, Jr. 2007. "The Black Letters on the Sign: W.E.B. Du Bois and the Canon." In *The Souls of Black Folk: The Oxford W.E.B. Du Bois, Volume 3*, edited by Henry Louis Gates Jr., xi–xxiv. Oxford: Oxford University Press.
Gaudry, Adam J. P . 2011. "Insurgent Research." *Wicazo Sa Review* 26(1): 113–36.
Geller, Pamela L. 2009. "Bodyscapes, Biology, and Heteronormativity." *American Anthropologist* 111(4): 504–16.
———. 2012. "Parting (with) the Dead: Body Partibility as Evidence of Commoner Ancestor Veneration." *Ancient Mesoamerica* 23(1): 115–30.
———. 2015. "Hybrid Lives, Violent Deaths: Seminole Indians and the Samuel G. Mor-

ton Collection." In *Disturbing Bodies: Perspectives on Forensic Anthropology*, edited by Zoë Crossland and Rosemary A. Joyce, 137–56. Santa Fe, NM: SAR Press.

———. 2017. *The Bioarchaeology of Socio-Sexual Lives: Queering Common Sense about Sex, Gender, and Sexuality*. New York: Springer.

———. 2020. "Building Nation, Becoming Object: The Bio-Politics of the Samuel G. Morton Crania Collection." *Historical Archaeology* 54(1): 1–19.

———. 2021. *Theorizing Bioarchaeology*. New York: Springer.

Geller, Pamela L., and Christopher Stojanowski. 2017. "The Vanishing Black Indian: Revisiting Craniometry and Historic Collections." *American Journal of Physical Anthropology* 162(2): 267–84.

Gibbon, Charles. 1878. *The Life of George Combe, Author of "The Constitution of Man."* London: Macmillan.

Gillett, Mary C. 1987. *The Army Medical Department, 1818–1865*. Washington, DC: Center of Military History, US Army.

Gilley, Brian Joseph. 2006. *Becoming Two-Spirit: Gay Identity and Social Acceptance in Indian Country*. Lincoln: University of Nebraska Press.

Ginsberg, Elaine. 1996. "Introduction: The Politics of Passing." In *Passing and the Fictions of Identity*, edited by Elaine K. Ginsberg, 1–18. Durham, NC: Duke University Press.

Glick, Leonard B. 1982. "Types Distinct from Our Own: Franz Boas on Jewish Identity and Assimilation." *American Anthropologist* 84(3): 545–65.

Gliddon, George. 1854. "Preface." In *Types of Mankind: Or, Ethnological Researches, Based upon the Ancient Monuments, Paintings, Sculptures, and Crania of Races, and upon Their Natural, Geographical, Philological and Biblical History*, edited by Josiah Nott and George Gliddon, ix–xiv. Philadelphia, PA: Lippincott, Grambo.

Gloucester Democrat. 1836. "Capt. Justin Dimmick." 24 June 1836, 3.

Godfrey, Mary. 1836. *An Authentic Narrative of the Seminole War; and of the Miraculous Escape of Mrs. Mary Godfrey, and Her Four Female Children. Annexed Is a Minute Detail of the Horrid Massacres of the Whites, by the Indians and Negroes, in Florida, in the Months of December, January, and February*. Providence, RI: D. F. Blanchard.

Goetzmann, William H. 1959. *Army Exploration in the American West, 1803–1863*. Lincoln: University of Nebraska Press.

Gould, D. Rae. 2017. "NAGPRA, CUI and Institutional Will." In *The Routledge Companion to Cultural Property*, edited by Jane Anderson and Haidy Geismar, 134–51. New York: Routledge.

Gould, Marcus T.C., ed. 1830. *The Quaker, Being a Series of Sermons by Members of the Society of Friends*. Philadelphia: 9th Street.

Gould, Stephen Jay. 1978. "Morton's Ranking of Races by Cranial Capacity." *Science* 200(4341): 503–9.

———. 1981. *The Mismeasure of Man*. New York: W. W. Norton.

Graff, Harvey J. 1995. *Conflicting Paths: Growing up in America*. Cambridge, MA: Harvard University Press.

Grant, Madison. 1916. *The Passing of the Great Race: The Racial Basis of European History*. New York: Charles Scribner's Sons.
Grant, William. 1852. *Sketch of the Life and Character of Samuel George Morton, M.D.: Lecture Introductory to a Course on Anatomy and Physiology in the Medical Department of Pennsylvania College*. Philadelphia: John Royer, Printer.
Gravlee, Clarence, H. Russell Bernard, and William R. Leonard. 2003a. "Boas's 'Changes in Bodily Form': The Immigrant Study, Cranial Plasticity, and Boas's Physical Anthropology." *American Anthropologist* 105(2): 326–32.
Gravlee, Clarence C., H. Russell Bernard, and William R. Leonard. 2003b. "Heredity, Environment, and Cranial Form: A Re-Analysis of Boas's Immigrant Data." *American Anthropologist* 105(1): 123–36.
Green, Rayna. 1975. "The Pocahontas Perplex: The Image of Indian Women in American Culture." *Massachusetts Review* 16(4): 698–714.
Grubb, Farley. 1988. "British Immigration to Philadelphia: The Reconstruction of Ship Passenger Lists from May 1772 to October 1773." *Pennsylvania History: A Journal of Mid-Atlantic Studies* 55(3): 118–41.
Gunn, John C. 1838. *Gunn's Domestic Medicine: Or, Poor Man's Friend; Describing, in Plain Language, the Diseases of Men, Women and Children, and the Latest and Most Approved Means Used in Their Cure; Designed Especially for the Use of Families. It Also Contains Descriptions of the Medical Roots and Herbs of the United States, and How They Are to Be Used in the Cure of Diseases. Arranged on a New and Simple Plan, by Which the Practice of Medicine Is Reduced to Principles of Common Sense*. Louisville, KY: Charles Pool.
Hacker, J. David. 2003. "Rethinking the 'Early' Decline of Marital Fertility in the United States." *Demography* 40(4): 605–20.
Hagerman, Edward. 1967. "From Jomini to Dennis Hart Mohan: The Evolution of Trench Warfare and the American Civil War." *Civil War History* 13(3): 197–220.
Haggard, Howard. 1929. *Devils, Drugs, and Doctors: The Story of the Science of Healing from Medicine-Man to Doctor*. London: William Heinemann (Medical Books).
Hall, Richard. 1993. *Patriots in Disguise: Women Warriors of the Civil War*. New York: Marlowe & Company.
Hall, Stuart. 1990. "Cultural Identity and Diaspora." In *Identity, Community, Culture, Difference*, edited by Jonathan Rutherford, 222–37. London: Lawrence and Wishart.
Hallowell, Benjamin. 1883. *Autobiography of Benjamin Hallowell*. Philadelphia: Friends' Book Association.
Halperin, Edward C. 2007. "The Poor, the Black, and the Marginalized as the Source for Cadavers in United States Anatomical Education." *Clinical Anatomy* 20(5): 489–95.
Hamilton, George. 1880. *Biographical Sketch of James Aitken Meigs, M.D., Late President of the Philadelphia County Medical Society. Read before the Members. February 25, 1880*. Philadelphia: Collins, Printers.
Hamilton, William. 1850. "Remarks on Dr. Morton's Tables on the Size of the Brain." *Edinburgh New Philosophical Journal* 98: 330–33.

Haraway, Donna. 1991. *Simians, Cyborgs, and Women: The Reinvention of Women*. London: Routledge.

Hardy, Dr. James Freeman Eppes. 1846. Letter to Samuel G. Morton, 13 July 1846. Association of American Geologists and Naturalists Papers. Academy of Natural Sciences, Philadelphia, PA.

Harlan, Richard. 1827. Letter to Samuel G. Morton, 3 August 1827. Samuel George Morton Papers, Series I—Correspondences 1819–1850. American Philosophical Society, Philadelphia, PA.

———. 1831. Letter to Samuel G. Morton, 9 December 1831. Samuel George Morton Papers, Series I—Correspondences 1819–1850. American Philosophical Society, Philadelphia.

———. 1835. *Medical and Physical Researches: Or, Original Memoirs in Medicine, Surgery, Physiology, Geology, Zoology, and Comparative Anatomy*. Philadelphia: Lydia R. Bailey.

Harley, Earl H. 2006. "The Forgotten History of Defunct Black Medical Schools in the 19th and 20th Centuries and the Impact of the Flexner Report." *Journal of the National Medical Association* 98(9): 1425–29.

Hartman, Saidiya. 2007. *Lose Your Mother: A Journey along the Atlantic Slave Route*. New York: Farrar, Straus and Giroux.

———. 2008. "Venus in Two Acts." *Small Axe: A Caribbean Journal of Criticism* 12(2): 1–14.

———. 2019. *Wayward Lives, Beautiful Experiments: Intimate Histories of Social Upheaval*. New York: W. W. Norton.

Haveman, Christopher D. 2018. *Bending Their Way Onward: Creek Indian Removal in Documents*. Lincoln: University of Nebraska Press.

Haviland, Margaret Morris. 2006. "Westtown's Integration: 'A Natural and Fruitful Enlargement of Our Lives.'" *Quaker History* 95(2): 19–33.

Haviland, William. 1994. "Wilton Marion Krogman: June 28, 1903–November 4, 1987." In *Biographical Memoirs: Volume 63*, edited by the National Academy of Sciences, 293–320. Washington, DC: National Academies Press.

Hayward, John. 1854. *Gazetteer of the United States of America*. Philadelphia: James L. Gihon.

Hemenway, Eric, Meredith E. Henry, and Amber L. Holt. 2012. *Finding Our Way Home: A Handbook for Tribes, Universities, Museums and Individuals Working toward Reparation under NAGPRA*. Harbor Springs, MI: Little Traverse Bay Bands of Odawa Indians in partnership with the National Park Service. Accessed 11 September 2023. https://coah-repat.com/digital-heritage/finding-our-way-home-handbook-tribes-universities-museums-and-individuals-working.

Herdt, Gilbert. 1997. "The Dilemmas of Desire: From 'Berdache' to Two-Spirit." In *Two-Spirit People: Native American Gender Identity, Sexuality, and Spirituality*, edited by Sue-Ellen Jacobs, Wesley Thomas, and Sabine Lang, 276–83. Urbana: University of Illinois Press.

Herrick, Francis Hobart. 1917. *Audubon the Naturalist: A History of His Life and Time*. Vol. 2. New York: D. Appleton & Company.

Hildebrandt, Sabine. 2016. *The Anatomy of Murder: Ethical Transgressions and Anatomical Science during the Third Reich*. New York: Berghahn Books.
Hodgkin, Thomas. 1824. Letter to John Norton. Samuel George Morton Papers, Series I—Correspondences 1819–1850. American Philosophical Society, Philadelphia, PA.
———. 1830. Letter to Samuel G. Morton, 12 May 1830. Samuel George Morton Papers, Series I—Correspondences 1819–1850. American Philosophical Society, Philadelphia, PA.
———. 1842. Letter to Samuel G. Morton, 1 March 1842. Samuel George Morton Papers, Series IV. American Philosophical Society, Philadelphia, PA.
Hogarth, Rana Asali. 2019. "The Myth of Innate Racial Differences between White and Black People's Bodies: Lessons from the 1793 Yellow Fever Epidemic in Philadelphia, Pennsylvania." *American Journal of Public Health* 109(10): 1339–41. https://doi.org/10.2105/AJPH.2019.305245.
Homans, Benjamin, ed. 1836. *The Army and Navy Chronicle*. Vol. 2. Washington, DC: B. Homans.
Horsman, Reginald. 1975. "Scientific Racism and the American Indian in the Mid-Nineteenth Century." *American Quarterly* 27(2): 152–68. https://doi.org/10.2307/2712339.
Howells, William W. 1989. *Skull Shapes and the Map: Craniometric Analyses in the Dispersion of Modern Homo*. Papers of the Peabody Museum of Archaeology and Ethnology, Vol. 79. Cambridge, MA: Harvard University.
Hrdlička, Aleš. 1911. Letter to Edward J. Nolan, 2 May 1911. Samuel George Morton Papers. American Philosophical Society, Philadelphia, PA.
———. 1914. "Physical Anthropology in America: An Historical Sketch." *American Anthropologist* 16(4): 508–54.
Hughes, Geoffrey. 2006. *An Encyclopedia of Swearing: The Social History of Oaths, Profanity, Foul Language, and Ethnic Slurs in the English-Speaking World*. Armonk, NY: M. E. Sharpe.
Hyrtl, Joseph. 1857. *Handbuch der Topagraphischen Anatomie und Ihrer Praktisch Medicinisch-chirurgischen Anwendungen*. Vol. 2. Vienna, Austria: Wilhelm Braumueller.
International Holocaust Remembrance Alliance. 2022. Spelling of Antisemitism. Accessed 4 January 2024. https://www.holocaustremembrance.com/antisemitism/spelling-antisemitism.
Jackson, Samuel. 1832. "Report Embracing a View of the Principal Facts Connected with the Prevalence of Malignant Cholera in Philadelphia in 1832, Made to the Consulting Medical Board." *Cholera Gazette* 1(15 & 16): 244–52.
Jacobs, Sue-Ellen, Wesley Thomas, and Sabine Lang. 1997a. "Introduction." In *Two-Spirit People: Native American Gender Identity, Sexuality, and Spirituality*, edited by Sue-Ellen Jacobs, Wesley Thomas, and Sabine Lang, 1–18. Urbana: University of Illinois Press.
———, eds. 1997b. *Two-Spirit People: Native American Gender Identity, Sexuality, and Spirituality*. Urbana: University of Illinois Press.

Jacobson, Matthew Frye. 1999. *Whiteness of a Different Color.* Cambridge, MA: Harvard University Press.

James, Sydney V. 1962. "Quaker Meetings and Education in the Eighteenth Century." *Quaker History* 51(2): 87–102.

Johnston, Carolyn. 2003. *Cherokee Women in Crisis: Trail of Tears, Civil War, and Allotment, 1838–1907.* Tuscaloosa: University of Alabama Press.

Jones, L. A. 2023. "Judge Tosses Opposition to Penn's Plan to Rebury Black Philadelphians in Morton Collection." *Philadelphia Inquirer,* 2 February 2023. Accessed 11 September 2023. https://www.inquirer.com/news/philadelphia/penn-museum-morton-cranial-collection-20230202.html.

Jones, R. 1839. "Army. Official. General, Orders, No. 15." *Army and Navy Chronicle* 8(7): 111–12.

Jordan, John Woolf, ed. 1911. *Colonial Families of Philadelphia.* Vol. 2. New York: Lewis.

Juzda, Elise. 2009. "Skulls, Science, and the Spoils of War: Craniological Studies at the United States Army Medical Museum, 1868–1900." *Studies in History and Philosophy of Science Part C: Studies in History and Philosophy of Biological and Biomedical Sciences* 40(3): 156–67. https://doi.org/10.1016/j.shpsc.2009.06.010.

Kakaliouras, Ann. 2008. "Leaving Few Bones Unturned: Recent Work on Repatriation by Osteologists." *American Anthropologist* 110(1): 44–52.

———. 2017. "NAGPRA and Repatriation in the Twenty-First Century: Shifting the Discourse from Benefits to Responsibilities." *Bioarchaeology International* 1(3/4): 183–90.

———. 2021. "Ignoble Trophies: The Samuel G. Morton Collection, Repatriation, and Redress for the 21st Century." *History of Anthropology Review* 45. Accessed 11 September 2023. https://histanthro.org/news/observations/ignoble-trophies/.

Karabel, Jerome. 2005. *The Chosen: The Hidden History of Admission and Exclusion at Harvard, Yale, and Princeton.* New York: Houghton Mifflin Company.

Kass, Amalie M., and Edward Harold Kass. 1988. *Perfecting the World: The Life and Times of Dr. Thomas Hodgkin 1798–1866.* New York: Harcourt Brace Jovanovich.

Katz, Alan R., and David M. Morens. 1992. "Severe Streptococcal Infections in Historical Perspective." *Clinical Infectious Diseases* 14(1): 298–307.

Keels, Thomas. 2003. *Philadelphia Graveyards and Cemeteries.* Charleston, SC: Arcadia.

Kelly, Howard Atwood. 1912. *A Cyclopedia of American Medical Biography: Comprising the Lives of Eminent Deceased Physicians and Surgeons from 1610 to 1910.* Vol. 2. Philadelphia: W. B. Saunders Company.

Kelly, Mary Louise, and Farah Eltohamy. 2021. "Cherokee Nation Strikes Down Language That Limits Citizenship Rights 'By Blood.'" *NPR WLRN,* 25 February 2021. Accessed 11 September 2023. https://www.npr.org/2021/02/25/971084455/cherokee-nation-strikes-down-language-that-limits-citizenship-rights-by-blood.

Kenny, Maurice. 1988. "Tinselled Bucks: A Historical Study in Indian Homosexuality." In *Living the Spirit: A Gay American Indian Anthology,* edited by Will Roscoe, 15–31. New York: St. Martin's Press.

Kerber, Linda K. 1988. "Separate Spheres, Female Worlds, Woman's Place: The Rhetoric of Women's History." *Journal of American History* 75: 9–39.

Kessel, William B., and Robert Wooster. 2005. *Encyclopedia of Native American Wars and Warfare*. New York: Book Builders.

King, Tiffany Lethabo. 2019. *The Black Shoals: Offshore Formations of Black and Native Studies*. Durham, NC: Duke University Press.

Kladky, William P. 2013. "Federal Reservations." In *Encyclopedia of American Indian Issues Today, Volume 2*, edited by Russell Lawson, 444–53. Santa Barbara, CA: Greenwood.

Klaus, Haagen. 2012. "Bioarchaeology of Structural Violence: Theoretical Model and Case Study." In *The Bioarchaeology of Violence*, edited by Debra L. Martin, Ryan P. Harrod, and Ventura R. Pérez, 29–62. Gainesville: University of Florida Press.

Klepp, Susan. 2004. "Malthusian Miseries and the Working Poor in Philadelphia, 1780–1830: Gender and Infant Mortality." In *Down and Out in Early America*, edited by Billy G. Smith, 63–92. University Park: Pennsylvania State University Press.

———. 2021. "Sarah Thorn Tyndale." In *Philadelphia Stories: People and Their Places in Early America*, by C. Dallett Hemphill, 243–69. Philadelphia: University of Pennsylvania Press.

Klos, George. 1989. "Blacks and the Seminole Removal Debate, 1821–1835." *Florida Historical Quarterly* 68(1): 55–78.

Knight, Lucian Lamar. 1917. *A Standard History of Georgia and Georgians*. Vol. 5. Chicago: Lewis.

Komar, Debra, and Jane E. Buikstra. 2008. *Forensic Anthropology: Contemporary Theory and Practice*. New York: Oxford University Press.

Kraus, Natasha Kirsten. 2008. *A New Type of Womanhood: Discursive Politics and Social Change in Antebellum America*. Durham, NC: Duke University Press.

Krogman, Wilton M. 1934. "The Racial Composition of the Seminole Indians in Florida and Oklahoma." *Journal of Negro History* 19(4): 412–30.

———. 1935a. *The Physical Anthropology of the Seminole Indians of Oklahoma*. Comitato Italians Per Lo Studie Dei Problemi Della Popolazions. Serie III, Vol. II. Rome: Failli.

———. 1935b. "Vital Data on the Population of the Seminole Indians of Florida and Oklahoma." *Human Biology* 7(3): 335–49.

———. 1936. "The Cephalic Type of the Full-Blood and Mixed-Blood Seminole Indians of Oklahoma." *Zeitschr Rassenk* 3(2): 176–90.

———. 1943. "Reviewed Work(s): Man's Most Dangerous Myth: The Fallacy of Race by M. F. Ashley Montagu." *American Anthropologist* 45(2): 292–93.

———. 1948. "The Racial Type of the Seminole Indians of Florida and Oklahoma." *Florida Anthropologist* 1(3–4): 61–74.

Lamb, D. S. 1917. A History of the United States Army Medical Museum, 1862 to 1917; compiled from the official records. United States Army Medical Museum, Washington, DC.

———. 1923. "The Army Medical Museum, Washington, DC." *Military Surgeon* 53(2): 89–140.

Lancaster, Jane F. 1994. *Removal Aftershock: The Seminoles' Struggles to Survive in the West, 1836–1866*. Knoxville: University of Tennessee Press.

Lander, James. 2010. *Lincoln and Darwin: Shared Visions of Race, Science, and Religion*. Carbondale: Southern Illinois University Press.

Lang, Sabine. 1997. "Various Kinds of Two-Spirit People: Gender Variance and Homosexuality in Native American Communities." In *Two-Spirit People: Native American Gender Identity, Sexuality, and Spirituality*, edited by Sue-Ellen Jacobs, Wesley Thomas, and Sabine Lang, 100–18. Urbana: University of Illinois Press.

Larsen, Clark Spencer, Alfred Crosby, Mark Griffin, Dale L. Hutchinson, Christopher B. Ruff, Katherine Russell, Margaret Schoeninger, Leslie Sering, Scott Simpson, Jeffry Takács, and Mark Teaford. 2002. "A Biohistory of Health and Behavior in the Georgia Bight." In *The Backbone of History: Health and Nutrition in the Western Hemisphere*, edited by Richard H. Steckel and Jerome C. Rose, 406–39. Cambridge: Cambridge University Press.

Latour, Bruno. 1999. *Pandora's Hope: Essays on the Reality of Science Studies*. Cambridge, MA: Harvard University Press.

Laudonnière, René Goulaine de. 1869. *History of the First Attempt of the French (the Huguenots) to Colonize the Newly Discovered Country of Florida*. New York: J. Sabin & Sons.

Lawrence, Charles. 1905. *History of the Philadelphia Almshouses and Hospitals*. Philadelphia: Charles Lawrence.

Laxson, D. D. 1954. "An Historic Seminole Burial in a Hialeah Midden." *Florida Anthropologist* 7(4): 111–18.

Lederer, Susan, and Susan Lawrence. 2022. "Rest in Pieces: Body Donation in Mid-Twentieth Century America." *Bulletin of the History of Medicine* 96(2): 151–81.

Leib, George C. 1841. Letter to Samuel G. Morton, 28 June 1841. Samuel George Morton Papers. American Philosophical Society, Philadelphia, PA.

Lemkin, Raphael. 1944. *Axis Rule in Occupied Europe: Laws of Occupation, Analysis of Government, Proposals for Redress*. Washington, DC: Carnegie Endowment for International Peace.

———. 1953. "Nature of Genocide: Confusion with Discrimination against Individuals Seen." *New York Times*, Sunday, 14 June 1953, 1, E.

Lerner, Gerda. 1971. "DOUGLASS, Sarah Mapps Douglass." In *Notable American Women: A Biographical Dictionary*, edited by Edward T. James, 511–13. Cambridge, MA: Harvard University Press.

———. 1972. *Black Women in White America: A Documentary History*. New York: Pantheon Press.

Levene, Mark. 1999. "The Chittagong Hill Tracts: A Case Study in the Political Economy of 'Creeping' Genocide." *Third World Quarterly* 20(2): 339–69.

Lewis, Jason, David DeGusta, Marc Meyer, Janet Monge, Alan Mann, and Ralph Holloway. 2011. "The Mismeasure of Science: Stephen Jay Gould versus Samuel George Morton on Skulls and Bias." *PLoS Biology* 9(6): e1001071.

Lewis, Morris J. 1914. "Memoir of Thomas G. Morton, M.D." *Transactions of the College of Physicians of Philadelphia* XXXVI: lxvii–lxxii.

Lieberman, Leonard, Andrew Lyons, and Harriet Lyons. 1995. "An Interview with Ashley Montagu." *Current Anthropology* 36(5): 835–44.

Liebmann, Matthew. 2008. "Postcolonial Cultural Affiliation: Essentialism, Hybridity, and NAGPRA." In *Archaeology and the Postcolonial Critique*, edited by Matthew Liebmann and Uzma Rizvi, 73–90. Lanham, MD: AltaMira Press.

———. 2015. "The Mickey Mouse Kachina and other 'Double Objects': The Hybridity in the Material Culture of Colonial Encounters." *Journal of Social Archaeology* 15(3): 319–41.

Lindhorst, Marie J. 1995. "Sarah Mapps Douglass: The Emergence of an African American Educator/Activist in Nineteenth Century Philadelphia." PhD dissertation, Department of Educational Theory and Policy, Pennsylvania State University.

Lindsay, Brendan. 2012. *Murder State: California's Native American Genocide, 1846–1873*. Lincoln: University of Nebraska Press.

Lippincott, Horace Mather. 1919. *The University of Pennsylvania, Franklin's College*. Philadelphia: J. B. Lippincott.

Little Hawk, Daniel. 1988. "Understanding Grandfather." In *Living the Spirit: A Gay American Indian Anthology*, edited by Will Roscoe, 193–94. New York: St. Martin's Press.

Lonsdale, Henry. 1870. *A Sketch of the Life and Writings of Robert Knox the Anatomist*. London: Macmillan.

Loren, Diana D. 2013. "Considering Mimicry and Hybridity in Early Colonial New England: Health, Sin and the Body 'Behung with Beades.'" *Archaeological Review from Cambridge* 28(1): 151–68.

Loudon, Irvine. 2000. *The Tragedy of Childbed Fever*. Oxford: Oxford University Press.

Lucas, Jeffery. 2011. "Dade's Massacre." In *The Encyclopedia of North American Indian Wars, 1607–1890: A Political, Social, and Military History. Volume 1: A–L*, edited by Spencer Tucker, 225–26. Santa Barbara, CA: ABC-CLIO.

Lynch, Bartholomew M. 1837–1839. Bartholomew Lynch Journal, 1837–1839. Florida Manuscript Materials. Special Collections & Archives, Florida State University Libraries, Florida State University, Tallahassee.

Lyons, Kristina, Juno Parreñas, and Noah Tamarkin. 2017. "Engagements with Decolonization and Decoloniality in and at the Interfaces of STS." *Catalyst: Feminism, Theory, Technoscience* 3(1): 1–47.

MacCauley, Clay. 1887. *Seminole Indians of Florida. Fifth Annual Report of the Bureau of Ethnology to the Secretary of the Smithsonian Institution, 1883–84*. Washington, DC: Government Printing Office.

MacFarland, Kathryn, and Arthur Vokes. 2016. "Dusting Off the Data: Curating and Rehabilitating Archaeological Legacy and Orphaned Collections." *Advances in Archaeological Practice* 4(2): 161–75.

Mach, Stephanie. 2021. "Affective Responses to Normalized Violence in Museums." *History of Anthropology Review* 45. Accessed 11 September 2023. https://histanthro.org/news/observations/affective-responses/.

Magalhães, Bruno, Simon Mays, and Ana Luisa Santos. 2020. "A New Approach to Recording Nasal Fracture in Skeletonized Individuals." *International Journal of Paleopathology* 30: 105–9.

Mahon, John. 1967. *History of the Second Seminole War, 1835–1842*. Gainesville: University Press of Florida.
Maillard, Kevin Noble. 2008. "Redwashing History: Tribal Anachronisms in the Seminole Nation Cases." *Freedom Center Journal* 1(1): 96–115.
Maldonado-Torres, Nelson. 2016. "Colonialism, Neocolonial, Internal Colonialism, the Postcolonial, Coloniality, and Decoloniality." In *Critical Terms in Caribbean and Latin American Thought: Historical and Institutional Trajectories*, edited by Yolanda Martínez-San Miguel, Ben Sifuentes-Jáuregui, and Marisa Belausteguigoitia, 67–78. New York: Springer.
Mantell, Gideon Algernon. 1832. Letter to Samuel G. Morton, 27 September 1832. Samuel George Morton Papers, Series I—Correspondences 1819–1850. American Philosophical Society, Philadelphia.
Marcou, Jules. 1896. *Life, Letters, and Works of Louis Agassiz, Volume 2*. New York: Macmillan.
Marks, Jonathan. 2011. "Plotz Biology." *Anthropomics* (blog). Accessed 11 September 2023. http://anthropomics.blogspot.com/2011/06/plotz-biology.html.
Martin, Emily. 1991. "The Egg and the Sperm: How Science has Constructed a Romance Based on Stereotypical Male-Female Roles." *Signs: Journal of Women in Culture and Society* 16(3): 485–501.
Martin, Jack B. 2011. *A Grammar of Creek (Muskogee)*. Lincoln: University of Nebraska Press.
Martin, Joel. 1838a. Letter to Samuel G. Morton, 16 May 1838. Samuel George Morton Papers. American Philosophical Society, Philadelphia, PA.
———. 1838b. Letter to Samuel G. Morton, 1 August 1838 Samuel George Morton Papers. American Philosophical Society, Philadelphia, PA.
Martin, Rudolf. 1928. *Lehrbuch der Anthropologie in Systematischer Darstellung mit Besonderer Berücksichtigung der Anthropologischen Methoden. Band 2: Kraniologie, Osteologie*. Jena, Germany: Gustav Fishcer.
Martínez-Fernández, Luis. 2002. *Protestantism and Political Conflict in the Nineteenth-Century Hispanic Caribbean*. New Brunswick, NJ: Rutgers University Press.
Mason, J. Alden. 1964. "H. Newell Wardle, 1875–1964." *Expedition* 6(4): 40.
Mato Nunpa, Chris. 2013. "Historical Amnesia: The 'Hidden Genocide' and Destruction of the Indigenous Peoples of the United States." In *Hidden Genocides: Power, Knowledge, Memory*, edited by Alexander Laban Hinton, Thomas La Pointe, and Douglas Irvin-Erickson, 97–125. New Brunswick, NJ: Rutgers University Press.
Mays, Simon, and Margaret Cox. 2000. "Sex Determination in Skeletal Remains." In *Human Osteology in Archaeology and Forensic Science*, edited by Margaret Cox and Simon Mays, 117–30. Cambridge: Cambridge University Press.
Mbembe, Achille. 2003. "Necropolitics." *Public Culture* 15(1): 11–40.
———. 2019. *Necropolitics*. Durham, NC: Duke University Press.
McCoy, Craig. 2021. "Controversy Flares over How Penn and Princeton Treated a MOVE Bombing Victim's Remains." *Philadelphia Inquirer*, 21 April 2021. Accessed 11 September 2023. https://www.inquirer.com/news/move-bombing-victim-remains-penn-philadelphia-princeton-20210421.html.

McDannell, Colleen. 1987. "The Religious Symbolism of Laurel Hill Cemetery." *Pennsylvania Magazine of History and Biography* 111(3): 275–303.

———. 1995. *Material Christianity: Religion and Popular Culture in America*. New Haven, CT: Yale University Press.

McElroy, Archibald. 1844. *McElroy's Philadelphia Directory for 1844*. Philadelphia: Edward C. Biddle.

———. 1849. *McElroy's Philadelphia Directory for 1849*. Philadelphia: Edward C. & John Biddle.

———. 1852. *McElroy's Philadelphia Directory, for 1852*. Philadelphia: Edward C. & John Biddle.

McFarland, Benjamin J., and Thomas Peter Bennett. 1997. "The Image of Edgar Allan Poe: A Daguerreotype Linked to the Academy of Natural Sciences of Philadelphia." *Proceedings of the Academy of Natural Sciences of Philadelphia* 147: 1–32.

McGuire, Hunter. 1893. "Original Communications. President's Address. Francis Marion Robertson, M.D." *North Carolina Medical Journal* XXXII(1): 16–20.

McIntosh, Tania. 2012. *A Social History of Maternity and Childbirth: Key Themes in Maternity Care*. New York: Routledge.

McKittrick, Katherine. 2021. *Dear Science and Other Stories*. Durham, NC: Duke University Press.

McLoughlin, William G. 1989. "The Reverend Evan Jones and the Cherokee Trail of Tears, 1838–1839." *Georgia Historical Quarterly* 73(3): 559–83.

McMillen, Sally. 2008. *Seneca Falls and the Origins of the Women's Rights Movement*. Oxford: Oxford University Press.

Medical Faculty of the University of Pennsylvania. 1839. *Catalogue of the Medical Graduates of the University of Pennsylvania; with an Historical Sketch of the Origin, Progress, and Present State of the Medical Department*. Philadelphia: Lydia R. Bailey.

Medicine, Beatrice. 2002. "Directions in Gender Research in American Indian Societies: Two Spirits and Other Categories." In *Online Readings in Psychology and Culture*, edited by Walter Lonner, Dale Dinnel, Susanna Hayes, and David Sattler, 1–11. Bellingham: Western Washington University Press.

Meigs, Charles D. 1838. *The Philadelphia Practice of Midwifery*. Philadelphia: J. Kay, Jun. & Brother.

———. 1847. *Lecture on Some of the Distinctive Characteristics of the Female: Delivered before the Class of the Jefferson Medical College, January 5, 1847*. Philadelphia: T. K. and P. G. Collins, Printers.

———. 1848. *Females and their Diseases: A Series of Letters to his Class*. Philadelphia: Lea and Blanchard.

———. 1849. *Obstetrics: The Science and the Art*. Philadelphia, PA: Lea and Blanchard.

———. 1851. *A Memoir of Samuel George Morton, M.D., Late President of the Academy of Natural Sciences of Philadelphia*. Philadelphia, PA: T. K. and P. G. Collins, Printers.

Meigs, James Aitken. 1857. *Catalogue of Skulls of Man and the Inferior Animals, in the Collection of Samuel George Morton, M.D.* Philadelphia, PA: J. B. Lippincott.

———. 1866. "Observations upon the Cranial Forms of the American Aborigines, based upon Specimens Contained in the Collection of the Academy of Natural Sciences of Philadelphia." *Proceedings of the Academy of Natural Sciences of Philadelphia* 18: 197–235.

Meindl, Richard, C. Owen Lovejoy, Robert Mensforth, and Lydia Don Carlos. 1985. "Accuracy and Direction of Error in the Sexing of the Skeleton: Implications for Paleodemography." *American Journal of Physical Anthropology* 68(1): 79–85.

Meindl, Richard S., and C. Owen Lovejoy. 1985. "Ectocranial Suture Closure: A Revised Method for the Determination of Skeletal Age at Death Based on the Lateral-Anterior Suture." *American Journal of Physical Anthropology* 68(1): 57–66.

Merrill, Lisa. 1999. *When Romeo Was a Woman: Charlotte Cushman and Her Circle of Female Spectators.* Ann Arbor, MI: University of Michigan Press.

Micco, Melinda. 2006. "'Blood and Money': The Case of Seminole Freedmen and Seminole Indians in Oklahoma." In *Crossing Waters, Crossing Worlds: The African Diaspora in Indian Country*, edited by Tiya Miles and Sharon P. Holland, 121–44. Durham, NC: Duke University Press.

Michael, John S. 1988. "A New Look at Morton's Craniological Research." *Current Anthropology* 29(2): 349–54.

Middleton, William Shainline. 1941. "Thomas Cadwalader and His Essay." *Annals of Medical History* 3(2): 101–13.

Mignolo, Walter, and Catherine Walsh. 2018. *On Decoloniality: Concepts, Analytics, Praxis.* Durham, NC: Duke University Press.

Miles, A. E. W. 2001. "The Miles Method of Assessing Age from Tooth Wear Revisited." *Journal of Archaeological Science* 28(9): 973–82.

Miles, Tiya. 2009. "'Circular Reasoning': Recentering Cherokee Women in the Antiremoval Campaigns." *American Quarterly* 61(2): 221–43.

Miller, Kerby A. 1985. *Emigrants and Exiles: Ireland and the Irish Exodus in North America.* Oxford: Oxford University Press.

Miller, Susan A. 2003. *Coacoochee's Bones: A Seminole Saga.* Lawrence: University Press of Kansas.

———. 2005. "Seminoles and Africans under Seminole Law: Sources and Discourses of Tribal Sovereignty and 'Black Indian' Entitlement." *Wicazo Sa Review* 20(1): 23–47.

Missall, John, and Mary Lou Missall. 2004. *The Seminole Wars: America's Longest Indian Conflict.* Gainesville: University Press of Florida.

Mock, Shirley Boteler. 2010. *Dreaming with the Ancestors: Black Seminole Women in Texas and Mexico.* Norman: University of Oklahoma Press.

Monge, Janet. 2008. "ORSA: The Open Research Scan Archive." *Expedition* 50(3). Accessed 9 January 2024. https://www.penn.museum/sites/expedition/orsa-the-open-research-scan-archive/.

Monge, Janet, and P. Thomas Schoenemann. 2011. "The Open Research Scan Archive (ORSA): A Massive Open-Access Archive of Research Quality Computed Tomography (CT) Scans." In *Pleistocene Databases: Acquisition, Storing, Sharing / Pleistozäne Datenbanken: Datenerwerb, Speicherung, Austausch*, edited by Ro-

berto Macchiarelli and Gerd-Christian Weniger, 61–67. Mettmann, Germany: Neanderthal Museum.
Montagu, Ashley. 1942. *Man's Most Dangerous Myth: The Fallacy of Race*. New York: Columbia University Press.
———, ed. 1964. *The Concept of Race*. New York: Free Press of Glencoe.
———. 1965. *The Idea of Race*. Lincoln: University of Nebraska Press.
———. 1970. *What We Know about Race*. New York: Anti-Defamation League of B'nai B'rith.
———, ed. 1975. *Race & IQ*. London: Oxford University Press.
———. 1997. *Man's Most Dangerous Myth: The Fallacy of Race*. Walnut Creek, CA: AltaMira Press.
Montagu, M. F. Ashley. 1944. "Aleš Hrdlička, 1869–1943." *American Anthropologist* 46(1): 112–17.
Montgomery, William. 1839. "Remarks of Mr. Montgomery." In *The Congressional Globe, Containing Sketches of the Debates and Proceedings of the Twenty-Fifth Congress*, edited by Francis P. Blair and John C. Rives, 268–70. Washington, DC: The Globe Office.
Moore, A. A. 1893. "Necrology: Francis Marion Robertson, M.D." *North Carolina Medical Journal* 32(1): 18–21.
Moore, Emily. 2010. "Propatriation: Possibilities for Art after NAGPRA." *Museum Anthropology* 33(2): 125–36.
Moore, J. Percy. 1946–1947. Moore's notes on the letters and drafts 1946–1947. J. Percy Moore Papers, 1847–1963. Academy of Natural Sciences, Philadelphia, PA.
Moore, John H. 1995. "Mvskoke Personal Names." *Names* 43(3): 187–212.
Moran, Rachel F. 2001. *Interracial Intimacy: The Regulation of Race and Romance*. Chicago: University of Chicago Press.
Morgensen, Scott Lauria. 2011. *Spaces between Us: Queer Settler Colonialism and Indigenous Decolonization*. Minneapolis: University of Minnesota Press.
Morton, George. 1774. Letter to Thomas Morton, June 1774. Morton and Allied Families includes Langstaffe, Latham, Morton, Moore and Others, Surnames L–M; Contributor Helen Kirkbride Morton. Historical Society of Pennsylvania, Philadelphia, PA.
———. 1784a. Letter to Margaret Cummings, 10 November 1784. Morton and Allied Families includes Langstaffe, Latham, Morton, Moore and Others, Surnames L–M; Contributor Helen Kirkbride Morton. Historical Society of Pennsylvania, Philadelphia, PA.
———. 1784b. Letter to Samuel Neale, 1784. Morton and Allied Families includes Langstaffe, Latham, Morton, Moore and Others, Surnames L–M; Contributor Helen Kirkbride Morton. Historical Society of Pennsylvania, Philadelphia, PA.
———. 1787. Letter to Jane Morton, 9 April 1787. Morton and Allied Families includes Langstaffe, Latham, Morton, Moore and Others, Surnames L–M; Contributor Helen Kirkbride Morton. Historical Society of Pennsylvania, Philadelphia, PA.
Morton, James. 1838. Letter to Samuel G. Morton, 17 November 1838. Morton and Allied Families includes Langstaffe, Latham, Morton, Moore and Others, Surnames

L–M; Contributor Helen Kirkbride Morton. Historical Society of Pennsylvania, Philadelphia, PA.

Morton, Samuel G. 1823. *Tentamen Inaugurale de Corporis Dolore*. Edinburgh: Excudebat P. Neill.

———. 1831. *Introductory Lecture to a Course of Demonstrative Anatomy*. Philadelphia: Miflin & Parry.

———. 1833. Letters and Memoranda of the Corresponding Secretary of the Academy of Natural Sciences of Philadelphia, 1832–1846 [Letter to J. J. Abert, 27 March 1833]. Coll. 80—ANSP Corresponding Secretary. Academy of Natural Sciences, Philadelphia, PA.

———. 1834. *Illustrations of Pulmonary Consumption: Its Anatomical Characters, Causes, Symptoms and Treatment. With Twelve Plates, Drawn and Coloured from Nature*. Philadelphia: Key & Biddle.

———. 1839. *Crania Americana: Or a Comparative View of the Skulls of Various Aboriginal Nations of North and South America*. Philadelphia: J. Dobson.

———. 1840a. *Catalogue of Skulls of Man, and the Inferior Animals, in the Collection of Samuel George Morton, M.D.* Philadelphia: Turner & Fisher.

———. 1840b. *Catalogue of Skulls of Man, and the Inferior Animals, in the Collection of Samuel George Morton, M.D.* Revised and extended. Coll. 30A. University of Pennsylvania Museum of Archaeology and Anthropology, Philadelphia, PA.

———. 1840c. Letter to John Jay Smith. John Jay Smith Recollections Library Company of Philadelphia, Philadelphia, PA.

———. 1841. *A Memoir of William Maclure, Esq*. Philadelphia: T. K. and P. G. Collins.

———. 1842. *Brief Remarks on the Diversities of the Human Species, and on Some Kindred Subjects: Being an Introductory Lecture Delivered Before the Class of Pennsylvania Medical College, in Philadelphia, November 1, 1842*. Philadelphia: Merrihew & Thompson, Printers.

———. 1844. *Crania Aegyptiaca; or Observations on Egyptian Ethnography, Derived from Anatomy, History and the Monuments*. Philadelphia: John Penington.

———. 1847. *Hybridity in Animals and Plants, Considered in Reference to the Question of the Unity of the Human Species*. New Haven, CT: B. L. Hamlen.

———. 1849a. *Catalogue of Skulls of Man and the Inferior Animals, in the Collection of Samuel George Morton*. Philadelphia: Merrihew & Thompson, Printers.

———. 1849b. Last Will and Testament of Samuel George Morton deceased [Copy]. Morton and Allied Families includes Langstaffe, Latham, Morton, Moore, and Others. Historical Society of Pennsylvania, Philadelphia, PA.

———. 1850a. "Letter to the Rev. John Bachman, D.D., on the question of hybridity in animals, considered in reference to the unity of the human species." *Charleston Medical Journal and Review* 5: 328–44.

———. 1850b. "Additional observations on hybridity in animals, and on some collateral subjects; being a reply to the objections of the Rev. John Bachman, D.D." *Charleston Medical Journal and Review* 5: 755–805.

———. 1850c. "Observations on the Size of the Brain in Various Races and Families of Man." *Edinburgh New Philosophical Journal* 98: 262–65.

———. 1850–1851. "On the Infrequency of Mixed Offspring between European and Australian Races." *Proceedings of the Academy of Natural Sciences of Philadelphia* 5: 173–75.

Morton, Thomas. 1774. Letter to George Morton, 25 June 1774. Morton and Allied Families includes Langstaffe, Latham, Morton, Moore and Others, Surnames L–M; Contributor Helen Kirkbride Morton. Historical Society of Pennsylvania, Philadelphia, PA.

———. 1785. Letter to George Morton, 24 May 1785. Morton and Allied Families includes Langstaffe, Latham, Morton, Moore and Others, Surnames L–M; Contributor Helen Kirkbride Morton. Historical Society of Pennsylvania, Philadelphia, PA.

———. 1800. Letter to Jane Morton, 27 July 1800. Morton and Allied Families includes Langstaffe, Latham, Morton, Moore and Others, Surnames L–M; Contributor Helen Kirkbride Morton. Historical Society of Pennsylvania, Philadelphia, PA.

———. 1803. Letter to Jane Morton, 1 November 1803. Morton and Allied Families includes Langstaffe, Latham, Morton, Moore and Others, Surnames L–M; Contributor Helen Kirkbride Morton. Historical Society of Pennsylvania, Philadelphia, PA.

———. 1804. Letter to Jane Morton, 30 June 1804. Morton and Allied Families includes Langstaffe, Latham, Morton, Moore and Others, Surnames L–M; Contributor Helen Kirkbride Morton. Historical Society of Pennsylvania, Philadelphia, PA.

Morton, Thomas George. 1864. Catalogue of the Mütter Museum, prepared by Tho. Geo. Morton, M.D., Curator (#000145085). CPP 7/002-02, Historical Medical Library of The College of Physicians of Philadelphia, PA.

Morton, Thomas George, and William Hunt. 1880. *Surgery in the Pennsylvania Hospital: Being an Epitome of the Practice of the Hospital Since 1756; Including Collations from the Surgical Notes, and an Account of the More Interesting Cases from 1873 to 1878; with Some Statistical Tables*. Philadelphia: J. B. Lippincott & Company.

Moser, Harold, David Hoth, and George Hoemann, eds. 1994. *The Papers of Andrew Jackson: Volume IV, 1816–1820*. Knoxville: University of Tennessee Press.

Moss, Michael, and David Thomas. 2021. *Archival Silences: Missing, Lost and, Uncreated Archives*. New York: Routledge.

Mossell, Nathan. 1941. Nathan Francis Mossell Biography. Mossell Papers. Archives of the University of Pennsylvania, Philadelphia, PA.

Mott, Lucretia. 1871. "Addresses." In *A History of the National Woman's Rights Movement*, edited by Paulina W. Davis, 31–32. New York: Journeymen Printers' Co-Operative Association.

Motte, Jacob Rhett. 1953. *Journey into Wilderness: An Army Surgeon's Account of Life in Camp and Field during the Creek and Seminole Wars, 1836–1838*. Gainesville: University of Florida Press.

Mullenix, Elizabeth Reitz. 2000. *Wearing the Breeches: Gender on the Antebellum Stage*. New York: St. Martin's Press.

Muller, Jennifer L., Kirsten Pearlstein, and Carlina de la Cova. 2017. "Dissection and Documented Skeletal Collections: Embodiments of Legalized Inequality." In *The

Bioarchaeology of Dissection and Autopsy in the United States, edited by Kenneth Nystrom, 185–201. New York: Springer.

Mulroy, Kevin. 2007. *The Seminole Freedmen: A History.* Norman: University of Oklahoma Press.

Nader, Laura. 1972. "Up the Anthropologist: Perspectives Gained from 'Studying Up.'" In *Reinventing Anthropology*, edited by Dell Hymes, 284–311. New York: Pantheon Books.

Nash, Gary B. 1972. "The Image of the Indian in the Southern Colonial Mind." *William and Mary Quarterly* 29(2): 197–230.

Nash, Stephen E., and Chip Colwell. 2020. "NAGPRA at 30: The Effects of Repatriation." *Annual Review of Anthropology* 49: 225–39.

Neale, Samuel. 1773. Letter to Israel Pemberton, 25 April 1773. Morton and Allied Families includes Langstaffe, Latham, Morton, Moore and Others, Surnames L–M; Contributor Helen Kirkbride Morton. Historical Society of Pennsylvania, Philadelphia, PA.

Necker, L. A. 1818. "Article X: Scientific Intelligence, and Notices of Subjects Connected with Science. Academy of Natural Sciences in Philadelphia." *Annals of Philosophy* 12: 385–86.

New-London Gazette. 1836. "The Florida Campaign." 10 November 1836.

Newman, Simon P. 2003. *Embodied History: The Lives of the Poor in Early Philadelphia*. Philadelphia: University of Pennsylvania Press.

Nichols, Catherine. 2014. "Lost in Museums: The Ethical Dimensions of Historical Practices of Anthropological Specimen Exchange." *Curator: The Museum Journal* 57(2): 225–36.

Nolan, Edward James. 1909. *A Short History of the Academy of Natural Sciences of Philadelphia*. Philadelphia: The Academy of Natural Sciences.

Norwood, William Frederick. 1970. "Medical Education in the United States before 1900." In *The History of Medical Education*, edited by C. D. O'Malley, 463–500. Los Angeles: University of California Press.

Novak, Shannon. 2017. "On the Stories of Men and the Substance of Women: Interrogating Gender through Violence." In *Exploring Sex and Gender in Bioarchaeology*, edited by Sabrina C. Agarwal and Julie K. Wesp, 129–64. Albuquerque, NM: University of New Mexico Press.

Novak, Shannon, and Alanna Warner-Smith. 2020. "Assembling Heads and Circulating Tales: The Doings and Undoings of Specimen 2032." *Historical Archaeology* 54(1): 71–91.

Novak, Shannon, and Wesley Willoughby. 2010. "Resurrectionists' Excursions: Evidence of Postmortem Dissection from the Spring Street Presbyterian Church." *Northeast Historical Archaeology* 39: 134–52.

Novy, Frederick G. 1908. "The Life of Professor Zina Pitcher." *Michigan Alumnus* 14: 295–305.

Nystrom, Kenneth, ed. 2017. *The Bioarchaeology of Dissection and Autopsy in the United States*. New York: Springer.

Nystrom, Kenneth C. 2014. "The Bioarchaeology of Structural Violence and Dissection in the 19th-Century United States." *American Anthropologist* 116(4): 765–79. https://doi.org/10.1111/aman.12151.

O'Brassill-Kulfan, Kristin. 2019. "'Severe Punishment for Their Misfortunes and Poverty': Philadelphia's Arch Street Prison, 1804–37." *Pennsylvania Magazine of History and Biography* 143(3): 247–69.

O'Brien, Thomas M., and Oliver Diefendorf. 1864. *General Orders of the War Department Embracing the Years 1861, 1862, & 1863. Adapted Specially for the Use of the Army and Navy of the United States. Chronologically Arranged in Two Volumes. With a Full Alphabetical Index.* Vol. 1. New York: Derby & Miller.

O'Donnell, Elizabeth A. 2013. "Quakers and Education." In *The Oxford Handbook of Quaker Studies*, edited by Stephen. W. Angell and Pink Dandelion, 409–15. Oxford: Oxford University Press.

Osborne, John B. 2008. "Preparing for the Pandemic: City Boards of Health and the Arrival of Cholera in Montreal, New York, and Philadelphia in 1832." *Urban History Review* 36(2): 29–42.

Owens, Deirdre Cooper. 2017. *Medical Bondage: Race, Gender, and the Origins of American Gynecology.* Athens: University of Georgia Press.

Palencia, Elaine Fowler. 1987. "The Cherokee Beloved Woman / War Woman: Then and Now." *Appalachian Heritage* 15(3): 24–31.

Palmer, Beverly Wilson, ed. 2002. *Selected Letters of Lucretia Coffin Mott.* Urbana: University of Illinois Press.

Palmié, Stephan. 2013. "Mixed Blessings and Sorrowful Mysteries: Second Thoughts about 'Hybridity.'" *Current Anthropology* 54(4): 463–82.

Paradise, Jordan, and Lori Andrews. 2007. "Tales from the Crypt: Scientific, Ethical, and Legal Considerations for Biohistorical Analysis of Deceased Historical Figures." *Temple Journal of Science, Technology & Environmental Law* 26: 223–99.

Parrish, Joseph. 1820. Letter from Joseph Parrish. Samuel George Morton Papers, Series I—Correspondences 1819–1850. American Philosophical Society, Philadelphia.

Paterson, Robert K. 2010. "Heading Home: French Law Enables Return of Maori Heads to New Zealand." *International Journal of Cultural Property* 17(4): 643–52. https://doi.org/10.1017/S0940739110000408.

Patterson, Henry S. 1854. "Memoir of the Life and Scientific Labors of Samuel George Morton." In *Types of Mankind: Or, Ethnological Researches, Based upon the Ancient Monuments, Paintings, Sculptures, and Crania of Races, and upon Their Natural, Geographical, Philological and Biblical History*, edited by J. C. Nott and George R. Gliddon, xvii–lvii. Philadelphia: Lippincott, Grambo.

Patterson, William, ed. 1951. *We Charge Genocide: The Historic Petition to the United Nations for Relief from a Crime of the United States Government against the Negro People.* New York: Civil Rights Congress.

Paxton, William McClung. 1897. *Annals of Platte County, Missouri.* Kansas City, MO: Hudson-Kimberly.

Peck, Robert McCracken, and Patricia Tyson Stroud. 2012. *A Glorious Enterprise: The Academy of Natural Sciences of Philadelphia and the Making of American Science.* Philadelphia: University of Pennsylvania Press.

Pennsylvania Senate. 1832–1833. "Monday, January 14, 1833. Alms House." *Journal of the Senate of the Commonwealth of Pennsylvania.* Harrisburg, PA: Henry Welsh.

Perdue, Theda. 1998. *Cherokee Women: Gender and Culture Change, 1700–1835.* Lincoln: University of Nebraska Press.

Perdue, Theda, and Michael D. Green. 2001 *The Columbia Guide to American Indians of the Southeast.* New York: Columbia University Press.

Pérez Ortega, Rodrigo. 2023. "Famously Creepy Mütter Museum Reckons with Its Past." *Science,* 21 July 2023. Accessed 5 January 2024. https://www.science.org/content/article/famously-creepy-mutter-museum-reckons-its-past.

Philadelphia Medical Examiner. 1851. "Samuel George Morton, M.D." *Boston Medical and Surgical Journal* XLIV: 398–401.

Philadelphia Yearly Meeting of the Religious Society of Friends. 1797. *Rules of Discipline and Christian Advices of the Yearly Meeting of Friends for Pennsylvania and New Jersey, First Held at Burlington in the Year 1681, and from 1685 to 1760, Inclusive, Alternately in Burlington and Philadelphia: and since at Philadelphia.* Philadelphia, PA: Samuel Sansom.

Phillips, Venia T. 1952. Letter to Mr. George Stuart (from Belmont Abbey Prep School in Belmont, NC), 29 February 1952. Collection 30. Morton, Samuel George, 1799–1851. Papers, 1825–1930. Academy of Natural Sciences of Philadelphia, Academy of Natural Sciences of Philadelphia, Philadelphia, PA.

Piper, Harry, Kenneth Hardin, and Jacquelyn Piper. 1982. "Cultural Responses to Stress: Patterns Observed in American Indian Burials of the Second Seminole War." *Southeastern Archaeology* 1(2): 122–37.

Pitcher, Zina. 1832. Letter to Samuel G. Morton, 13 June 1832. Correspondence ("Official"), 1812–1920. Collection 567. Academy of Natural Sciences, Philadelphia, PA.

———. 1834. Letter to Samuel G. Morton, 4 March 1834. Samuel George Morton Papers. American Philosophical Society, Philadelphia, PA.

Pittman, Hannah D. 1903. *Americans of Gentle Birth and their Ancestors. Volume 1.* St. Louis: Buxton & Skinner.

Pleins, J. David. 2013. *The Evolving God: Charles Darwin on the Naturalness of Religion.* New York: Bloomsbury Academic.

Polak, Rabbi Joseph A., William Seidelman, Lilka Elbaum, and Sabine Hildebrandt. 2021. "The Vienna Protocol: Recommendations/Guidelines for the Handling of Future Discoveries of Remains of Human Victims of Nazi Terror 'Vienna Protocol' for when Jewish or Possibly-Jewish Human Remains are Discovered." *Journal of Biocommunication* 45(1): 74–86. https://doi.org/10.5210/jbc.v45i1.10829.

Porter, Kenneth W. 1943. "Florida Slaves and Free Negroes in the Seminole War, 1835–1842." *Journal of Negro History* 28(4): 390–421.

———. 1944. "Seminole Flight from Fort Marion." *Florida Historical Quarterly* 22(3): 113–33.

———. 1996. *The Black Seminoles: History of a Freedom-Seeking People*, revised and edited by Alcione M. Amos and Thomas P. Senter. Gainesville: University Press of Florida.

Portnoy, Alisse. 2005. *Their Right to Speak: Women's Activism in the Indian and Slave Debates*. Cambridge, MA: Harvard University Press.

Potter, Woodburne. 1836. *The War in Florida: Being an Exposition of Its Causes, and an Accurate History of the Campaigns of Generals Clinch, Gaines, and Scott*. Baltimore: Lewis and Coleman.

Prichard, James Cowles. 1835. *A Treatise on Insanity and Other Disorders Affecting the Mind*. London: Sherwood, Gilbert, and Piper.

———. 1839–1840. "On the Extinction of Human Races." *Edinburgh New Philosophical Journal* 28: 166–170.

Proctor, Robert. 1988. *Racial Hygiene: Medicine under the Nazis*. Cambridge, MA: Harvard University Press.

Pyle, Gerald F. 1969. "The Diffusion of Cholera in the United States in the Nineteenth Century." *Geographical Analysis* 1(1): 59–75.

Rabinow, Paul, and Nikolas Rose. 2006. "Biopower Today." *BioSocieties* 1(2): 195–217.

Rankin-Hill, Lesley M. 1997. *A Biohistory of 19th-Century Americans: The Burial Remains of a Philadelphia Cemetery*. Westport, CT: Bergin & Garvey.

Red Earth, Michael. 1997. "Traditional Influences on a Contemporary Gay-Identified Sisseton Dakota." In *Two-Spirit People: Native American Gender Identity, Sexuality, and Spirituality*, edited by Sue-Ellen Jacobs, Wesley Thomas, and Sabine Lang, 210–16. Urbana: University of Illinois Press.

Redman, Samuel J. 2016. *Bone Rooms: From Scientific Racism to Human Prehistory in Museums*. Cambridge, MA: Harvard University Press.

Renschler, Emily, and Janet Monge. 2008. "The Samuel George Morton Cranial Collection: Historical Significance and New Research." *Expedition* 50(3): 30–38.

Richardson, Ruth. 1987. *Death, Dissection and the Destitute*. London: Routledge & Kegan.

Richmond Enquirer. 1836. "Domestic." 31 May 1836. Accessed 11 September 2023. https://chroniclingamerica.loc.gov/lccn/sn84024735/1836-05-31/ed-1/seq-2/.

Rivers, Larry E., and Canter Brown. 1997. "'The Indispensable Man': John Horse and Florida's Second Seminole War." *Journal of the Georgia Association of Historians* 18: 1–23.

Roberts, Mary Louise. 2002. "True Womanhood Revisited." *Journal of Women's History* 14(1): 150–55.

Robertson, Francis Marion. 1841. Letter to Samuel G. Morton, 29 June 1841. Samuel George Morton Papers, Series IV. American Philosophical Society, Philadelphia, PA.

———. 1842. Letter to Samuel G. Morton, 13 August 1842 Samuel George Morton Papers, Series IV. American Philosophical Society, Philadelphia, PA.

Robertson, Thomas Heard, Jr. 2002. "The Richmond Blues in the Second Seminole War: Letters of Capt. Francis Marion Robertson, M.D." *Military Collector & Historian* 54(2): 51–63.

———. 2015. *Resisting Sherman: A Confederate Surgeon's Journal and the Civil War in the Carolinas, 1865*. El Dorado Hills, CA: Savas Beatie.

Rohner, Ronald P. 1969. *The Ethnography of Franz Boas: Letters and Diaries of Franz Boas Written on the Northwest Coast from 1886–1931*. Translated by Hedy Parker. Chicago: University of Chicago Press.

Romans, Bernard. 1776. *A Concise Natural History of East and West Florida*. New York: R. Aitken, Bookseller.

Roque, Ricardo. 2010. *Headhunting and Colonialism: Anthropology and the Circulation of Human Skulls in the Portuguese Empire, 1870–1930*. New York: Palgrave Macmillan.

Roscoe, Will. 1988a. "North American Tribes with Berdache and Alternative Gender Roles." In *Living the Spirit: A Gay American Indian Anthology*, edited by Will Roscoe, 217–22. New York: St. Martin's Press.

———. 1988b. "Strange Country This: Images of Berdaches and Warrior Women." In *Living the Spirit: A Gay American Indian Anthology*, edited by Will Roscoe, 48–76. New York: St. Martin's Press.

———. 1991. *The Zuni Man-Woman*. Albuquerque: University of New Mexico Press.

———. 1998. *Changing Ones: Third and Fourth Genders in Native North America*. New York: St. Martin's Press.

Rose, Jerome, Thomas Green, and Victoria Green. 1996. "NAGPRA Is Forever: Osteology and the Repatriation of Skeletons." *Annual Review of Anthropology* 25(1): 81–103.

Rosenberg, Charles E. 1962. *The Cholera Years: The United States in 1832, 1849, and 1866*. Chicago: University of Chicago Press.

———. 1977a. "And Heal the Sick: The Hospital and the Patient in 19th-Century America." *Journal of Social History* 10: 428–47.

———. 1977b. "The Therapeutic Revolution: Medicine, Meaning, and Social Change in Nineteenth-Century America." *Perspectives in Biology and Medicine* 20(4): 485–506.

———. 1982. "From Almshouse to Hospital: The Shaping of Philadelphia General Hospital." *Health and Society* 60(1): 108–54.

Rothstein, William G. 1987. *American Medical Schools and the Practice of Medicine: A History*. New York: Oxford University Press.

Rotman, Deborah. 2009. *Historical Archaeology of Gendered Lives*. New York: Springer.

Rozema, Vicki. 2003. *Voices from the Trail of Tears*. Winston Salem, NC: John F. Blair.

Rubenstein, William. 1996. *A History of the Jews in the English-Speaking World: Great Britain*. New York: St. Martin's Press.

Ruschenberger, William Samuel Waithman. 1852. *A Notice of the Origin, Progress, and Present Condition of the Academy of Natural Sciences of Philadelphia*. Philadelphia: T. K. and P. G. Collins, Printer.

Rush, Benjamin. 1794. *An Account of the Bilious Remitting Yellow Fever as It Appeared in the City of Philadelphia in the Year 1793*. Philadelphia: Thomas Dobson.

———. 1809. *Medical Inquiries and Observations*. 4 vols. Philadelphia: Carey et al.

Ryan, Mary P. 1975. *Womanhood in America: From Colonial Times to the Present.* New York: New Viewpoints.

Sanitary Board. 1832. *Report of the Commission Appointed by the Sanitary Board of the City Councils to Visit Canada for the Investigation of the Epidemic Cholera, Prevailing in Montreal and Quebec.* Philadelphia: Mifflin & Parry.

Sappol, Michael. 2002. *A Traffic of Dead Bodies: Anatomy and Embodied Social Identity in Nineteenth-Century America.* Princeton, NJ: Princeton University Press.

Scharf, John Thomas, and Thompson Westcott. 1884. *History of Philadelphia, 1609–1884, Volume 3.* Philadelphia: L. H. Everts & Company.

Schoenemann, P. Thomas, James Gee, Brian Avants, Ralph Holloway, Janet Monge, and Jason Lewis. 2007. "Validation of Plaster Endocast Morphology through 3D CT Image Analysis." *American Journal of Physical Anthropology* 132(2): 183–92.

Seidelman, William, Lilka Elbaum, and Sabine Hildebrandt, eds. 2017. *How to Deal with Holocaust Era Human Remains: Recommendations Arising from a Special Symposium (Yad Vashem, May 2017).* Boston: Elie Wiesel Center for Jewish Studies, Boston University. Accessed 9 January 2024. https://www.bu.edu/jewishstudies/files/2018/06/Final-How-to-Deal-with-Holocaust-Era-Human-Remains.pdf.

Shannon, Gary, and Robert Cromley. 1982. "Philadelphia and the Yellow Fever Epidemic." *Urban Geography* 3(4): 355–70.

Shapin, Steven. 1975. "Phrenological Knowledge and the Social Structure of Early Nineteenth-century Edinburgh." *Annals of Science* 32(3): 219–43.

Shepley, Carol Ferring. 2008. *Movers and Shakers, Scalawags and Suffragettes: Tales from Bellefontaine Cemetery.* St. Louis: Missouri History Museum.

Shipman, Pat. 1994. *The Evolution of Racism: Human Differences and the Use and Abuse of Science.* New York: Simon & Schuster.

Shire, Laurel Clark. 2016. *The Threshold of Manifest Destiny: Gender and National Expansion in Florida.* Philadelphia: University of Pennsylvania Press.

Silliman, Stephen W. 2013. "What, Where, and When Is Hybridity?" In *The Archaeology of Hybrid Material Culture,* edited by Jeb J. Card, 486–500. Carbondale: Southern Illinois University Press.

———. 2015. "A Requiem for Hybridity? The Problem with Frankensteins, Purées, and Mules." *Journal of Social Archaeology* 15(3): 277–98.

Simmons, William Hayne. 1822. *Notices of East Florida: With an Account of the Seminole Nation of Indians.* Charleston, SC: A. E. Miller.

Smith, Anna Bustill. 1925. "The Bustill Family." *Journal of Negro History* 10(4): 638–44.

Smith, Billy G. 1995. "Philadelphia: The Athens of America." In *Life in Early Philadelphia: Documents from the Revolutionary and Early National Periods,* edited by Billy G. Smith, 1–26. University Park: Pennsylvania University Press.

Smith, Billy G., and Cynthia Shelton. 1985a. "The Daily Occurrence Docket of the Philadelphia Almshouse, 1800." *Pennsylvania History: A Journal of Mid-Atlantic Studies* 52(2): 86–116.

———. 1985b. "The Daily Occurrence Docket of the Philadelphia Almshouse: Selected Entries, 1800–1804." *Pennsylvania History: A Journal of Mid-Atlantic Studies* 52(3): 183–205.

Smith, Jeffrey E. 2020. "Till Death Keeps Us Apart: Segregated Cemeteries and Social Values in St. Louis, Missouri." In *Till Death Do Us Part: American Ethnic Cemeteries as Borders Uncrossed*, edited by Allan Amanik and Kami Fletcher, 157–81. Jackson: University Press of Mississippi.

Smith, John Jay. 1872. A Legacy for My Descendants. John Jay Smith Recollections. Library Company of Philadelphia, Philadelphia, PA.

———. 1892. *Recollections of John Jay Smith*. Philadelphia, PA: J. B. Lippincott Company.

Smith, Lizzie. 2013. "Dehumanising Sex Workers: What's 'Prostitute' Got to Do with It." *Conversation*, 29 July 2013. Accessed 11 September 2023. https://theconversation.com/dehumanising-sex-workers-whats-prostitute-got-to-do-with-it-16444.

Smith, Rachel Pearsall. 1835. Letter to Albanus and Elizabeth Pearsall Smith, February 1835. Smith Family Papers, 1678–1937; Series II John Jay Smith Papers, a. General Correspondence. Historical Society of Pennsylvania, Philadelphia, PA.

Smith, Sidney. 1838. *The Principles of Phrenology*. Edinburgh: William Tait.

Smithers, Gregory D. 2014. "Cherokee 'Two Spirits': Gender, Ritual, and Spirituality in the Native South." *Early American Studies* 12(3): 626–51.

———. 2022. *Reclaiming Two-Spirits: Sexuality, Spiritual Renewal, and Sovereignty in Native America*. New York: Beacon Press.

Smith-Rosenberg, Carroll. 1985. *Disorderly Conduct: Visions of Gender in Victorian America*. Oxford: Oxford University Press.

Snow, Edward Rowe. 1935. *Islands of Boston Harbor*. Carlisle, MA: Commonwealth Editions.

Sparks, Corey, and Richard Jantz. 2002. "A Reassessment of Human Cranial Plasticity: Boas Revisited." *Proceedings of the National Academy of Sciences* 99(23): 14636–39.

———. 2003. "Changing Times, Changing Faces: Franz Boas's Immigrant Study in Modern Perspective." *American Anthropologist* 105(2): 333–37.

Spencer, Frank. 1983. "Samuel George Morton's Doctoral Thesis on Bodily Pain: The Probable Source of Morton's Polygenism." *Transactions & Studies of the College of Physicians of Philadelphia* 5(4): 321–38.

Spencer-Wood, Suzanne M. 1999. "The World Their Household: Changing Meanings of the Domestic Sphere in the Nineteenth Century." In *The Archaeology of Household Activities*, edited by Penelope Allison, 162–89. New York: Routledge.

Sprague, John Titcomb. 1848. *The Origin, Progress, and Conclusion of the Florida War*. New York: D. Appleton.

Squires, Kirsty, Charlotte A. Roberts, and Nicholas Márquez-Grant. 2022. "Ethical Considerations and Publishing in Human Bioarcheology." *American Journal of Biological Anthropology* 177(4): 615–19.

Stantis, Chris, Carlina de la Cova, Dorothy Lippert, and Sabrina Sholts. 2023. "Biological Anthropology Must Reassess Museum Collections for a More Ethical Future." *Nature Ecology & Evolution* 7(6): 786–89.

Stanton, Elizabeth Cady. 1848. "Declaration of Sentiments. Woman's Rights Convention, Seneca Falls, NY, 19–20 July 1848." Accessed 11 September 2023. http://awpc.cattcenter.iastate.edu/2017/03/09/the-declaration-of-sentiments-july-19-1848/

Stanton, William. 1960. *The Leopard's Spots: Scientific Attitudes toward Race in America, 1815–1859.* Chicago: University of Chicago Press.

Starn, Orin. 2004. *Ishi's Brain: In Search of America's Last "Wild" Indian.* New York: W. W. Norton.

Steinweis, Alan. 2006. *Studying the Jew: Scholarly Antisemitism in Nazi Germany.* Cambridge, MA: Harvard University Press.

Stengers, Isabelle. 2018. *Another Science Is Possible: A Manifesto for Slow Science.* Translated by Stephen Muecke. Medford, MA: Polity Press.

Stephens, Lester D. 2014. "Centers of Creation: John Perkins Barratt's Biogeographical Theory of Racial Origins." *Journal of Southern History* 80(2): 259–86.

Stillé, Alfred. 1846. *Medical Education in the United States: An Address Delivered to the Students of the Philadelphia Association for Medical Instruction at the Close of the Session of 1846.* Philadelphia: Isaac Ashmead, Printer.

Stocking, George W., Jr. 1987. *Victorian Anthropology.* New York: The Free Press.

Stojanowski, Christopher, and William Duncan. 2017. "Defining an Anthropological Biohistorical Research Agenda: The History, Scale, and Scope of an Emerging Discipline." In *Studies in Forensic Biohistory: Anthropological Perspectives*, edited by Christopher Stojanowski and William Duncan, 1–28. Cambridge: Cambridge University Press.

———, eds. 2017. *Studies in Forensic Biohistory: Anthropological Perspectives.* Cambridge: Cambridge University Press.

Stone, Witmer. 1906. "Dr. Samuel W. Woodhouse, '47 M." *Alumni Register (University of Pennsylvania)* 9(1): 105–9.

Strachey, Barbara. 1980. *Remarkable Relations: The Story of the Pearsall Smith Women.* New York: Universe Books.

Sturtevant, William C., and Jessica Cattelino. 2004. "Florida Seminole and Miccosukee." In *Southeast*, Vol. 14 of *Handbook of North American Indians*, edited by Raymond Fogelson, 429–49. Washington, DC: US Government Printing Office.

Sundquist, Matthew L. 2010. "Worcester v. Georgia: A Breakdown in the Separation of Powers." *American Indian Law Review* 35(1): 239–55.

Swanton, John R. 1928. "Aboriginal Cultures of the Southeast." In *Forty-Second Annual Report of the Bureau of American Ethnology to the Secretary of the Smithsonian Institution, 1924–1925*, edited by Jesse Walter Fewkes, 673–726. Washington, DC: Government Printing Office.

Takaki, Ronald. 1993. *A Different Mirror: A History of Multicultural America.* Boston: Little, Brown.

TallBear, Kimberly. 2003. "DNA, Blood, and Racializing the Tribe." *Wicazo Sa Review* 18(1): 81–107.

———. 2013. *Native American DNA: Tribal Belonging and the False Promise of Genetic Science.* Minneapolis: University of Minnesota Press.

Tattersall, Ian. 2013. "Stephen J. Gould's Intellectual Legacy to Anthropology." In *Stephen J. Gould: The Scientific Legacy*, edited by Gian Antonio Danieli, Alessandro Minelli, and Telmo Pievani, 115–27. New York: Springer.

Tepper, Michael, ed. 1986. *Passenger Arrivals at the Port of Philadelphia, 1800–1819: The Philadelphia Baggage Lists.* Baltimore: Genealogical Pub. Co.

Tharps, Lori. 2014. "The Case for Black with a Capital B." *New York Times*, 18 November 2014, Opinion. Accessed 11 September 2023. https://www.nytimes.com/2014/11/19/opinion/the-case-for-black-with-a-capital-b.html.

Thayer, Theodore. 1943. *Israel Pemberton, King of the Quakers.* Philadelphia: Historical Society of Pennsylvania.

The Diversity Style Guide. 2019. "White, White." Accessed 11 September 2023. https://www.diversitystyleguide.com/glossary/white-white/.

Theriot, Nancy M. 1996. *Mothers and Daughters in Nineteenth-Century America: The Biosocial Construction of Femininity.* Lexington: University Press of Kentucky.

Thomas, David, Simon Fowler, and Valerie Johnson, eds. 2017. *The Silence of the Archive.* London: Facet.

Thomas, David Hurst. 2000. *Skull Wars: Kennewick Man, Archaeology, and the Battle for Native American Identity.* New York: Basic Books.

Thomas, Jayne-Leigh, and Krystiana L. Krupa. 2021. "Bioarchaeological Ethics and Considerations for the Deceased." *Human Rights Quarterly* 43(2): 344–54.

Thomas, Wesley, and Sue-Ellen Jacobs. 1999. "'. . . And We are Still Here': From Berdache to Two-Spirit People." *American Indian Culture and Research Journal* 23(2): 91–107.

Timberlake, Henry. 1765. *The Memoirs of Lieut. Henry Timberlake, Who Accompanied the Three Cherokee Indians in the Year 1762.* London: J. Ridley.

Toomey, Noxon. 1917. *Proper Names from the Muskhogean Languages.* St. Louis: Hervas Laboratories.

Townsend, John Kirk. 1835. Letter to Samuel G. Morton, 20 September 1835. Samuel George Morton Papers. American Philosophical Society, Philadelphia, PA.

Tremblay, Lori A., and Sarah Reedy, eds. 2020. *The Bioarchaeology of Structural Violence: A Theoretical Framework for Industrial Era Inequality.* New York: Springer.

Tribal Legal Development Clinic. 2020. "The Need for Confidentiality within Tribal Cultural Resource Protection." Tribal Legal Development Clinic, UCLA School of Law. Accessed 6 July 2023. https://law.ucla.edu/sites/default/files/PDFs/Native_Nations/239747_UCLA_Law_publications_Confidentiality_R2_042021.pdf.

Tronchetti, Carlo, and Peter van Dommelen. 2005. "Entangled Objects and Hybrid Practices: Colonial Contacts and Elite Connections at Monte Prama, Sardinia." *Journal of Mediterranean Archaeology* 18(2): 183–209.

Trouillot, Michel-Rolph. 1995. *Silencing the Past: Power and the Production of History.* Boston: Beacon Press.

Tsui, Bonnie. 2006. *She Went to the Field: Women Soldiers of the Civil War.* Guilford, CT: Globe Pequot Press.

Tulchinsky, Theodore H. 2018. *Case Studies in Public Health.* London: Academic Press.

Tumin, Remy. 2022. "Penn Museum to Bury Skulls of Enslaved People." *New York Times*, 9 August 2022. Accessed 11 September 2023. https://www.nytimes.com/2022/08/09/us/university-pennsylvania-black-skulls-burial.html.

Turnbull, Laurence. 1881. *Memoir of James Aitken Meigs, A.M., M.D: Professor of the Institutes of Medicine and Medical Jurisprudence in Jefferson Medical College, Philadelphia.* Philadelphia, PA: Pugh Madeira.

United States Congress. 1850. "The Seventh Census." *Congressional Globe.* 31st Congress, 1st Session (43): 671–77. Accessed 11 September 2023. https://memory.loc.gov/ammem/amlaw/lwcglink.html#anchor31.

United States Surgeon-General's Office. 1883. *Death Announcement of Joseph K. Barnes.* Washington, DC: Surgeon General's Office.

University of Pennsylvania. 1891. *Catalogue and Announcements, 1890–91.* Philadelphia: Printed for the University.

Valentine, Lonnie. 2013. "Quakers, War, and Peacemaking." In *The Oxford Handbook of Quaker Studies,* edited by Stephen W. Angell and Pink Dandelion, 363–76. Oxford: Oxford University Press.

van Dommelen, Peter. 2005. "Colonial Interactions and Hybrid Practices: Phoenician and Carthaginian Settlement in the Ancient Mediterranean." In *The Archaeology of Colonial Encounters: Comparative Perspectives,* edited by Gil Stein, 109–41. Santa Fe, NM: SAR Press.

Velpeau, Alfred Armand Louis Marie. 1831. *Elementary Treatise on Midwifery, or, Principles of Tokology and Embryology.* Translated by Charles Meigs. Philadelphia: Grigg & Elliot.

Virkus, Frederick A., ed. 1925. *Abridged Compendium of American Genealogy: The Standard Genealogical Encyclopedia of the First Families of America, Volume I.* Chicago: F. A. Virkus & Company.

Vogt, Carl. 1864. *Lectures on Man: Place in Creation, and in the History of the Earth.* London: Longman, Green, Longman, and Roberts.

Wagner, Frederick B., Jr. 1989. "Part III: Clinical Departments and Divisions Continued—Chapter 32: Department of Surgery." In *Thomas Jefferson University—Tradition and Heritage, Paper 31,* edited by Frederick B. Wagner, 505–79. Accessed 11 September 2023. http://jdc.jefferson.edu/wagner2/31.

Waite, Frederick C. 1935. "Birth of the First Independent Proprietary Medical School in New England, at Castleton, Vermont, in 1818." *Annals of Medical History* 7(3): 242–52.

Walker, James R., ed. 1980. *Lakota Belief and Ritual.* Lincoln: University of Nebraska Press.

Waldenmaier, Nellie Protsman. 1944. *Some of the Earliest Oaths of Allegiance to the United States of America.* Lancaster, PA: Privately printed.

Walker, Mark, and Chris Cameron. 2021. "After Denying Care to Black Natives, Indian Health Service Reverses Policy." *New York Times,* 8 October 2021. Accessed 11 September 2023. https://www.nytimes.com/2021/10/08/us/politics/indian-health-service-freedmen.html.

Walker, Phillip. 1995. "Problems of Preservation and Sexism in Sexing: Some Lessons from Historical Collections for Palaeodemographers." In *Grave Reflections: Portraying the Past through Cemetery Studies,* edited by Shelley Saunders and Ann Herring, 31–47. Toronto: Canadian Scholars' Press.

Walker, Phillip, Rhonda Bathurst, Rebecca Richman, Thor Gjerdrum, and Valerie Andrushko. 2009. "The Causes of Porotic Hyperostosis and Cribra Orbitalia: A Reappraisal of the Iron-Deficiency-Anemia Hypothesis." *American Journal of Physical Anthropology* 139(2): 109–25.

Wall, Diana DiZerega. 1991. "Sacred Dinners and Secular Teas: Constructing Domesticity in Mid-19th-Century New York." *Historical Archaeology* 25: 69–81.

Wardle, H. Newell. 1929. "Wreck of the Archeological Department of the Academy of Natural Sciences of Philadelphia." *Science* 70(1805): 119–21.

Warner-Smith, Alanna. 2022. "Working Hands, Indebted Bodies: Embodiment of Inequality and Labor in an Era of Progress." PhD dissertation, Department of Anthropology, Syracuse University.

———. 2024. "Global Mobilities, Intimate Movements: Embodying Nineteenth-Century Domestic Labor." In *The Routledge Handbook of Feminist Anthropology*, edited by Pamela L. Geller. New York: Routledge.

Warren, Edward. 1860. *The Life of John Collins Warren, M.D. Compiled Chiefly from His Autobiography and Journals, Vol. 2.* Boston: Ticknor and Fields.

Warren, Leonard. 1998. *Joseph Leidy: The Last Man Who Knew Everything.* New Haven, CT: Yale University Press.

Warrington, Joseph. 1839. *The Nurse's Guide: Containing a Series of Instructions to Females Who Wish to Engage in the Important Business of Nursing Mother and Child in the Lying-in Chamber.* Philadelphia: Thomas, Cowperthwait.

Washington, Harriet A. 2006. *Medical Apartheid: The Dark History of Medical Experimentation on Black Americans from Colonial Times to the Present.* New York: Doubleday Books.

Wasserman, Adam. 2010. *A People's History of Florida, 1513–1876: How Africans, Seminoles, Women, and Lower Class Whites Shaped the Sunshine State.* Sarasota, FL: A. Wasserman.

Watkins, Joe. 2004. "Becoming American or Becoming Indian? NAGPRA, Kennewick and Cultural Affiliation." *Journal of Social Archaeology* 4(1): 60–80.

Watkins, Rachel J. 2008. "Knowledge from the Margins: W. Montague Cobb's Pioneering Research in Biocultural Anthropology." *American Anthropologist* 109(1): 186–96.

———. 2012. "Biohistorical Narratives of Racial Difference in the American Negro: Notes toward a Nuanced History of American Physical Anthropology." *Current Anthropology* 53(S5): S196–S209. https://doi.org/10.1086/662416.

———. 2018. "Anatomical Collections as the Anthropological Other: Some Considerations." In *Bioarchaeological Analyses and Bodies*, edited by Pamela K. Stone, 27–47. New York: Springer.

Watkins, Rachel J., and Jennifer Muller. 2015. "Repositioning the Cobb Human Archive: The Merger of a Skeletal Collection and Its Texts." *American Journal of Human Biology* 27(1): 41–50.

Watson, William. 2009. "The Sisters of Charity, the 1832 Cholera Epidemic in Philadelphia and Duffy's Cut." *U.S. Catholic Historian* 27(4): 1–16.

Weaver, Karol K. 2016. "'Painful Leisure' and 'Awful Business': Female Death Workers in Pennsylvania." *Pennsylvania Magazine of History and Biography* 140(1): 31–55.

Weeber, Christine. 2020. "Why Capitalize 'Indigenous'?" *Sapiens*, 19 May 2020. Accessed 11 September 2023. https://www.sapiens.org/language/capitalize-indigenous/.

Weik, Terrance. 1997. "The Archaeology of Maroon Societies in the Americas: Resistance, Cultural Continuity, and Transformation in the African Diaspora." *Historical Archaeology* 31(2): 81–92.

———. 2009. "The Role of Ethnogenesis and Organization in the Development of African-Native American Settlements: An African Seminole Model." *International Journal of Historical Archaeology* 13(2): 206–238.

Weisberg, Michael. 2014. "Remeasuring Man." *Evolution & Development* 16(3): 166–78.

Weisman, Brent R. 1989. *Like Beads on a String: A Culture History of the Seminole Indians in North Peninsular Florida*. Tuscaloosa: University of Alabama Press.

———. 1999. *Unconquered People: Florida's Seminole and Miccosukee Indians*. Gainesville: University Press of Florida.

———. 2007. "Nativism, Resistance, and Ethnogenesis of the Florida Seminole Indian Identity." *Historical Archaeology* 41(4): 198–212.

Welcker, Hermann. 1862. *Untersuchungen über Wachstum und Bau des Menschlichen Schädels*. Leipzig: Wilhelm Engelmann-Verlag.

Wells, Susan. 2001. *Out of the Dead House: Nineteenth-Century Women Physicians and the Writing of Medicine*. Madison: University of Wisconsin Press.

Welter, Barbara. 1966. "The Cult of True Womanhood: 1820–1860." *American Quarterly* 18(2): 151–74.

Wertz, Richard, and Dorothy Wertz. 1977 *Lying-in: A History of Childbirth in America*. New Haven, CT: Yale University Press.

Westerman, Gwen, and Bruce White. 2012. *Mni Sota Makoce: The Land of the Dakota*. St. Paul: Minnesota Historical Society.

Wetherill, John Price, Samuel G. Morton, and George B. Ellis. 1826. "Observations on the Geology, Mineralogy, &c., of the Perkiomen Lead Mine in Pennsylvania." *Journal of the Academy of Natural Sciences of Philadelphia* 5: 305–16.

Wheeler, Ryan, Jaime Arsenault, and Marla Taylor. 2022. "Beyond NAGPRA/Not NAGPRA." *Collections* 18(1): 8–17.

White, Frank F., Jr. 1950. "A Journal of Lt. Robert C. Buchanan during the Seminole War." *Florida Historical Quarterly* 29(2): 132–51.

White, George. 1855. *Historical Collections of Georgia: Containing the Most Interesting Facts, Traditions, Biographical Sketches, Anecdotes, etc. Relating to Its History and Antiquities, from Its First Settlement to the Present Time*. New York: Pudney & Russell.

Whooley, Owen. 2013. *Knowledge in the Time of Cholera: The Struggle over American Medicine in the Nineteenth Century*. Chicago: University of Chicago Press.

Wickman, Patricia. 2006. *Osceola's Legacy*. Tuscaloosa: University of Alabama Press.

Wilkie, Laurie. 2003. *The Archaeology of Mothering: An African-American Midwife's Tale*. New York: Routledge.

Williams, John Lee. 1837. *The Territory of Florida: Or Sketches of the Topography, Civil and Natural History, of the Country, the Climate, and the Indian Tribes, from the*

First Discovery to the Present Time, with a Map, Views, &c. New York: A. T. Goodrich.

Williams, Lucy Fowler, Stacey O. Espenlaub, and Janet Monge. 2016. "Twenty-Five Years of NAGPRA at the Penn Museum." *Expedition* 58(1): 28–37.

Williams, Walter L. 1985. "Persistence and Change in the Berdache Tradition among Contemporary Lakota Indians." *Journal of Homosexuality* 11(3–4): 191–200.

———. 1986. *The Spirit and the Flesh: Sexual Diversity in American Indian Culture.* Boston: Beacon Press.

Willoughby, Christopher D. E. 2022. *Masters of Health: Racial Science and Slavery in US Medical Schools.* Chapel Hill: University of North Carolina Press.

Wilson, James Grant, ed. 1888. *Appleton's Cyclopaedia of American Biography, Vol. II: Crandall-Grimshaw.* New York: D. Appleton.

Wilson, James Grant, and John Fiske, eds. 1887. *Appleton's Cyclopaedia of American Biography, Vol. I: Aaron-Crandall.* New York: D. Appleton.

Wilson, Thomas. 1825. *The Philadelphia Directory and Stranger's Guide, for 1825; Containing a Diagram of the City and Suburbs.* Philadelphia: Thomas Wilson & Wm. D. Vanbaun, Jobn. Bioren.

Winch, Julie. 1999. "Douglass, Sarah Mapps." In *American National Biography* online. Accessed 11 September 2023. https://doi.org/10.1093/anb/9780198606697.article.1500187

Winsberg, Morton D. 1993. "The Advance of Florida's Frontier as Determined from Post Office Openings." *Florida Historical Quarterly* 72(2): 189–99.

Winter, Thomas. 2004. "Cult of Domesticity." In *American Masculinities: A Historical Encyclopedia*, edited by Bret Carroll, 120–22. New York: Sage Publications.

Wojczuk, Tana. 2020. *Lady Romeo: The Radical and Revolutionary Life of Charlotte Cushman, America's First Celebrity.* New York: Avid Reader Press.

Wood, George B. 1840. *A Memoir of the Life and Character of the Late Joseph Parrish, M.D.* Philadelphia: Lydia R. Bailey.

———. 1853. *A Biographical Memoir of Samuel George Morton, M.D.* Philadelphia: T. K. and P. G. Collins.

Woodhouse, Samuel W. 1992. *A Naturalist in Indian Territory: The Journals of S. W. Woodhouse, 1849–1850.* Edited by John S. Tomer and Michael J. Brodhead. Norman: University of Oklahoma Press.

Woolford, Andrew, Jeff Benvenuto, and Alexander Laban Hinton, eds. 2014. *Colonial Genocide in Indigenous North America.* Durham, NC: Duke University Press.

Wright, James R., Jr. 2016. "The Pennsylvania Anatomy Act of 1883: Weighing the Roles of Professor William Smith Forbes and Senator William James McKnight." *Journal of the History of Medicine and Allied Sciences* 71(4): 422–46.

Wright, Joseph J. B. 1841. "Art. I.—Army Medical Reports." *American Medical Intelligencer* 1(6): 113–20.

Yee, Andrew, Ema Zubovic, Jennifer Yu, Shuddhadeb Ray, Sabine Hildebrandt, William Seidelman, Rabbi Joseph Polak, Michael Grodin, J. Henk Coert, and Douglas Brown. 2019. "Ethical Considerations in the Use of Pernkopf's Atlas of Anatomy: A Surgical Case Study." *Surgery* 165(5): 860–67.

Young, Hugh, Mark F. Boyd, and Gerald M. Ponton. 1934. "A Topographical Memoir on East and West Florida with Itineraries of General Jackson's Army, 1818." *Florida Historical Society Quarterly* 13(1): 16–50.

Younging, Gregory. 2018. *Elements of Indigenous Style: A Guide for Writing by and about Indigenous Peoples*. Edmonton: Brush Education.

Zeuske, Michael. 2002. "Hidden Markers, Open Secrets: On Naming, Race-Marking, and Race-Making in Cuba." *New West Indian Guide / Nieuwe West-Indische Gids* 76(3–4): 211–41.

Zipursky, Alvin. 2002. "A History of Pediatric Specialties." *Pediatric Research* 52(5): 617. https://doi.org/10.1203/00006450-200211000-00002.

INDEX

Page numbers in *italics* indicate illustrations and tables.

Abadie, Eugene Hilarian: biography, 82, 125; death of, 108; skull collector, 96–98, 100, 114, 124, 137–38, 139–40, 165, 217n10, 218n13; US Army surgeon, 83–84, 95
Abert, John James, 87, *96*, 112, 115–20, 213n2, 219nn3–5
Aborigines' Protection Society, 20, 75–77, 216n22
Abortion, 148
Academy of Natural Sciences: ANS Ledger, 161; correspondents and members of, 36, 76, 82, 86, 94, 117, 132, 133, 213n2, 216n23; history, 13, 55, 179, 209n1, 221n12, 223n3; Morton Collection, 1, 17, 84, 103, 105, 146, 167, 176–77, 180, 186–87, 190, 223n4; Samuel Morton's involvement, 44, 78, 175
African-American Burial Grounds Preservation Act, 202, 227n37
Agassiz, Louis, 129–30, 132–33
Aliens Act of 1905, UK, 182
Ambition, 3, 4, 20, 53, 60, 67, 88, 151
American Indian: citizenship, 172; "Five Civilized Tribes," 13, 83, 210n12; "friendly" or "hostile," 7, 22, 92, 111–14, 98, 102, 123, 136; genocide, 193; legislation, 216n3, 218–19n20 (*see also* Indian Removal Act of 1830, US; Native American Graves Protection and Repatriation Act); relationship with Black Americans, 23, 134–39; Southeastern US, 12, 14, 163–65; stereotypes, 28. *See also* Cherokee; Choctaw; Creek; Odawa (Little Traverse Bay Band of Odawa Indians of Michigan); Osage; Seminole; Sioux; Two-Spirits

American Medical Association, 69, 148
American Museum of Natural History, 178
American Revolution, 28–29
Anatomical museum. *See* Pathological cabinet
Anatomy Act of 1883 (Pennsylvania), 59, 184, 215n9, 224n12
Anti-miscegenation. *See* Miscegenation
Antisemitism, 46, 182–83, 190, 193, 224n10
Archives, 15–16, 66, 126, 144, 194, 204, 206
Arch Street Prison, 64–65
Army Corps of Topographical Engineers, US, 22, 113, 116–17, 119, 168, 219n4
Army Medical Museum, 106, 218n19
Athlaha Ficksa, 86, *87*, 125, 126. *See also* Creek
Audubon, John James, 1, 64, 209n2
Autopsy, 43, 58, 173–74, 214n7. *See also* Dissection

Bachman, John, 133–34
Barnes, Joseph K., 105–6, 218n18
Barratt, John Perkins, 131–32
Becoming object: effects of, 21, 42, 104, 127; Achille Mbembe on, 9, 218n16; process of, 58, 102–3, 116, 123, 171, 186–87, 206. *See also* Mbembe, Achille
Biography, 2–3, 21, 125, 127, 174, 186, 194
Biohistorical analysis, 10–12, 160
Biomedical bodyscape, 10–11, 142
Biopolitics, 6, 12, 18, 53, 63, 142, 147–48, 170, 197
Biopower, 6–8, 10, 53, 147. *See also* Biopolitics; Necropolitics
Black Dirt. *See* Foke Luste Hadjo
Black Indians: Black Seminole, 23, 98, 135, 137–39, 196–98, 225nn25–26; Cherokee Freedmen, 197. *See also* Hybridity; Miscegenation
Black Lives Matter (BLM), 200–201, 226n30

272 · Index

Black Philadelphians, 184, 201–2, 226nn33–34, 227n35
Blockley Almshouse. *See* Philadelphia Almshouse
Blumenbach, Johann, 72, 128
Boas, Franz, 177–79, 182–83, 190, 223nn5–7
Body politic: exclusion, 16, 22, 194; heterogeneity, 4, 10, 132; inclusion, 3, 21, 54, 107, 129, 140, 182; women's second-class status, 24, 141, 180
Boston Tea Party, 27–28
British and Foreign Aborigines Protection Society. *See* Aborigines' Protection Society
Brown, Corinna, 114–15, 135, 219n2
Burke and Hare scandal, 59, 78, 214–15n8
Butler, Judith, 7, 17–18. *See also* Precarity; "Ungrievable lives"

Canguilhem, Georges, 6
Captivity narratives, 135–37, 140, 221n15
Catalogue of Skulls of Man, and the Inferior Animals, in the Collection of Samuel George Morton, M.D., The: Creeks, 86; Euchee, 84; formatting, 214nn5; "idiots" and "lunatics," 57–78, 63, 156, 214n6; by James Aitken Meigs, 222n7; mixed races, 128, 221n13; named individuals, 124–27; Potawatomie, 219n5; Seminoles, 139, 165, 218n13
Cavallo, John, 98–99, 138–39. *See also* Coacoochee
Cemeteries: Bellefontaine Cemetery, 108; cemetery beautiful movement, 107; Eden Cemetery, 202, 224n13; Laurel Hill Cemetery, 109–10, 168, 170, 174, 205, 224n12; Lebanon Cemetery, 184; Magnolia Cemetery, 108
Census taking, 129–31, 187–88, 219n3, 221n14, 224–25n17
Cherokee, 47, 87–91, 118, 164, 197, 210n12, 216nn3,5, 217n6, 225n27. *See also* American Indians; Black Indians
Choctaw, 128, 164, 210n12. *See also* American Indians
Cholera: epidemic of 1832, 20, 53, 61–62, 68; etiology and symptoms, 215nn13,14; racialization of, 65; response in Philadelphia, 63–64, 66. *See also* Epidemics

"Circular No. 2," 105–6
Cisneros, José Rodriguez, 203–4, 209n5
Citizenship: of American Indians, 24, 172; "participatory," 186; second-class for women, 141; tribal, 196–97. *See also* Body politic
Coacoochee, 98–99, 138–39, 139, 218n14. *See also* Cavallo, John
Cobb, W. Montague, 188. *See also* Legacy collections
College of Physicians of Philadelphia, 30, 175, 210n13, 212nn12–13, 220n8. *See also* Legacy collections: Mütter Museum
Combe, George: Charlotte Cushman and, 223n10; Frederick Douglass and, 73–75; Edinburgh Phrenological Society, 50; Samuel Morton and, 20, 78; Lucretia Mott and, 154–55, 222n9; James Cowles Prichard and, 77
Consent, 5, 25, 43, 58, 174, 185–87, 193, 202, 204, 207, 210n14, 212nn10,12
"Considerate" colonialism, 51, 75
Consumption: in the almshouse, 55, 125; *Illustrations of Pulmonary Consumption*, 7, 50, 56, 82; racialized, 81, 84, 188
Crania Aegyptiaca, 175, 189, 203
Crania Americana: Athlaha Ficksa, 86, 126; George Combe's appendix, 75; dedication to James Cowles Prichard, 77; Justin Dimick's heroism, 122–23 (*see also* Dimick, Justin); financial burden, 78, 167, 177; Johann Blumenbach's influence, 72; responses to, 101, 152, 175, 181, 189; scientific racism, 104, 128, 203; "Sioux warrior of bad character," 161, *162*, 195
Craniometry: development of, 72, 75; in biohistoric analysis, 13, 137, 210n11, 221n16; racial categorization by Morton, 9, 22, 24, 54, 104; sex differences, 140, 152
Creek: Morton Collection decedents, 86–88, 226n27; removal, 83–84, 95, 118; slavery, 135, 138; ties to Seminole, 92–93, 114; Two-Spirits, 164. *See also* Athlaha Ficksa
Cribra orbitalia, 14, 18, 90, 95, 97, 98, 139, 163, 165, 211n16. *See also* Precarity
Critical fabulation, 15, 16, 25, 126, 194, 196. *See also* Hartman, Saidiya

Croom, Hardy, 92–94, *96*
Cropper, James, 51
Cultural evolution, 24, 28, 75–76, 182, 185
Cushman, Charlotte, 146, 157, *158*, 223n10

Darwin, Charles, 23, 46, 133
Delirium tremens. See Mania à potu
Desilver's Philadelphia Directory and Stranger's Guide, 117, 213n1
Dimick, Justin, 22, *96*, 112, 121–24, 135, 141, 159, 182, 220nn7,8
Dissection, 9, 36, 40–41, 43, 46, 48, 49, 56, 58–59, 214n7. *See also* Autopsy; Medical education, nineteenth century
Douglass, Frederick, 73–74, 153, 175–76; 223n2. *See also* Combe, George
Douglass, Sarah Mapps, 16, 34–36, 212n8
Du Bois, W.E.B., 223n1, 227n34

Eakins, Thomas, 15, 41, 212n10
Egyptian skulls, 128, 151, 189, 203
Emerson, Gouverneur, *96*, 123, 215n16, 220n8
Endnotes, 18–19
Enslavement: abolition, 51, 56, 73, 154, 216n4; archival documentation, 16; biohistorical study of, 11–12; evidence in Morton Collection, 175, 201, 203–4, 226n31; Native practice of, 25, 83, 90, 97, 196–97, 210n12; necropolitics, 2, 8, 18, 130, 149; precarity, 135–36, 138–39; Quaker position on, 34–35; resistance to, 7, 98, 121, 123, 134–35, 137
Eoklo-Emathla, 22, *96*, 124, 126–27, 138
Epidemics, 5, 20, 30–31, 72, 200, 216n5. *See also* Cholera; Puerperal fever; Scarlet fever; Whooping cough; Yellow fever
Episcopal church, 48, 71, 145, 168, 174
Ethnology, 4, 20, 54, 71–73, 75, 78, 175, 179
Ethos, 5, 25, 205, 226n33. *See also* Consent
Eugenics, 7, 185, 193

Fabian, Ann, 3, 54, 223nn2,5
Female masculinity, 159–60
Flexner Report, 67
Foke Luste Hadjo, *96*, 98, *99*, 113–14, 218n13
Footnotes, 18–19
Forbes, William S., 184
Forts: Fort Brooke, 97; Fort Cass, 90; Fort Gardiner, *96*, 217n10,12; Fort Gibson, 81–84, 86, 87
Foucault, Michel: biopower, 5–7, 11, 53, 209n6; biohistory, 10; birth of the clinic, 50; history of the present, 194; medical gaze, 41, 212n10

Genocide, 9, 192–93
Gliddon, George, 175, 203
Gould, Stephen Jay, 188–89, 190, 225n19
Grave robbing, 42, 59, 184
Great Depression, 179, 184
Grimké sisters, Angelina and Sarah, 16
Gummere Academy, 36
Gunn's Domestic Medicine, 70

Hamann, Carl, 187. *See also* Legacy collections
Hardy, James, *89*, 91, 225n27
Harlan, Richard, 54–55, 59–61, 62, 64–66, 71. *See also* Arch Street Prison; Cholera
Hartman, Saidiya, 15, 16, 112, 126, 171, 194, 206, 212n10, 220n10, 227n34. *See also* Critical fabulation
Hicks, Elias, 41, 154
Hildebrandt, Sabine, 9
Hippocratic oath, 7, 21
Historical Society of Pennsylvania, 13, 78, 210n13, 220n8
Hodgkin, Thomas, 21, 46–48, 49, 50, 51, 67, 75–76, 213n14. *See also* Aborigines' Protection Society
Holocaust, 9, 193, 204, 209n8
Homeopathy, 68–71
Hrdlička, Aleš, 177–78, 181
Hybridity: anti-miscegenation, 129, 134, 185; Franz Boas's study of, 178–79; hybrid lives, 34–35, 99, 100, 135, 137–38, 140, 143, 196; Samuel Morton's study of, 112, 131–34, 188; multiple meanings, 22–23. *See also* Black Indians; Miscegenation

Ideology of separate spheres, 36, 146–47, 153, 157, 160. *See also* True womanhood
Immigration, 27, 51, 62, 82, 129, 145, 166, 178, 182–83, 221n14
Indian Appropriations Act, US, 172, 218n20
Indian Removal Act of 1830, US, 14, 20–21, 47, 72, 80, 92, 113, 178, 216nn2–3

Indian Territory, 81–82, 87–88, 91, 98, 127, 137, 138–39
Indigenous sex/gender systems, 143, 160, 164, 170
Insanity, 7, 57–58, 63, 156, 213n4, 214n6. See also Mania à potu
Ireland: British colonialism, 28; domestic labor, 145; emigration to US, 27; James Morton sent to, 31–32; Samuel Morton visits, 45. See also Immigration

Jackson, Andrew, 20, 47, 79–80, 82–83, 95, 111, 119, 216nn1–3. See also Indian Removal Act of 1830, US
Jesup, Thomas S., 136–37
John Horse. See Cavallo, John

Knox, Robert, 19, 48–50, 214n8
Krogman, Dr. Wilton (Bill) Marion, 185, 187, 188, 225n18

Laënnec, René-Théophile-Hyacinthe, 41–42, 50
Lanier, Melanie, 159
Layers out of the dead. See Watchers of the dead
Legacy collections: concept of, 12, 25, 186, 193, 198, 206, 224n15; Hamann-Todd Osteological Collection, 187–88, 224nn16–17; Huntington Anatomical Collection, 227n38; Moore Collection, 179; Morton Collection as, 190, 205; Mütter Museum, 212n12; W. Montague Cobb Human Skeletal Collection, 188
Lemkin, Raphael, 192–93. See also Genocide
Library Company of Philadelphia, 13, 210nn10,13, 216n20
Love letters, 29, 66, 144
Lunatic. See Insanity
Lyell, Charles, 133

Maintaining object, 9, 13, 14, 105, 186
Making future dead, 9, 21, 91, 95, 102, 124
Mania à potu, 57, 156, 213n4, 214n6
Manifest destiny, 14, 22, 80, 106, 113, 119
Mapmaking, 111, 113, 115, 119, 219n1
Martin, Joel, 88–91, 216n5

Mbembe, Achille, 8, 9, 104, 105, 209n7, 218n16. See also Becoming object; Necropolitics
McKittrick, Katherine, 18–19, 22
Medical Department at the University of Pennsylvania, 39, 54, 80, 82, 86–87, 105, 128, 161, 184, 216n21. See also Medical schools
Medical education, nineteenth century: apprenticeship, 38, 54; curriculum, 36, 39, 43, 148; dissection, 40, 41; preceptorship, 44, 215n18, 226n31; proprietary medical schools, 60, 67–68; sourcing cadavers, 42, 56–57, 184, 186 (see also Anatomy Act of 1883); study abroad, 45–46, 49. See also Medical schools; Pathological cabinet
Medical gaze, 41, 50, 212n10. See also Foucault, Michel
Medical schools: Female Medical College of Pennsylvania, 35–36, 211n8; Hahnemann Medical College, 183; Jefferson Medical College, 41, 68, 150, 151, 177, 184; Ladies Institute of Pennsylvania Medical University, 212n8; Medical College of South Carolina, 101, 109, 115; Medical Department at the University of Pennsylvania, 5, 39, 54, 80, 212n9, 215n17 (see also University of Pennsylvania); Pennsylvania Medical College, 67, 212n8, 215n19; Philadelphia Association for Medical Instruction, 60, 67, 69, 72; University of Edinburgh, 19, 39, 45–46
Meigs, Charles, 36, 60, 63, 96, 150–52, 160, 175–76, 179, 215n16, 222nn1,7. See also Cholera; Obstetrics and gynecology; Puerperal fever
Meigs, James Aitken, 1, 177, 222n7, 223n4
Memoir writing, 174–75
Miccosukee Tribe of Indians of Florida. See Seminole
Midwifery, 23, 39, 147–50, 174
Miscegenation, 23, 112, 133–35, 178, 188, 196, 221n13. See also Black Indians; Hybridity
Mixed races. See Miscegenation
Monogenism, 76–77. See also Polygenism
Montagu, M. F. Ashley, 180–83, 185, 190
Moore, Clarence B., 179
Moore, J. Percy, 180–81
Mortality rates: American Indians, 65, 97; Black Americans, 12, 188; impacted by epi-

demics, 5, 53, 64; infant and childhood, 30, 71, 83 (*see also* Scarlet fever); maternal, 149

Morton, Anna (sister of Samuel), 31, 32, 37, 38

Morton, George (father of Samuel), 5, 27–31

Morton, James (brother of Samuel), 31–32

Morton, James (uncle of Samuel), 31–32, 44, 45, 78

Morton, James St. Clair (son of Samuel), 67, 145, 167, 168, *169*

Morton, Jane (née Cummings): births Samuel, 30; marries George Morton, 29, 66, 145; marries Thomas Rogers, 33; Quaker religion, 31–32; death, 38

Morton, Rebecca (née Grellet Pearsall): death, 168, 169, *170*; dutiful wife and mother, 1, 67, 141–42, 145, 150; kin relations, 70, 143; view of Morton Collection, 1, 146, 167, 176–77; marriage to Samuel, 38, 48, 66, 144–45; Society of Friends, 154; "true womanhood," 24, 147, 155

Morton, Thomas (grandfather of Samuel), 27–29, 30–32, 211nn1–2

Morton, Thomas George (son of Samuel), 42–43, 66–67, 144, 167, 168, 210n13, 212n11

Mott, Lucretia, 24, 35–36, 142, 153–56, 222n9

Motte, Jacob Rhett, 122, 137

Museum of the American Indian, Heye Foundation, 179, 224n8. *See also* Legacy collections: Moore Collection

Nader, Laura, 4, 19

Naming, 17, 122, 124–27, 182, 220n10

National Museum of Natural History, 178, 218n19

Native American. *See* American Indian

Native American Graves Protection and Repatriation Act of 1990, US (NAGPRA), 25, 172, 190, 196, 198–99, 201–2, 204, 225nn22,24, 226n29

Native "Beloved" women, 24, 160, 163–66, 206

Natural history: medicine and, 4, 7, 20, 39, 46, 54, 102; military officers, 80, 88; museums and societies, 176, 178, 179, 224n16; Samuel Morton and, 3, 44, 51, 78, 110, 171, 175

Necropolitics: disenrollment of Black Seminoles, 225n26 (*see also* Black Indians); human remains and, 11, 104–5, 193; nation-building, 3, 16, 21–22, 24, 80–81, 139, 166, 194, 200, 204, 218n20; necropower, 8, 110, 126; naturalists' and physicians' complicity, 47, 86, 91, 95, 119, 124, 149, 178, 190, 206, 226n33; theorizing about, 9, 197, 209n7. *See also* Mbembe, Achille

Nott, Josiah, 175

Nuremberg Code, 185, 193, 224n14

Obstetrics and gynecology, 23–24, 68, 142, 148–51, 174. *See also* Midwifery

Odawa (Little Traverse Bay Band of Odawa Indians of Michigan), 199–200

Okeechobee Battlefield Historic State Park (Florida), 198

Ontological insecurity, 80, 82, 88, 135, 140, 190, 197, 199

Osage, 81, 85. *See also* American Indian

Osteobiography, 11, 14

Pancoast, Joseph T., 86, *87*

Parrish, Joseph, 38–39, 42, 44, 54, 56, 60, 215n16

Pathological cabinet, 42–43, 50, 102, 174, 212n12. *See also* Medical education

Pearsall, Robert, Jr., 34, 38, 70, 143, 144–45

Penn & Slavery Project, 201, 226n31

Penn Museum: Morton Collection curation, 1, 17, 103, 187, 190, 225nn22,24; MOVE controversy, 226n33; repatriation, 25, 195–96, 198, 199–202, 225n27, 227n36; research conducted at, 13, 188

Pennsylvania Hospital, 39, 42

Pernkopf's Atlas, 9, 209n8

Philadelphia Almshouse: cholera epidemic of 1832, 63–64, 66; inmates, 24, 156, 214n6; location, 213n3; medical staff, 7, 20, 53, 55–56, 60, 86, 106; source of cadavers and skulls, 42, 57–59, 97, 123, 184, 194

Phrenology: anti-slavery evidence, 154; Central Phrenological Society, 51, 213nn16–17; George Combe on, 73–75; Phrenological Society (Edinburgh), 50; pseudoscience, 77, 103, 175, 178; skull collection and, 94, 101–2. *See also* Combe, George; Douglass, Frederick; Mott, Lucretia

Physick, Philip Syng, 40–41, 43–45, 51, 56

Pitcher, Zina, 84–85
Polygenism, 20, 49, 77, 131–34, 175, 177, 181. *See also* Monogenism
Post offices, 103
Precarity: American Indians and, 21, 65, 80–82, 84, 88, 95, 97, 118, 135, 216n5; Black Americans and, 187; concept of, 17; epidemics and, 63; pathological evidence for, 18, 90, 98, 139–40, 163. *See also* Butler, Judith
Prichard, James Cowles, 20, 76–77, 216n23
Propaganda. *See* Captivity narratives
Propatriation, 199
Prostitutes, 24, 42, 55, 146, 156
Puerperal fever, 149, 151. *See also* Meigs, Charles; Obstetrics and gynecology

Quakerism. *See* Society of Friends
Queer Indigeneity, 170, 194–95

Racism: anti-Black racism, 35, 40, 108, 188, 197, 202; antisemitism, 182, 193, 224n10; Michel Foucault on, 7; scientific racism, 2, 8, 49, 172, 175–76, 189, 197, 218n17, 225n19
Red Earth, Michael, 195
Reparations, 10, 25, 197, 202, 204, 207. *See also* African-American Burial Grounds Preservation Act; Repatriation
Repatriation: decolonial work, 25, 199; international, 26, 203–4; at Penn Museum, 25, 195–96, 198, 200–201, 225nn24,27, 226n29. *See also* Native American Graves Protection and Repatriation Act of 1990, US; Propatriation
Robertson, Francis Marion, 96, 100–102, 108–9
Rogers, Thomas, 31, 33–34, 37
Ruschenberger, William, 3
Rush, Benjamin, 5–6, 7, 45, 56, 68. *See also* Yellow fever

Scarlet fever, 5, 20, 31, 34, 69–71. *See also* Epidemics
Seminole: assimilation, 210n12; ethnogenesis, 92; gender relations, 165; mortuary practices, 95, 97, 100, 217n11; naming patterns, 127; repatriation, 198; slavery, 97, 134–35, 137, 196–97, 225n25 (*see also* Black Indians). *See also* Seminole Wars

Seminole Wars: Aborigines' Protection Society on, 75–76; Battle of Lake Okeechobee, 99–100; Black alliances during, 135, 137–38; Dade's Massacre, 101–2; impacts on Native life, 165; Justin Dimick's exploits, 22, 121–22; duration, 91–92, 217n9; mapping during, 119, *120*; Native resistance, 98, 114, 121, 123; propaganda, 136 (*see also* Captivity narratives); rape by US soldiers, 166; government reparations, 197; US Army scorched earth policy, 95; White settlers during, 92–94, 114–15, 219n2; White Wars, 198
Seneca Falls Convention of 1848 (New York), 153
Shippen, William, 40, 45, 148
Sioux, 161–63, 195, 225n23
Skull: fetishization, 11, 17, 81; pathology displayed, 13–14, 18, 97–98, 139–40, 165; textual surfaces, 17, 84, 139, 221n17; trauma displayed, 12–13, 18, *87*, 89, *96*, 100, 119, 124
Smith, Gulielma, 20, 69–70, 109, 110
Smith, John Jay: brother-in-law of Samuel Morton, 3, 34, 37–38; death of daughters, 20, 69–70; family archives, 66, 143, 168, 216n20; Laurel Hill Cemetery, 109–10; Library Company of Philadelphia, 13
Smith, Rachel (née Pearsall), 20, 66, 69, 70, 143, *144*, 144–45
Society of Friends: abolitionism and, 38, 40; American Indians and, 73; boarding schools, 19, 31, 32–36, 66; disownment, 30, 145; death and, 32, 41, 109, 110; in Edinburgh, 46, 48; pacifism, 8; racism, 34–35 (*see also* Douglass, Sarah Mapps); Rebecca Morton and, 145; Samuel Morton and, 20, 37, 41, 45, 50, 51, 71, 80, 222n2; Lucretia Mott and, 24, 154
"Studying up," 4

Todd, T. Wingate, 187–88. *See also* Legacy collections
Treaty of Moultrie Creek of 1823, 92, *93*, 155
Treaty of Payne's Landing of 1832, 92
Trouillot, Michel-Rolph, 15, 17, 112, 123–24
True womanhood, 24, 140, 142, 146–47, 151, 155, 157, 174. *See also* Ideology of separate spheres

Tuberculosis. *See* Consumption
Two-Spirits, 25, 159–60, 162–66, 194–95, 223n12

UNESCO Statements on Race, 185
"Ungrievable lives," 7, 84, 140. *See also* Butler, Judith
University of Edinburgh, 19, 39, 45–46, 51, 55
US Army surgeons, 80–84, 86, 88, 105–6, 139, 165, 198, 216n4. *See also* Abadie, Eugene Hilarian; Barnes, Joseph K.; Martin, Joel; Motte, Jacob Rhett; Pitcher, Zina; Walker, Joseph
US National Museum. *See* National Museum of Natural History
Utilitarianism, 25, 42, 56–57, 59, 184, 185, 190, 205, 227n38

Walker, Joseph, 86–87, *96*, 216n4
Watchers of the dead, 174
Westtown School, *33*, 34, 37, 70, 143
Whooping cough, 5, 31, 34, 90
Wild Cat. *See* Coacoochee
Winkte, 161, 195, 223n12. *See also* Sioux; Two-Spirits
Wistar, Caspar, 38–39, 41–42, 45, 56
Wood, George, 60, 66, 69, 71, 175
Woodhouse, Samuel, 87

Yellow fever, 5–6, 30–31, 62, 65. *See also* Epidemics
Young, Hugh, 111–13, 115, 119
"Your Obedient Servant," 4, 21, 75

Pamela L. Geller is associate professor of anthropology at the University of Miami. She is the author of *Theorizing Bioarchaeology* and *The Bioarchaeology of Social-Sexual Lives* and coeditor of the contributed volume *Feminist Anthropology: Past, Present, and Future*. She is also editor of the Routledge book series "The Archaeology of Gender and Sexuality." In addition to the numerous academic journal articles and book chapters she has written, her opinion essays have appeared in *Slate, Miami Herald,* and the *New York Times.*

www.ingramcontent.com/pod-product-compliance
Lightning Source LLC
Chambersburg PA
CBHW030818230426
43667CB00008B/1277